See What Others Have Said About
The Complete Idiot's Guide to T'ai Chi & QiGong, Acclaimed Primer and Reference Used by Top T'ai Chi, QiGong, and Health Professionals

"[I was] living an extremely unhealthy lifestyle ... taking numerous medications for arthritis, depression, and pain. ... Then one day while browsing in the library I discovered a book ... *The Complete Idiot's Guide to T'ai Chi and QiGong*. I was so impressed that I ordered Bill's videos. ... Now that I am practicing T'ai Chi and QiGong daily. I am off most of my medications. People keep telling me I look 'different' and that I look happy. Well, I am happy and I feel great! ... Thank you! Thank you! Thank you!"

—Dave Long, Washington

"Visionary! If you only buy one book on T'ai Chi, *then this is the book*. This book is all you ever needed to know to change your life. I have taught T'ai Chi for several decades myself, yet I have now read Bill's book from cover to cover *seven times*, and *still* get something new from it each time."

—Dr. Michael Steward Sr., DMA, PhD, MA, Senior Coach for Team USA, Inductee of the World Sports Medicine and World Martial Arts Hall of Fame

"I highly recommend this book to all seeking to enhance their physical, mental, and spiritual potential. Quantum Physics and leading-edge cell biology emphasize the primal role of energy in our lives. In a user-friendly and meaningful style, Bill Douglas offers a compelling and easy-to-understand description of ancient Asian energy exercises that effectively reduce stress and improve health."

—Bruce H. Lipton, PhD, Cellular Biologist and best-selling author of *The Biology of Belief: Unleashing the Power of Consciousness, Matter & Miracles*

"I had the privilege of studying T'ai Chi with this book's author, Bill Douglas. As a practicing physician, there are certainly times when stress can seem to be the norm. I found T'ai Chi to be profoundly beneficial in reducing stress, increasing mental clarity, and improving my emotional as well as physical health. Where else can you find such a highly effective tool to achieve these worthwhile goals without fancy equipment or complicated formulas? If T'ai Chi can help with stress in an ER room where lives often hang in the balance, imagine what it can do for everyone else!"

—John D. Hernandez, MD, Integrative Medicine

"Sometimes Chinese culture can be difficult to explain. Sifu Bill Douglas successfully uses American culture to explain the art of T'ai Chi Chuan. He simplifies difficult concepts, making them easier to understand. This book takes the best parts of T'ai Chi and makes them understandable [to Westerners] without requiring a grounding in Chinese culture and history."

—Sifu Yijiao Hong, USA All-T'ai Chi Grand Champion and USA Team member; Certified International Coach and Judge, International Wushu Federation

"Douglas has achieved for QiGong what Apple did for the computer. He's brought it to the people ... great place to start for beginners. ... Teachers may also find this an excellent manual on how to explain these concepts to the general public ...."

—R. Poccia, stress management instructor, *Beyond Anonymous*, San Francisco

"It has been a year since I began practicing T'ai Chi under the teaching of the author of this book, Bill Douglas, and his associate instructor, Erik Feagans. This span of time certainly allows me to evaluate the result of this gentle 'martial art,' not only as stress-management therapy, but, more impressively, with regard to its effect on my physical health.

"Suffering for years from chronic neck pain consequent to a whiplash injury, and also suffering from a limited motion of the right shoulder, I approached the T'ai Chi course with some skepticism. The course was initiated after unsuccessful sessions of physical therapy, including mobilization, ultrasounds, heat application, etc. After two months of T'ai Chi, the pain in the cervical region disappeared while the range of motion of my right shoulder returned completely to normal. This achievement remained unchanged during the past winter up until now.

"I would not hesitate to recommend T'ai Chi to individuals suffering from the same ailments, as well as to mature persons who are seeking to maintain or improve their health and to remain free of chronic pain due to the aging process."

—Loredana Brizio-Molteni, MD, FACS

"After leaving my very first T'ai Chi class with the author of this book, I remember driving home, and it was as if someone had opened up every one of my senses. It was an overwhelming sense of happiness that swept over me. It was at that very moment I knew T'ai Chi is something I want in my life forever."

—Lisa Shikles, Shawnee, Kansas

"Because of my practice of T'ai Chi and QiGong, my barometer for detecting 'dis-ease' within myself earlier allows me to prevent serious infection and speed up healing. I feel T'ai Chi is a wonderful part of a revolution in healthcare, whereby each of us takes much more responsibility for our own health and healing."

—Susan Norman, CIMT

W9-ABE-898

"I found you by accident while looking for an alternative to back surgery … with three ruptured discs in my lower back. … I read your book from cover to cover. … I am also now over halfway through your second tape, and my range of motion is better than it has been in years. I have also managed to lose a few pounds. … Recently, I went to my regular medical doctor. … [H]e told me he was very pleased with my range of motion and my attitude. … He was so intrigued by my description of your program that he has borrowed my book and the tapes I have finished."

—Mark Herndon, Georgia

"Since beginning Bill Douglas's T'ai Chi program, I have taught the exercises I learned for the past five years in our Pain Management multidisciplinary program at Research Medical Center. My clients have found improved breathing, larger mobility, better posture, improved balance and coordination, flexibility, increased endurance and strength, and relaxation."

—Berni Wheeler, occupational therapist

"I have found so many health benefits since beginning Bill Douglas's T'ai Chi program, which I began during a nervous breakdown with panic, chest pains, fatigue, and chronic migraines. I saw Bill's T'ai Chi and QiGong program information, and I gave it a try. I felt sudden and immediate benefits. My chest pains started to go away, my heavy fatigue went away, my nervousness calmed. My migraines are now nonexistent, as is the severe hay fever I'd had since childhood. And if that isn't enough, I have also lost my craving for fatty foods I once used to soothe my stress, and am now losing weight."

—Tina Webb, Shawnee, Kansas

"As a physical therapist assistant, I believe that these techniques that are taught by Bill through his book and tapes will become one of the essential tools to be utilized in medical facilities as an adjunct to standard therapy.

"Not a day goes by when I am not able to help an individual find pain control using Bill's QiGong techniques, and many find increased balance and coordination, even after a small taste of T'ai Chi, seeing an automatic difference. Personally, tests show me with a 90 percent improvement in overall balance and in one test a 105 percent improvement in balance since beginning T'ai Chi."

—Joyce Rupp, physical therapist assistant, Hays, Kansas

"From the perspective of a health psychologist serving patients who are coping with chronic illness and stressful life events, I see the gentle mindfulness exercises of T'ai Chi and QiGong relaxation therapy as potentially useful for a broad spectrum of people. The author of this book, Bill Douglas, explains the complexities of T'ai Chi and QiGong in the form of an invitation, easing his students into a greater understanding of the usefulness and purpose of this ancient form of meditative movement."

—Kristy Straits-Troster, PhD, clinical psychologist, Primary Care Medicine

"Dizziness is one of the more common reasons for a doctor visit, particularly in patients over the age of 50. Because the causes of dizziness can range from benign, self-limiting conditions to potentially life-threatening ones, a thorough medical evaluation is essential before embarking on any form of therapy. Persistent dizziness certainly has a distinct impact on the quality of life and emotional well-being of the patient. Falls, hip fractures, and lack of confidence in public often create a feeling of helplessness.

"In over 20 years of experience as a clinical neurologist, I find that extensive and expensive medical evaluation, including CAT scans, MRI scans, and vascular imaging studies, as well as prescription medications, add little to alleviating the problem. I have found vestibular rehabilitation exercises in the form of T'ai Chi classes to be a cost-effective mode of therapy. Many of my patients have opted for this nonmedication approach to treatment and have developed a sense of self-confidence through this form of exercise. In short, as a traditional medical practitioner, I frequently recommend T'ai Chi for my patients with dizziness and disequilibrium."

—Charles D. Donohoe, MD, neurologist

"Since beginning Bill's T'ai Chi program, my resting heart rate has gone from 81 to 61. It's amazing!"

—Anne Bauman, Kansas

"I found the energy work (Sitting QiGong) and breath work learned in Bill's T'ai Chi program to be calming and to have that effect on those around me as well, including a returning patient who was hallucinating and having panic attacks. By walking with him and breathing deeply, the patient eventually calmed and lay down breathing evenly to await the doctor."

—Psychotherapist, Kansas City area

"Rx: Continue T'ai Chi.—Dx: Hypertension."

—An actual physician's prescription for a patient to continue in Bill Douglas's hospital T'ai Chi and QiGong classes

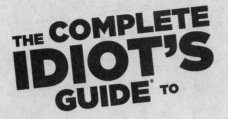

THE **COMPLETE IDIOT'S GUIDE** TO

T'ai Chi & QiGong

Illustrated

Fourth Edition

by Bill Douglas and Angela Wong Douglas

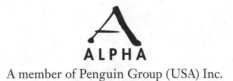

ALPHA

A member of Penguin Group (USA) Inc.

In loving memory of my father, William Edward Douglas Sr., a man who endured the horror of war and hardship like few others … yet from that experience hungered for a world of justice and peace for all peoples of the world. Your Herculean efforts to heal your life serve as an example, enabling me to open to the profound healing T'ai Chi and QiGong offer me and the world. I hope you are up there enjoying the sight of Germans and Americans, Jews and Arabs, all playing T'ai Chi together every year. I dedicate World T'ai Chi and QiGong Day to your memory.

ALPHA BOOKS

Published by Penguin Group (USA) Inc.

Penguin Group (USA) Inc., 375 Hudson Street, New York, New York 10014, USA • Penguin Group (Canada), 90 Eglinton Avenue East, Suite 700, Toronto, Ontario M4P 2Y3, Canada (a division of Pearson Penguin Canada Inc.) • Penguin Books Ltd., 80 Strand, London WC2R 0RL, England • Penguin Ireland, 25 St. Stephen's Green, Dublin 2, Ireland (a division of Penguin Books Ltd.) • Penguin Group (Australia), 250 Camberwell Road, Camberwell, Victoria 3124, Australia (a division of Pearson Australia Group Pty. Ltd.) • Penguin Books India Pvt. Ltd., 11 Community Centre, Panchsheel Park, New Delhi—110 017, India • Penguin Group (NZ), 67 Apollo Drive, Rosedale, North Shore, Auckland 1311, New Zealand (a division of Pearson New Zealand Ltd.) • Penguin Books (South Africa) (Pty.) Ltd., 24 Sturdee Avenue, Rosebank, Johannesburg 2196, South Africa • Penguin Books Ltd., Registered Offices: 80 Strand, London WC2R 0RL, England

Publisher: *Mike Sanders*

Executive Managing Editor: *Billy Fields*

Senior Acquisitions Editor: *Tom Stevens*

Development Editor: *Mark Reddin*

Senior Production Editor: *Janette Lynn*

Copy Editor: *Jan Zoya*

Cover Designer: *William Thomas*

Book Designers: *William Thomas, Rebecca Batchelor*

Indexer: *Johnna VanHoose Dinse*

Layout: *Ayanna Lacey*

Proofreader: *John Etchison*

ALWAYS LEARNING   PEARSON

Contents

Introduction

Before I began T'ai Chi and QiGong classes, my stress was unbearable, and depression and anxiety were almost a way of life. I actually thought at the time that that's just the way life was. It's funny what we'll settle for, when all the while there are powerful and exciting opportunities to change—just waiting for us to reach out and grab them. Back then, I returned home every night from a job I didn't like and used greasy food, overspending, too much TV, or whatever else could help me handle the stress of a life I didn't really feel too good about. I really didn't see much hope for finding any real joy in my life.

Then a friend suggested a T'ai Chi class. From that day, my life began to change, to loosen, to expand and open, becoming more than I ever dreamed possible. Today I travel the world, sharing the most exciting life possibilities with fascinating people all seeking to expand their lives into more than they ever imagined.

This book will demystify the esoteric aspects of T'ai Chi and QiGong so that even the more mystical sides become congruous with physics. Team U.S.A. Senior Coach and Martial Arts Hall of Famer Dr. Michael Steward Sr., after reading this book several times over, called it "visionary," and "life changing." Why?

This book's combination of highly effective how-to instructions, augmented with a treasure trove of Web Video Support, is unequaled. However, what sets this book apart, and what makes it popular with even long-time T'ai Chi and QiGong teachers and professionals, is its insights into the deeper *inner* aspect of these arts. The inner aspect is most profound, because T'ai Chi and QiGong are considered *Internal Arts*. The profound health, performance, and sports improvement benefits these arts will give you will only be reflections of the deep *internal* changes you will be achieving *beneath the surface*. Teachers worldwide have used this book as a teaching tool to help them enable their students to dive deep into these inner realms, which vastly expands their grasp of the physical aspects of T'ai Chi and QiGong as well.

This book has been acclaimed by many of the world's top T'ai Chi and QiGong masters as well as by those who are new to these ancient arts, for one simple reason: In the words of U.S. T'ai Chi Forms Grand Champion Sifu Hong Yijiao, "Sometimes Chinese culture can be difficult to explain … [*The Complete Idiot's Guide to T'ai Chi & QiGong*] successfully uses American culture to explain the art of *T'ai Chi Ch'uan* … simplifying difficult concepts, making them easier to understand."

Here's an example. You might be surprised to know that even if you have never heard of QiGong (pronounced chee gong), you have been practicing a simple form of it for years. Each time you yawn, you are practicing an effective QiGong, or breathing, exercise. You feel better after you yawn, right? Imagine how good you are going to feel as you delve deeper into these ancient gifts from the East, providing life-tools that will rock your world so intensely as to appear *magical*.

T'ai Chi enabled me to let go of my tight, rigid grip on what I thought was possible in life. As it taught me to breathe deeply and allow my body's rigid muscles to let go and relax, my mind and heart began to do so as well. An open mind and open heart expanded outward into an open world. When we begin to live for what we love, the world begins to love us for it. T'ai Chi and QiGong help us loosen up so the love within us can expand outward into all aspects of our lives. This is how we become "lovely" in the truest sense of the word. There is such beautiful potential awaiting all of us, and I am so proud and so grateful that this book has been a part of so many people's expansion—just as T'ai Chi and QiGong have been a part of mine. Enjoy!

How This Book Is Organized

Although some chapters of this book use particular T'ai Chi styles to give readers an experience of T'ai Chi and QiGong, the majority of this book and its Web Video Support are profoundly useful to anyone interested in any style of T'ai Chi or QiGong and are used by teachers worldwide, from many different styles, as a primer and textbook for their students. Its easygoing, accessible style has helped T'ai Chi and QiGong teachers find fresh, user-friendly explanations to help students "get" T'ai Chi or QiGong more quickly and easily by relaxing into it.

This book is divided into six parts, plus the supporting Web Video. Each part's information will prepare you for the next, opening your mind and imagination to concepts that will unlock your ability to expand your awareness of T'ai Chi and QiGong even more. The Web Video supports many sections of the book's chapters with carefully selected visual information that text and illustrations simply cannot convey.

Here's what you get:

The Web Video Support, *Visual Support for This Book's Instruction*, is a powerful new addition, with exhibitional inserts to support the text and illustrated instruction and general information throughout this book. The Web Video Support is created from excerpts of two of my acclaimed, fully instructional DVD programs that total well over five hours in content (Appendix C). Carefully selected excerpts were chosen to powerfully augment the information and instructions provided within the book. As you read through the book's six parts, you'll be directed at appropriate points to view the Web Video Support provided with this book to expand your understanding of the book's instructions and information. As various sections of the book refer you to these video excerpts, you'll discover a multidimensional quality to the Web Video Support, encouraging you to see T'ai Chi and QiGong's many subtle aspects and qualities.

Part 1, T'ai Chi: Relax into Raw Power, explains how T'ai Chi and QiGong can change every part of your life for the better, with visual enhancement of the Web Video Support. Part 1 concludes by explaining how T'ai Chi and QiGong work by introducing you to Traditional Chinese Medicine (TCM) and explaining how modern Western science is now beginning to understand how this ancient wisdom works.

Part 2, Suiting Up and Setting Out, prepares you to dive into T'ai Chi and QiGong big time or little time, depending on how much of T'ai Chi's magic you want to experience. In this part, you learn the nuts and bolts of how classes are taught (with Web Video visuals), along with T'ai Chi etiquette, terms, wardrobe, and all the things that will enable you to choose the best class for you. You also discover the underlying tenets of T'ai Chi and QiGong, which will dramatically enhance the benefit you get from class or video instruction beyond this book's voluminous resources.

Part 3, Starting Down the QiGong Path to T'ai Chi, explains how QiGong works and then leads you into an experience that is exquisite beyond words. Part 3 ends with an introduction to Moving QiGong exercises, including the warm-ups that prepare your mind and body to dive into an ocean of T'ai Chi experience (with references to the Web Video Support). T'ai Chi literally means "the supreme ultimate," so hold on for an incredible ride!

Part 4, Learning a T'ai Chi Long Form, illuminates the history of T'ai Chi and how the Kuang Ping Yang style was brought to the West by Master Kuo Lien Ying. Then you are led through the entire 64 postures of this powerful, ancient form (with video support for each one of the 64 postures' instructions and an entire exhibition of the T'ai Chi long form with a QiGong Breathing tutorial). Instructions include the specific benefits of some movements, and rich details on weight shift, energy flow, and more. Yet remember, the benefits are endless, and because this book is bound by its covers, to discover them you must experience them yourself as they unfold beautifully within you every day for the rest of your life.

Part 5, T'ai Chi's Buffet of Short, Sword, and Fan Styles, exposes you to the many incredibly beautiful forms of T'ai Chi (with Web Video Support) available to you today. Remember that only about 30 years ago, these arts were secrets of China, so we are very lucky to have these exquisite art forms available to us now in our lifetimes. Part 5 gives you a small yet delicious taste of what is available. If you seek, ye shall find.

Part 6, Life Applications, shows that T'ai Chi is much more than just a "physical exercise." T'ai Chi can help heal every aspect of our lives, our relationships, and our world (Web Video Support complements these points). To that end, Part 6 explains how T'ai Chi and/or QiGong can be used to help treat almost any illness or physical malady. It also explains to what extent T'ai Chi can be a powerful adjunct therapy for many mental or emotional problems, as well as a powerful tool that helps you increase your productivity and creativity in your professional life. But even beyond healing, you will see how T'ai Chi can help the world realize a much more expansive vision of possibility for our ever-evolving future.

Extras

Throughout this book, I've included five types of extra information for your enlightenment:

OUCH!

These boxes alert you to any caution you should observe in T'ai Chi practice. There won't be many of these; T'ai Chi injuries are nearly nonexistent when done correctly.

KNOW YOUR CHINESE

These boxes give you definitions for Chinese medical and philosophical terms related to T'ai Chi and QiGong, including pronunciation aids.

A T'AI CHI PUNCH LINE

These boxes are full of fun anecdotes and trivia about the fascinating world of T'ai Chi and QiGong, modern and old.

T'AI SCI

These boxes provide you modern scientific terms and insights into the world of T'ai Chi's ancient discoveries.

SAGE SIFU SAYS

These boxes offer you tips on living the principles of T'ai Chi and maximizing your understanding of T'ai Chi's subtle layers to help you get the most out of it. Sifu (pronounced see-foo) means "one who has mastered an art"—but not only martial arts; a master chef or artist might also be a sifu.

But Wait! There's More!

We've included tons of additional Web Video Support content. Bookmark or add to your favorites www.idiotsguides.com/taichi for ongoing Web Video Support of most chapters in this book and enjoy!

Acknowledgments

A great thanks to the many dedicated Chinese creators of T'ai Chi who've spent lifetimes developing this wonderful art and health science the world now has access to. T'ai Chi and QiGong are great gifts the Chinese culture has provided for the world, and I offer the creators a deep and heartfelt thank you. Their efforts leave me convinced that every culture on this planet has treasures to offer the rest, and I hope we all can open our hearts and minds to truth and value, no matter where it comes from.

A profound thanks to my teacher, Master Jennifer Booth; her teacher, Gil Messenger; their teacher, Russell Schofield; and our grandmaster, Kuo Lien Ying, who made the daunting journey from China to San Francisco, as did many other courageous masters of other styles of T'ai Chi and forms of QiGong. Their courage in migrating to strange lands made it possible for millions of people in many nations to have access to the beauty and power of Kuang Ping Yang T'ai Chi Ch'uan and the other wonderful forms, including Chen, Yang, Wu, Sun, Mulan, and others. I would further like to thank my teacher, Ms. Booth, for focusing intensely on the healing aspects of T'ai Chi and QiGong and for imparting that importance to me.

My mother-in-law, Shun Oi Wong, was an integral part of my T'ai Chi journey, and my father-in-law, Bonwyn Wong, embodied the humility and infinite wisdom Chinese people are known for. My children, Isaac, Andrea, and Michael, led me to the doorway of change through their innocent examples of wisdom, and my parents, Evelyn and William Douglas, showed me that even the harshest tests can produce pearls in us beautiful creatures known as human beings.

Thanks to Mulan Quan instructors Angela Wong Douglas and Andrea Mei-Wah Douglas for their wonderful exhibitions and insights into the elegant art form of Mulan Quan basic, Fan, and Sword style. Angela has been a treasure trove of insight into understanding Chinese culture, which is woven throughout the principles of T'ai Chi and QiGong's elegant philosophy and science.

With the modern stress plague ravaging the world, I want to thank the visionary educators beginning to incorporate T'ai Chi and QiGong into education systems worldwide. When every graduating senior is a T'ai Chi master, how much less drug and alcohol abuse, and how much less violence and fewer children in prisons will there be? Thank you all for your courage, vision, and open-heartedness, to see the profound value of these tools even though they come from another culture. Thanks to all the innovative T'ai Chi teachers who are discovering new ways to teach these ancient arts, to make them fun and contemporary so modern children (and adults) in all societies can learn to love them. All the T'ai Chi and QiGong teachers working to educate the world on the last Saturday of April each year on World T'ai Chi and QiGong Day (and all year) are pioneers whose health education work will benefit the world in ways we cannot yet even imagine.

I'd like to thank illustrator Jenny Hahn for her brilliant insightful work on the more than 200 instructional sketches and her dedication to this project. Ms. Hahn is an extraordinary artist with an ability to capture complex and even internal T'ai Chi concepts in her illustrations. Her work has set a new standard for T'ai Chi book instruction. Also, thanks to Jessica Kincaid for her computer graphics and to master photographer David Larson for his brilliant photos.

And lastly, thank you Tom Stevens, Janette Lynn, and Mark Reddin, for your clarifying insights, attention to detail, and brilliant and elegant T'ai Chi–like approach to the editing of this book.

Special Thanks to the Technical Reviewer

The Complete Idiot's Guide to T'ai Chi & QiGong was reviewed by an expert who double-checked the accuracy of what you'll learn here, to help us ensure that this book gives you everything you need to know about T'ai Chi and QiGong. Special thanks are extended to Master Jennifer Booth.

Trademarks

All terms mentioned in this book that are known to be or are suspected of being trademarks or service marks have been appropriately capitalized. Alpha Books and Penguin Group (USA) Inc. cannot attest to the accuracy of this information. Use of a term in this book should not be regarded as affecting the validity of any trademark or service mark.

T'ai Chi: Relax into Raw Power

In This Part

Part 1 explains why a simple, easy-to-do, 2,000-year-old Chinese martial art is the most popular exercise in the world today and is practiced in corporations, hospitals, living rooms, and backyards just like yours around the world.

If you want to find a calm center in the middle of life's storm of change while also toning your muscles and healing your mind and body, T'ai Chi and QiGong are just what the doctor ordered—literally. *Ask your doctor!* Whether you seek a simple, easy-to-do exercise, a stress-management tool, or a profoundly healthy philosophy of life, T'ai Chi may just be what you've been looking for.

This edition's new CIG Web Video Support webpages contain video exhibitions that bring this book's richly detailed illustrations and written instructions to life! Throughout many parts of the book you will be directed to video links, enabling you to see the text explanations in action. You will happily discover that this book's triangular approach of illustrated graphics, and text explanations, coupled with video support, offers an unequaled, easygoing user-friendly approach to T'ai Chi instruction. Some video nodes include special effects enabling you to see "inside the body," giving this book an unequaled and profound "internal" approach to the internal-energy arts of T'ai Chi and QiGong.

Why Practice T'ai Chi and QiGong?

In This Chapter

- The reasons behind T'ai Chi's exploding popularity
- The mental and emotional challenges to learning T'ai Chi and QiGong
- A brief history of T'ai Chi
- Powerful benefits from *all* styles of T'ai Chi
- Web Video Support: *Overview of Book's Web Video Support*

T'ai Chi Ch'uan (pronounced *tie chee chwan*), sometimes spelled Taijiquan, means "supreme ultimate fist," or "highest martial art." But because most people now practice it for health, it is often simply called T'ai Chi, for *supreme ultimate experience.*

T'ai Chi is paradoxically as simple as pie, and as deep as an ocean in unfolding complexity. I have worked with T'ai Chi and QiGong teachers all over the planet and found that it is rare that two T'ai Chi teachers will agree on exactly what T'ai Chi is. This is because these arts are such expansively multi-dimensional experiences that offer breakthroughs in health, mental and emotional growth, creativity, and other areas that often defy description. But in the end, all styles of T'ai Chi can provide similarly profound benefits, and this book has been very useful to anyone studying, or teaching, any style of T'ai Chi or QiGong.

A Harvard Medical University Publication referred to T'ai Chi as "medication in motion," and Oprah's Book Club selected author Eckart Tolle (*A New Earth*), wrote that T'ai Chi and QiGong would be a major part of *global awakening*. So what are these ancient arts? Practical health and fitness sciences, or are they esoteric life-altering consciousness-expanding practices? The answer is all of the above, and so much more. This chapter begins with two amazing exercises that will prove to you just how physically empowering and esoterically life expanding these tools can be.

The Chinese call life energy Qi (pronounced *chee*). The character for Qi is also the character for air or breath. QiGong means "breathing exercise," but also means "life energy" exercise. There are about 7,000 QiGong exercises in the Chinese Book of Medicine, and T'ai Chi is among the most effective of the Moving QiGong exercises.

We begin by exposing you to two T'ai Chi and QiGong techniques that will take you far beyond mentally comprehending the power of these ancient arts, by enabling you to actually *feel* that power and expansion.

First, we'll take a peek ahead to enjoy Chapter 9's *Sitting QiGong* meditation, or by using the Web Video Support (top of Chapter 1's listed videos, at www.idiotsguides.com/taichi). Ease back into a comfortable chair, and listen as I lead you through a soothing, mind-expanding QiGong meditation. If you can't access the internet, you can use the text version in Chapter 9.

This QiGong meditation will enable you to actually *feel* the subtle energy that is your life energy, or Qi, which T'ai Chi and QiGong are based upon. If you don't sense it the first time, don't give up. You will eventually!

Second, do the following exercise on the power of completing your Microcosmic Orbit. After these two experiences, whether you are a rank beginner or an advanced teacher, you'll understand the tremendous potential T'ai Chi and QiGong offer. However, this is only a taste of what these pages offer in what is hoped to be your continuing lifelong T'ai Chi and QiGong journey of self-discovery and personal expansion.

Subtle Adjustments Equal Powerful Changes

During T'ai Chi and QiGong exercises, the tip of the tongue lightly touches the roof of the mouth. Why?

There are two reasons for this: First is that by placing the tip of the tongue lightly touching the gum line just behind the top front teeth, it changes the throat structure. Research shows that long, gradual breaths are the most effective, rather than rapid inhales and exhales. When the mouth is open, the throat is open. When the tongue touches the roof of the mouth, the throat canal narrows some, causing your breaths to be longer and more gradual, thereby maximizing their healthful effects. See the Web Video Support *QiGong Breathing Tutorial*.

SAGE SIFU SAYS

Remember to bookmark or add to your list of favorite sites the Web Video Support address (www.idiotsguides.com/taichi) and enjoy the benefits of the videos along with each chapter.

But the second reason is an energetic-engineering one. You'll learn more in the next chapter about T'ai Chi's connection with Traditional Chinese Medicine's Acupuncture energy meridians. As you see in the following figure, the curved lines on the image on the left show how the energy from what's called *the Microcosmic Orbit* flows up your back and down your front.

The Microcosmic Orbit flows up from your perineum through the center of your back, over your head, and ends in the roof of your mouth. This is called your Governing Vessel. The energy flow of the Conception Vessel is represented by the curved line from the perineum up the center of your frontal body to end in the lower jaw. The Microcosmic Orbit is interrupted by the mouth.

But when you touch the tip of the tongue to the roof of the mouth, you complete this energy circuit, and this can profoundly affect your body's solidity and power. Here's an easy exercise to feel that effect.

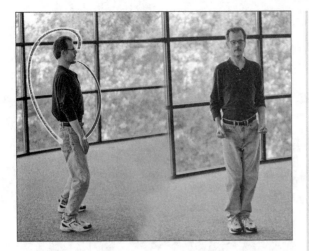

The Microcosmic Orbit energy channel is illustrated by the left figure. The right figure is the stance used to test the power of completing the Microcosmic Orbit, with the help of a friend pressing down on your resisting fist to draw you off balance.

Here's how to do this exercise:

Note: This illustrated instruction is augmented in a Web Video Support feature in Chapter 1's video section, *Subtle Adjustment Equal Powerful Changes.*

1. See in the figure to the right of the Microcosmic Orbit example with the feet close together, and fists upturned. Stand this way.

2. Have someone push down on one of your upturned fists. (Note: If you have any arm, shoulder, or back injuries, you may want to skip this exercise.) Use resistance so that they will pull you off balance. Notice how that felt as you began to lose your balance.

3. Now, smash your tongue up against the roof of your mouth, and have them push down on your upturned fist again.

4. You should notice that it is much more difficult, if not impossible, for them to pull you off balance by pushing down on your resisting fist this time.

Yeah, mind-blowing, isn't it? I learned this technique from Grandmaster Jianye Jiang while at the Zhang San Feng Festival in New York, where Angela and I were presented with our 2009 Internal Arts Hall of Fame Induction. I had been doing T'ai Chi for nearly 30 years at the time I discovered this. This gives you an idea of just how deep and wide your T'ai Chi journey will become, as you continually learn new and profound aspects of T'ai Chi and QiGong even after decades of study.

Realize that this technique is just to illustrate the power of completing the Microcosmic Orbit, and to highlight how subtle physical adjustments make huge differences. But in T'ai Chi and QiGong, you don't actually move around with your tongue smashed up against the roof of the mouth. They are done in a relaxed way, with the tip of the tongue just *lightly* touching the gum line near the roof of the mouth, because you should always be relaxed.

Where This Journey Can Lead

T'ai Chi and QiGong are both practical *no-nonsense* calorie-burning fitness routines and esoteric transcendental experiences. They are extremely low impact, and accessible to *anyone*. To give you a perspective of their breadth and depth, realize that T'ai Chi is the product of about 1,200 years of Chinese mind-body medical research, and QiGong is about 2,000 years in the making.

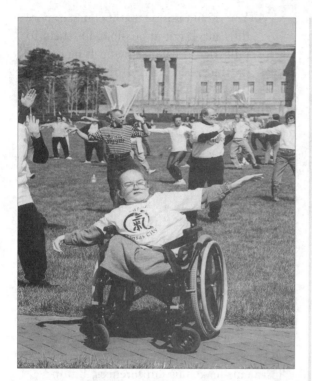

T'ai Chi is becoming increasingly popular for a wide range of practioners!

T'ai Chi or QiGong are at the cutting edge of health science and are perhaps the most effective stress-management exercises in the world—which is saying a lot in an overstressed world where 70 to 85 percent of *all illnesses* are caused by stress (Kaiser Permanente study). However, T'ai Chi and QiGong are so much more.

T'ai Chi and QiGong are *mind-body* tools. Therefore, for your body to get maximum benefit, it is critical to wrap your mind around the vast breadth of possibility they offer you, so you can then deeply relax into the process without having to second-guess the intellectual foundation of the practices.

T'ai Chi comes in several excellent styles. While some chapters in this book relate to particular T'ai Chi styles, you'll find it to be a valuable resource to anyone exploring any form of T'ai Chi or QiGong.

This book will help you hit the ground running. Appendix A helps you locate local teachers or schools anywhere around the world, while Appendix C describes effective DVD programs.

Relaxing the Mind, the Body, and Our Lives

When I began T'ai Chi and QiGong 30 years ago, I mistakenly thought that T'ai Chi was *hard*. I used to joke, "It's amazing how hard it is to move effortlessly." With the help of this book, you will learn to relax through the biggest hurdles you'll encounter in learning these mind-body arts—the mental and emotional challenges.

At their core, T'ai Chi and QiGong are all about letting go and loosening your grip on your body, your consciousness, and your life. In this book, you'll learn techniques like "the unbendable arm," which are not only great party tricks, but illustrate the effortless power these tools will bring into every aspect of your life. Your athletic prowess will increase exponentially as you dive into this world.

You may begin your T'ai Chi or QiGong journey to improve your health, calm your mind, or improve your golf game, but in the end you will look back and see how these life tools not only untangled many of your mental-physical knots and problems, but also expanded your potential, creativity, and love of life.

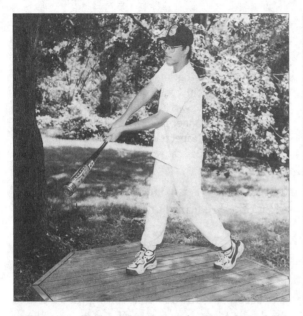

This photo illustrates how a loose frame sends the full force of the dan tien's motion up through your relaxed body, out the bat, and through the ball. Notice how the batter's back foot turns as the dan tien turns into the ball he's hitting.

Unfurl Your Constricted Creativity

My own T'ai Chi journey has been a testament to this potential of creativity expansion, resulting not only in my writing this best-selling T'ai Chi book that is published worldwide in several languages, but by my multiple-award-winning novels and essays, and by my having founded a global event now held annually in over 70 nations each year. None of this would have happened had I not been lucky enough to stumble into that T'ai Chi and QiGong class 30 years ago, where I began this journey of untangling the mental and emotional stress knots that had kept my potential constricted and limited. You may one day look back on when you first picked up this book and started your own classes with this same fondness.

Getting Centered Makes Life Magical

This book will help you understand that these exercises are celebrations of life, and an act of thankfulness for these wonderful bodies we've been given. You may start them in order to look more fit or beautiful, but in the end, how you look won't matter at all because you will "feel gorgeous inside and realize that you have been beautiful all along," and discover that is the only beauty that really matters.

You may start T'ai Chi and QiGong to become more creative and get an edge in business in order to become more wealthy, but in the end you will find these tools have helped you understand that every breath, everyone, and everything you see in this life is a treasure and that you are blessed to have this life you've been given already—and your desire for wealth will become less of a source of angst and pressure. That appreciation of self and life will shine through you, causing people to want to be around you, and success after success can follow.

You may be running after things by pursuing T'ai Chi and QiGong, but as they slow you and the merry-go-round you call your life down, you will ultimately find that all the things you really needed have been around you all along. You will become aware of the miraculous in the mundane.

Now, as mentioned before, T'ai Chi and QiGong are very practical no-nonsense mind-body tools that can address many basic issues, and the more you understand how these tools work, the more you'll be able to relax into the process and get the maximum benefit. That will enable you to transcend analytical thought and be immersed in the pleasures and sensations that are much wider and deeper experiences than can be described intellectually.

So let's expand on your intellectual understanding of these arts, before moving on to the application of these tools.

T'ai Chi and QiGong as Physical Engineering Principles

T'ai Chi and QiGong are based on physical engineering principles. You'll learn how the "vertical axis" and the "dan tien" are at their core, not only esoteric energy concepts, but practical engineering systems that these physical sciences are built upon. They will teach you how to align your body for maximum performance with the least amount of effort. They will teach you how to untangle your knots physically, mentally, and emotionally so that the maximum amount of power and energy can flow through this vessel you call your body.

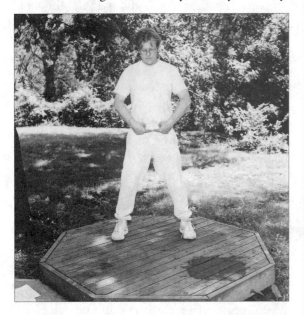

The dan tien is located about 1¹/₂ to 3 inches below the navel, near the center of the body, slightly toward the front.

SAGE SIFU SAYS

T'ai Chi and QiGong are effortless, and should always feel good. Don't strain at them. They may seem hard at first, but when you look back, you'll realize it was never hard; it was just that you were *making it hard* unnecessarily. This realization will make other aspects of your life become more effortless, as well.

The vertical axis is your postural alignment. Most of us are leaning forward, always in a hurry to get somewhere else, always feeling five steps behind the rushing world. This postural dysfunction causes many problems. For example, the tight shoulders we often feel are largely due to the head leaning forward all day long. That 8- or 9-pound melon we call our head, held out of alignment, causes those little muscles in the shoulders to overwork all day long as the head leans forward in a rush to get somewhere else all the time. As T'ai Chi teaches you to align your posture day after day, a lot of that chronic shoulder tension will dissipate over time. You'll feel some relief right away, but the full effect may take some time. In the end it will amaze you how much pressure it will unload off of your body!

Lower-back issues will often disappear as well, because stress causes lower-back muscles to tighten up, causing an over-curvature of the back, pressure on the vertebrae, and thereby back pain. The physical adjustment will result in a mental shift, as you stop propelling forward and stand in the center of yourself, noticing the world around you rather than anxiously rushing to a place you can never quite get to.

OUCH!

T'ai Chi's *spinal lengthening* offers the opposite of what high heels do to your back, because high heels cause your back to over-curve, putting stress on the lower vertebrae. T'ai Chi will give you great legs, so you won't need to torture your back with high heels to look good!

T'ai Chi and QiGong posture lengthens the spine, stacking up the vertebrae in alignment, and taking enormous pressure off the back, shoulders, head, and more.

Getting Daily Biofeedback Untangles Life Issues

T'ai Chi and QiGong's slow, gentle, inner-mindful movements are unlike any other exercise, in that they give you the opportunity to go within to see issues beneath the physical ones. This can be a powerful therapy on several levels, enabling T'ai Chi's engineering align-ments to untangle mental and emotional knots.

T'ai Chi and QiGong as Biofeedback

T'ai Chi and QiGong show us that the entire body is a connected whole, not individual parts. Fixing your posture can help eliminate chronic headaches, etc. We've all heard, "the head bone's connected to the neck bone; the neck bone's connected to the ...." It's true, and the biofeedback element of T'ai Chi and QiGong will help all these parts relax into a loosening flow of motion that will untangle many knots beyond the places you begin to align, loosen, and relax.

T'AI SCI

Biofeedback uses a computer program to train people how to deeply relax. Leading biofeedback specialist Dr. Gary Green refers to T'ai Chi as "biofeedback without the computer."

As far as chronic pain issues, you will discover that your bones are often not the problem, but rather that *muscle tension* was *pulling the bones out of alignment.* So your stress levels, or in other words, the accumulated unmanaged mental-emotional stress that we collect or grip in our cells, is at the root of most of our physical problems (see Chapter 18).

Therefore, the physical engineering of T'ai Chi and QiGong *will* take stress off the bones and connective tissue, as taught by the "unbendable arm" phenomenon taught in Chapter 3—an exercise meant to show students how they can be much more powerful by relaxing. Yes, that sounds like a paradox, but as you progress through the exercises in this book and later in a live class, hopefully you will feel that relaxed power expanding through you.

OUCH!

Never force yourself through motions when doing T'ai Chi and QiGong. The biofeedback slow-mindfulness quality will enable you to be aware of your body's limits, and ease up against those limits in a way that feels good. Your range will increase over time.

As you learn to move from the dan tien (which will be expanded on later), lengthen your spine, and relax around this elongated posture, you'll actually learn how to let the earth beneath you take most of the pressure caused by work or exercise. Your relaxed body, through a series of subtle release visualizations, will pass all the strain down through your body to the earth under your feet.

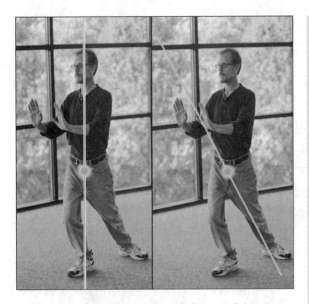

This image illustrates the vertical axis and dan tien in alignment (left), and how you will learn to allow the force of your effort, in this case a push, to transfer through your relaxed body (see Unbendable Arm in Chapter 3) into the earth below you.

The new way you will begin to approach mowing the grass, shoveling snow, pushing a shopping cart, or hitting a golf ball will greatly reduce strain on your lower back, while adding much more power to your actions.

After a few months of T'ai Chi, because of this subtle internal biofeedback-like awareness, next time you shovel snow or rake leaves, you'll feel much less sore than you did the year before, because of these small core adjustments in posture and movement.

Yet, there is an even more important lesson to be found in this physical loosening. You will realize that the world does not fall apart when you let go of the tendency to feel like the world is on your shoulders. The physical letting go of effort and strain will translate into a mental and emotional letting go. This doesn't mean you'll become an uncaring sloth who is of no value to the world. Quite the opposite; you'll discover that the fewer burdens you grip

in your muscles, mind, and heart, the more energy you will be able to access by allowing it to "flow through you." Most T'ai Chi and QiGong practitioners find themselves becoming more caring people, more relaxed, creative, and effective workers, and basically better at everything—clearer, happier, and more fun to be around. (Notice the unhurried, relaxed flow of T'ai Chi's flowing forms in Chapter 1's *Soothing Unhurried Flow of T'ai Chi*.)

Seeing the Physical and Mental Health Link

So, the physical engineering of the body mentioned above is inextricably related to your mental and emotional states. As QiGong meditation/visualization and breathing techniques begin to relax your mind and emotional state, the muscles will relax and the bones will align.

Our muscles are like a thermometer, in that they show you what you can't see. The tension we hold in our muscles is an indicator of the tension we've held beneath the surface in our mind and heart, and in the field of energy that we are when we get down to the tiny subatomic bits that make us up.

In the classic golf movie *The Legend of Bagger Vance*, actor Will Smith's character spoke a quintessential T'ai Chi line: "The way you hold your club is the way you hold your life." When we get challenged in life, we tend to hold our breath, and that causes us to tighten up, which causes us to get more rigid emotionally and mentally.

T'ai Chi is a form of Moving QiGong (pronounced *chee gong*). QiGong means "breathing exercise." By practicing these breathing techniques that include what the Chinese call "the sinking" or the "letting go of our entire being on each exhale," our entire body relaxes more, and our life relaxes more, as we let the "vertical axis" hold us up and everything else *lets go*. See Chapter 1's video *Sinking Your Qi*.)

T'AI SCI

This book's author is the T'ai Chi expert for famed naturopathic physician and best-selling author Dr. Andrew Weil's popular website. Dr. Weil has written that most of our health problems are caused by *poor breathing habits*.

So, as you are fixing your physical tension issues, you will often discover that the depression and anxiety issues we face in this fast-paced modern world begin to dissipate as well through our T'ai Chi and QiGong practice. In the medical research in the next chapter, you'll see that this assertion has been validated by studies again and again.

OUCH!

When you catch yourself trying *too hard* or notice your head and shoulder muscles tightening—just stop. Take some deep breaths, and on each sighing exhale think of every one of your 50 trillion cells absolutely letting go of everything they are squeezing on to. Feel your entire being lightening up on itself, permeated by a silken effortless-ness that expands through you. Feel the weight of the world lift off your shoulders. Go ahead! Do it right now; don't wait. And repeat this several times. Now, doesn't that feel nice?

One amazing benefit you will realize over time is that as your muscles relax and your bones align, you will find that you not only move through life more effortlessly, but more powerfully as well. Your sports performance will dramatically improve, and sometimes

quite quickly. A student in one of my classes, a psychologist who later authored a book that advocated T'ai Chi for mental-emotional issues, reported to me that after only a few months of T'ai Chi and QiGong classes he had increased his golf drive by *100 yards*, adding happily, "I don't have to swing nearly as hard now, so my drives are more accurate, too!" In a recent major pro golf tournament the champion of the event was asked how he did it, and he replied, "I relaxed out of the way of my swing." This is the essence of T'ai Chi and QiGong.

As T'ai Chi and QiGong fix your physical and mental/emotional issues, they will also become a powerful medical tonic that will expand through your life, heading off or even treating many health challenges you may encounter. This isn't meant to replace your physician. It's mentioned so that you can bring it to your doctor's attention. Many major medical schools in America are now training medical students in T'ai Chi and QiGong, not only to prescribe to their patients but to use for themselves to help them cope and be more effective in the high-stress career they are pursuing.

T'ai Chi and QiGong are Powerful Life Medicine

In 2009 I was invited to speak at what was to be the National Institutes of Health's first-ever Mind-Body Week event in Washington. The event was later postponed to 2012, but the winds of change for American healthcare began then. I was later commissioned by the world-renowned health journal *Prevention Magazine* to create the T'ai Chi tutorial for their December 2010 issue article titled, "Boost Your Immune System Naturally with T'ai Chi."

If a pill could do what T'ai Chi and QiGong can do, it would be the top-selling drug in the world. But in spite of what profound health tools they are, you won't be bombarded with T'ai Chi and QiGong TV advertising because there is no fortune to be made in teaching these arts—therefore, no massive advertising budgets. So hang on to this book and keep it by your remote control and when TV ads come on, hit the mute button and pick up this book again and again. And tell people you care for about T'ai Chi and QiGong, because research shows when you help others it makes you healthier.

T'AI SCI

Harvard Health publication recently wrote that T'ai Chi might more accurately be called "medication in motion," because of all the myriad health issues it is now proving to prevent or treat, according to mounting medical research.

T'ai Chi and QiGong use breathing/visualization relaxation techniques in combination with effortless gentle movements to loosen up all the collected stress grit in the body, and, as you read previously, in the mind and heart as well. This has a profound impact on the various health systems, which are all integrated together. At the core of our health is stress management. When the physical body practices poor postural habits, poor breathing habits, and poor mental/emotional habits, this weakens the immune system. You may be wondering, how is that?

T'AI SCI

T'ai Chi and QiGong are part of Traditional Chinese Medicine, as is acupuncture. The gentle motions of these exercises help massage and stimulate the 361 main acupuncture points through the body to facilitate a healthful flow of Qi, or *life energy*.

Reboot Your Nervous System for Clarity

The body, mind, and heart (or emotional body) are made of energy, as is all of existence when you get down to the subatomic bits. Chinese researchers began exploring this energy aspect of us millennia ago, and found that a radiant flow of energy moves through us all the time, but is constricted when we hold on to stress loads. It is like static interrupting all the minute, subtle signals powering all the health communication networks and systems in our being, and especially our immune system.

These tools' ability to help us unload that accumulated stress on a daily basis has profound implications. It's exactly like when you've overstrained your computer by running multiple programs and it becomes intermittently paralyzed by multiple conflicting signals (as when stressed thoughts spin through our minds chaotically), until you reboot by turning it off to let the circuits clear. When you turn it on, programs run more efficiently and smoothly. This is exactly how the hard drive of your mind, the electrical pulses of your nervous system, and the hardware of your muscle and organ tissue are slowed down, cleared out, and reinvigorated by T'ai Chi and QiGong's slow, contemplative breathing, motion, and visualization techniques.

OUCH!

Nearly one third of adult Americans have chronic high-blood pressure, while over 70 million suffer chronic sleep disorders. Medical research shows T'ai Chi and QiGong can help with both, which can also un-gnarl, or head off, many other related problems.

Just to give you an example of what a powerful health science T'ai Chi is, take a recent study from UCLA that showed T'ai Chi practitioners boosted their Helper T cell count by 50 percent over the control groups not practicing T'ai Chi. These T cells are the foundation of the immune system, consuming virus, bacteria, and even cancer cells. T'ai Chi profoundly boosted the practitioners' immune system. You will be stunned to learn of the growing number of major health issues medical research is now showing T'ai Chi and QiGong can help with.

The next chapter covers some of those medical benefits. As mentioned before, T'ai Chi and QiGong are *mind-body* exercises. The mind-set that you approach them with will make all the difference in how effective the actual exercises are. So by knowing and believing that these tools work, you actually enhance their effectiveness. But before moving on to that, let's look at a couple of other life issues T'ai Chi and QiGong can help with—beginning with career success.

T'ai Chi and QiGong for Career Enhancement

You should show this book to your company's human resources wellness director—especially Chapter 20, "T'ai Chi as Corporate Wellness"—for it is estimated that U.S. business is losing upwards of $300 billion per year due to employee stress (that's $7,500 per employee per year). You may be able to get your company to spring for T'ai Chi and QiGong classes at your workplace. It'll save them money and make the work environment so much more pleasant. Trust me, I was an HR administrator for years before becoming a T'ai Chi teacher full time. I finally made the decision to spend my life teaching people tools to manage stress, rather than expending all my energy refereeing internal stress-driven squabbles between edgy employees.

T'ai Chi and QiGong can also help you advance your career. While that may sound like a stretch, as your practice expands over coming months, you'll quickly realize that we don't practice T'ai Chi and QiGong to get better at T'ai Chi and QiGong—we practice to become better at *everything*.

Here's an example. At the time I began learning T'ai Chi and QiGong I had no real training or education in business, for I'd been an art major in school. My first serious job after college was as an entry-level temporary office clerk who went from company to company entering data at very low pay. But my practice of these meditative arts had so de-stressed me that I became a much more affable person to be around. It was because of this that one of the companies where I temped hired me on as their 401k/payroll administrator, dramatically boosting my salary, and getting me out of a cubicle and into a corner office *with a window*. With zero business background, I was nevertheless hired for this administrator position over all the accounting clerks in the department, simply because of being more enjoyable to be around. T'ai Chi and QiGong then helped me manage the enormous stress of learning in a few weeks what these people had spent years preparing for, and I did it successfully, doing payroll, related taxes, and managing retirement funds for five international corporations for several years! These powerful stress-reduction tools very literally *changed my life!*

We tend to think of "professionals" as very analytical people who check every detail on our resumé, etc., to find the most highly qualified people to employ. But the real world is filled with real human beings who much prefer spending their days around those that they can *enjoy* working with.

Of course, you need to be competent as well, which you definitely are, or you wouldn't be reading a book meant to improve your life and make you more efficient. While your mental and emotional flexibility and affability is an enormous part of *getting* that job you seek, T'ai Chi and QiGong will enable you to be effective at actually *performing* that job successfully, because the same loosening of the muscles, body, heart, and mind that makes you easier to get along with also makes you more creative and flexible in dealing with challenges.

Psychologists have written that T'ai Chi is a perfect microcosmic working model for understanding how we handle the macrocosm of our lives. As you learn T'ai Chi, you quickly realize that the more you breathe and release all your tight efforts to learn, the more easily your mind and body can absorb information. As you learn how to relax into the learning of T'ai Chi, you are also discovering how to *relax into learning* new computer programs or changing business systems, and so on.

Multi-Tasking: Meditation, Fitness, and Massage

Meditation is a powerful health and self-improvement tool. There are many wonderful forms of meditative practices. However, T'ai Chi and QiGong offer something no other meditations, other than perhaps yoga, do—a *physical-ization* of the meditative state. Several meditations use a repeated word or phrase, known as a chant or a mantra, to keep the mind occupied enough not to worry or wander, but simple enough so that the mind can transcend analytical thought, and sink into a deeper alpha brain-wave state of mind. Chinese masters over all these many centuries have evolved a "physical meditation" system that uses the "pleasure sensations" of our body as the mantra. In our

fast-paced lives, to get the benefits of meditation while also getting physical fitness benefits can be a huge time-saver.

Now, there are standing or sitting forms of QiGong meditation that don't involve movement (see Chapter 9), but even those use this physical-awareness mantra to focus the mind and clear the heart. Using these still forms can greatly enhance your moving practices by cultivating a deep inner awareness of your state of mind and physical sensations. As you delve into these practices, you will discover that emotional and mental blocks or discomforts also have a physical sensation related to them, and as you utilize the powerful threefold combination of breathing, visualization, and gentle motion to relax and untangle the physical sensations, the mental and emotional issues beneath them will also begin to dissipate.

As you relax into these gentle forms of movement, your internal relaxed awareness becomes like a massaging of all the 50 trillion cells of your being, as you let your center move your bones, causing your relaxed muscles to be massaged by the motion. This may sound too good to be possible, and it's really impossible to convey in words. You'll just have to dive into it. You'll feel benefits right away, but this will expand for a lifetime as you continue your T'ai Chi or QiGong journey.

Styles of T'ai Chi

There are many T'ai Chi styles, and even more subsets of those styles, and many QiGong styles. As a beginner, finding a teacher who is *right for you* is more important than pursuing any given style. The question often arises, "How do I know if a T'ai Chi or QiGong class or teacher is a good one?" This author's stock answer is this: if you feel better after class than you did when you went in, then it's a good one. Those who dive into these arts often find they want to try many styles and teachers, and Appendix A will help you connect with teachers worldwide of all different styles.

> **OUCH!**
>
> Although most styles of T'ai Chi are slow, some are faster and more demanding, and all can be modified. So if you have physical limitations, talk to your prospective teacher to learn how to make T'ai Chi accessible to your condition. T'ai Chi should *always* feel good.

Most (but not all) of the main T'ai Chi styles reflect the family names of who created them: Yang, Kuang Ping Yang, Chen, Wu, Sun, Wu Hao, and Mulan styles are among the more common styles.

The Chen style was the original style of T'ai Chi, founded by Chen Chang-hsing. The Yang style was founded by Yang Lu-chan, who studied under the original T'ai Chi master Chen Chang-hsing. The Kuang Ping Yang style (exhibited in the Long Form in Chapter 13) was brought to the United States by Kuo Lien-ying, who studied under Yang Pan-hou, son of the Yang style founder. The Wu style was founded by Wu Quan-yu, student of the originator of the Yang style and his son. The Sun style was developed by Sun Lu-t'ang. The Mulan Quan (Chapters 14, 15, and 16) is the only major old style that was created by a woman master, Sifu Mei Fing Ying, although since there have been other great women masters who've created styles.

Years ago I saw T'ai Chi history being made when I attended the International T'ai Chi Symposium at Vanderbilt University. Six grandmasters, descendants of the original Chinese T'ai Chi creators, came together and stated

that "all" T'ai Chi styles offer the same benefits when done properly. This was a testament to the *non-contending humanity* T'ai Chi cultivates in practitioners, to see these men who one would have thought might see one another as "competitors," embracing the value and wisdom of each other, and considering the other style grandmasters as "compatriots" with one common goal—expanding world health.

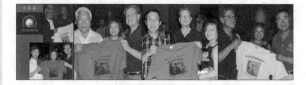

Authors Bill Douglas and Angela Wong-Douglas met with the six grandmasters of the major T'ai Chi styles at the International T'ai Chi Symposium at Vanderbilt University, all direct descendants of the Yang, Wu, Chen, and Sun family styles.

(Photo courtesy of Rod Ferguson, Australian Academy of T'ai Chi.)

If you aren't excited yet about your new or continuing T'ai Chi and QiGong journey, you should be. Think about it. This is pretty heady stuff: increasing your personal power on many levels, and cleansing your mind and heart of stress; boosting your health and mental acuity to become more creative and effective at everything you do, and doing all of this with just one easy, low-impact exercise system. Whether you are a rank beginner, a long-time enthusiast, or even a teacher, the profound depth and breadth of T'ai Chi & QiGong's multidimensional benefits, when illuminated as they are in this book, can take your (or your students') practice to a whole new level. Now, let's further enhance your intellectual awareness of T'ai Chi and QiGong's potential in the next chapter on T'ai Chi and QiGong as medical therapy.

The Least You Need to Know

- Everyone can do T'ai Chi or QiGong.
- T'ai Chi and QiGong are highly effective mental/emotional therapies.
- T'ai Chi and QiGong are powerful performance enhancers: sports, business, and more.
- T'ai Chi and QiGong are "medication in motion," preventing or healing many health challenges.
- T'ai Chi and QiGong should feel easy and good, without strain or pain.

Medical T'ai Chi & QiGong: The Prescription for the Future

In This Chapter

- T'ai Chi is *powerful* medicine
- Unlocking your healing mind using the T'ai *Key*
- Exploring the links between acupuncture and T'ai Chi
- Western medicine is now sold on T'ai Chi and QiGong
- Understanding how T'ai Chi and QiGong have integrated with modern medicine
- Web Video Support: *Horse Stance and Resistance-Free motion*

The great American inventor Thomas Alva Edison wrote: "The doctor of the future will prescribe no medicine, but will interest his patients in the care of the human frame." This encapsulates the essence of what T'ai Chi and QiGong are all about, as well as the profound shift that these tools are helping to create in modern healthcare.

T'ai Chi and QiGong's medical benefits have been studied for nearly 2,000 years in China and for only about 30 years in the West. However, Western medical research is now discovering what Chinese medicine has long realized—that T'ai Chi and QiGong provide more medical benefits than any other single exercise. That's why these ancient Chinese exercises are now not only at the cutting edge of modern medical research, but increasingly are a part of modern healthcare. (See Chapter 2's T'ai Chi Medical Research Library link: www.idiotsguides.com/taichi.)

We are very lucky to live at a time when these wonderful tools are available to us in the West. We are also lucky to be able to see scientific proof that they work because as practitioners of Traditional Chinese Medicine (TCM) understood centuries ago, *our faith is the greatest healer*. So if we know in our minds that T'ai Chi and QiGong work, our bodies will allow them to do their magic, and we will be the big winners.

The Health Benefits of T'ai Chi and QiGong

We live in a stressful world; only recently has Western medical research come to recognize that stress is at the root of most health problems. Therefore, the health crisis that stress is causing in the West has actually created a great opportunity for us because it is opening us up to the wonders of TCM and tools like T'ai Chi and QiGong. In fact, the following list of T'ai Chi's measurable health benefits indicates how this opening to T'ai Chi may save us from our healthcare crisis. T'ai Chi and QiGong can …

- Boost the immune system

- Reduce or eliminate chronic pain issues

- Slow the aging process

- Reduce anxiety, depression, and overall mood disturbance

- Lower high blood pressure

- Alleviate stress responses

- Enhance the body's natural healing powers, such as recovering from injury

- Increase breathing capacity

- Reduce asthma and allergy reactions

- Improve balance and coordination *twice* as well as the best balance-conditioning exercises in the world

- Help ensure full-range mobility far into old age

- Provide the lowest-impact weight-bearing exercise known

However, before adding T'ai Chi or QiGong to your physical therapy program, consult your physician to see if they might affect your medication levels. For example, many with high blood pressure find that their blood pressure lowers after playing T'ai Chi for a while. Your physician should know if T'ai Chi can alter your current therapy for such conditions and then can lower your medication safely. (See Chapter 18 for other conditions T'ai Chi or QiGong may benefit, and show it to your doctor.)

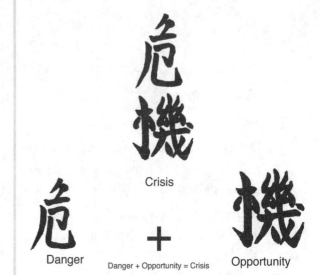

The Chinese character for "crisis" is a combination of two other characters—one for "danger" and the other for "opportunity."

Mind Over Matter

The Chinese realized that our mind or consciousness is the root of who we are. Our health and our lives are merely reflections of our state of mind. T'ai Chi's mindful quality incorporates the mind and body into a powerful healing force. See Chapter 2's Web Video Support's *QiGong and T'ai Chi bring the mind … inside the body.*

Interestingly, Western science now sees that TCM's ancient insights were right on the money. A new science called *psychoneuroimmunology* has found that our mind constantly communicates to every cell of our body.

Emotional chemicals, known as neuropeptides, flow throughout our bodies, communicating every feeling to the entire body. So when hitting every red light on the street aggravates us or we become anxious in every line we stand in, we walk around in a state of perpetual panic. This negatively affects our heart, brain, and entire circulatory system. In fact, those effects, in turn, affect other organs, which can cause a breakdown of the entire system over time. The state of perpetual panic ends up causing such extremes as kidney failure, heart enlargement, and hardening of the arteries.

T'ai Chi helps us do just the opposite. We can decide to let issues slide right off us, literally breathing fears out with every sigh and yawn. As we sit in QiGong meditation or move in T'ai Chi's soothing postures, we let a nourishing, healing flow of Qi, or life energy, fill every cell of our body.

Don't try too hard to memorize any of these details on TCM or Western medicine. Rather, let the concepts wash over your relaxed mind. The important stuff will stick, and you can always go back and look up details later.

To fully appreciate T'ai Chi's medical benefits, it may be helpful to understand how TCM views the body. TCM has known for centuries what Western science is only now discovering—that the mind and body are two inseparable things. There's a joke in TCM that "the only place the mind, body, emotions, and spirit are separate is in textbooks." In real life and T'ai Chi, it just isn't so. T'ai Chi's slow, mindful movements are the epitome of this union of mind and body. Now Western medicine is convinced of it as well."

So when your body's muscles are rigid, your thinking will likely be more rigid, too. Likewise, if your thinking is harsh and rigid, in time this will be reflected in stiffness in your muscular frame. This stiffness impedes the flow of Qi, which diminishes your health. Therefore, your mind and your thoughts are just as important to your health as the food you eat and the exercise you get.

I have students regularly come into my class with a headache or stiff neck, and discover after we complete the Sitting QiGong technique that their headache or neck-ache has disappeared. Its because cranial or other muscular tension was at the core of their pain, so by letting the energetic fibers of the mind and body relax through a mindful, nonphysical meditation— their physical pain went away. Enjoy the *Sitting QiGong* meditation daily, or even twice per day. (See Chapter 2's Web Video Support section *Sitting QiGong.*)

Energy meridians, or *jing luo*, link all the organs and the entire physical body to the mind and emotional systems. This explains how T'ai Chi and QiGong's mind/body exercises integrate all aspects of the self into a powerful self-healing system. See Chapter 2's Web Video Support *T'ai Chi and the Acupuncture Meridians.*

KNOW YOUR CHINESE

The body's energy meridians, or **jing luo,** are a network of channels that move Qi through the body. *Jing* literally means "to move through," and luo means "a net."

What are these energy meridians that T'ai Chi and QiGong help unblock? Qi flows through and powers every cell in your body, the way electricity powers your house. Without Qi, the cell would be dead, for Qi is the life force. Qi radiates in your cells via the meridians. You can't see these meridians; you can only detect the energy that moves through them, just as you cannot see an ocean current in the water, but you can detect its motion. (See Chapter 2's Web Video Support, *The 3 Dan Tiens.*)

Ancient maps of these meridians, made thousands of years ago by traditional Chinese doctors, show 14 main energy meridians that carry Qi throughout the body internally and externally. These meridians' flow of energy is opened and balanced by T'ai Chi and QiGong practice. It is not necessary to mentally memorize or locate them to enjoy the benefits. However, for your intellectual curiosity, their names are listed here, first by the modern acupuncture abbreviation, then by the English name, and a few followed by the Chinese name in italics:

- CV = Conception Vessel, or *Ren Mai*
- CX = Pericardium Channel
- GB = Gallbladder Channel
- GV = Governing Vessel, or *Du Mai*
- HE = Heart Channel
- KI = Kidney Channel
- LI = Large Intestine Channel
- LU = Lung Channel
- LV = Liver Channel
- SI = Small Intestine Channel
- SP = Spleen-Pancreas Channel
- ST = Stomach Channel
- TW = Triple Warmer, or *San Jiao* Channel
- UB = Urinary Bladder Channel

Acupuncture and T'ai Chi

Three aspects make up Traditional Chinese Medicine (TCM): acupuncture, herbal medicine, and T'ai Chi/QiGong. All three share a common premise that Qi radiates through the body and our health is diminished when the energy flow gets blocked or squeezed off.

So whether an acupuncturist is treating you with needles, an herbalist is prescribing herbs, or you are practicing T'ai Chi, you are trying to balance the imbalances, or unblock the energy that flows throughout your body. Millions of Americans now use alternative therapies like acupuncture and herbs. If you practice T'ai Chi or QiGong daily, your relaxed state will help herbs or acupuncture work even more effectively.

The energy meridians, which flow throughout the interior of the body, have 361 points that surface at the skin. These are the most common treatment points acupuncturists use. But the whole body and even the mind can be treated with acupuncture because the meridians that surface at the skin also flow inside the body, through the brain and other organs.

T'AI SCI

Modern acupuncturists often call the Qi meridians *bioenergetic circuits*.

T'ai Chi and QiGong affect the same energy flow that acupuncture does, although acupuncture can be better for acute problems, whereas T'ai Chi is a daily tune-up. Acupuncturists may recommend T'ai Chi to their patients, and T'ai Chi teachers may recommend acupuncture to their students with chronic or acute conditions as a supplement to the students' standard medical treatments. T'ai Chi, QiGong, and acupuncture are very complementary.

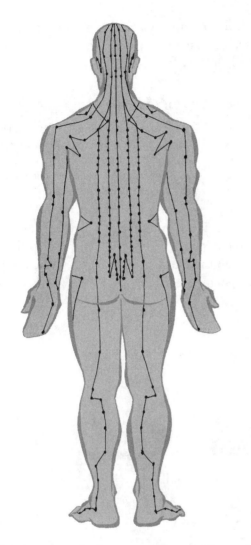

Here is an example of an acupuncture meridian map. The lines represent the meridians, or energy channels, flowing through the body. The dots on the lines are the acupuncture points, which are often the places of least electrical resistance on the skin.

A T'AI CHI PUNCH LINE

There are also acupuncture maps for animals. In fact, some racing horses have their own personal acupuncturists. Many veterinarians use acupuncture as part of their practice.

It is mind-boggling when you consider that many modern acupuncturists find acupuncture points with electronic equipment, not unlike an Ohmmeter, a device used to measure electrical resistance. What's more amazing is that acupuncture maps were made long before electronics was developed. How did they know where those points were back then? They might have felt them. As you practice T'ai Chi and QiGong, you will eventually begin to feel the Qi flowing from your hands or in your body.

Acupuncture sees the body holistically, meaning that each small part of the body contains connections to the whole body. Therefore, an acupuncturist can treat any problem in the whole body through, for example, the ears. Likewise, any part of the body, or even the mind, can be treated through the hands or the feet.

One of the powerful health benefits T'ai Chi provides is a daily acupuncture tune-up. Because T'ai Chi is so slow and the weight shifts are so deliberate, with the body very relaxed the feet are massaged by the earth during a T'ai Chi exercise. The bottoms of the feet have acupuncture points that affect the entire body as well as the mind. The acupressure foot massage you get during a T'ai Chi session stimulates all the acupuncture points on the foot, treating the whole body. This type of slow, relaxed motion makes T'ai Chi unique in providing you an acupuncture tune-up each time you do your daily exercise.

View *Soothing Unhuried Flow of T'ai Chi* on Chapter 2's Web Video Support to visually understand the flow and effortless slowness of the forms that result in stimulating the acupressure points on the feet and throughout the entire body. *No other exercise provides this.*

Zang Fu: Massaging Internal Organs for Health

Another profound benefit T'ai Chi provides is a gentle massaging of the internal organs. Because T'ai Chi moves the body in about 95 percent of the possible motions it can go through, it not only clears the joints of calcium deposits, but it also gently massages the internal organs. See Chapter 2's Web Video Support's *Your Rotating Dan Tien Massages Your Organs*.

In TCM, this is a powerful therapy for optimum health. TCM recognizes that the body is an integrated whole, whereby all the parts are connected by the flow of Qi. In fact, the Chinese system of medicine is built upon a *Zang Fu* graph, which shows how organs interact with and depend on one another for good, healthy function.

KNOW YOUR CHINESE

Literally translated, **Zang Fu** means "solid hollow." Organs within the body considered to be hollow, like the stomach or large intestines, are Fu organs, while the solid organs, such as liver and lungs, are Zang organs.

Because T'ai Chi massages all the organs through its gentle, full rotations, it helps balance all the integrating activities of the Zang Fu systems.

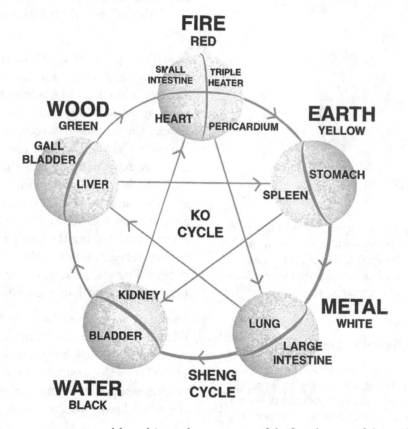

The Zang Fu system uses a memory model, applying each organ to one of the five elements of the earth. The Chinese see the world as made of earth, metal, water, wood, and fire. The energy flow affects different organs through the Sheng Cycle and the Ko Cycle. This figure shows how organs are interactive and interdependent on one another for healthful function.

Your Organs Are Related to Your Emotions

Acupuncture, herbal medicine, and T'ai Chi/ QiGong use the Zang Fu system to understand how the body, mind, and emotions integrate. A problem with a particular organ may have emotional symptoms. Likewise, a chronic emotional state may have a physical impact on the organs. The following list explains the Zang Fu connection between organs and emotions commonly related to imbalances with those organs or their energy channels:

- Liver = depression, anger

- Heart = excess joy (such as manic behavior), excess mental function

- Spleen = obsession

- Lung = anguish, grief, melancholy

- Kidney = fear, fright

SAGE SIFU SAYS

If you go to a traditional Chinese physician, he or she may likely ask you about your emotions as well as your physical symptoms because emotional states may help lead him or her to understand which organ's energy is deficient or in excess.

T'ai Chi benefits the mental and emotional states, not only by encouraging us to let go of the day's problems by focusing on breath and movement, but in other ways as well. T'ai Chi stimulates the organs with gentle massage, while stimulating the acupressure points on the feet and throughout the body with its gentle, relaxed postures. The breathing in T'ai Chi is full, yet effortless, encouraging internal releases of mental and emotional blocks that also help the internal Zang Fu systems become less

restricted, more free-flowing, and more healthful on mental, emotional, and physical levels. (Chapter 3 explains how T'ai Chi and QiGong can provide mental and emotional healing.)

Increase Flexibility

T'ai Chi increases flexibility not only by regularly stretching the muscles very gently, but through the Zang Fu system as well. As we age—especially but not exclusively men—we often find a depletion in our kidney energy. The kidney energy is responsible for the function of the liquid systems of the body. Therefore, the decrease in kidney energy that accompanies aging causes our connective tissue, such as tendons, to become brittle. We are then much more likely to tear or otherwise injure our bones or joints when we stumble or fall.

The tremendous balance improvements T'ai Chi offers are only part of why T'ai Chi practitioners are much less likely than other people to suffer falling injuries. The improved performance of all organ functions enhances the entire physical body's health. In fact, in this way, Sitting QiGong may also increase flexibility, even though it is a nonphysical exercise.

Western Medicine's Research on T'ai Chi and QiGong

After reading this section, you should be satisfied beyond a doubt that *T'ai Chi works*. When you get to the QiGong and T'ai Chi exercises in Parts 3, 4, and 5, you won't have to think about their benefits. The mind is the greatest healer; if you believe in the value of your therapy, it will be much more effective for you.

Stress Is the Root of Your Health Issues

By now you know that stress is the chief cause of illness in the modern world. As Western medicine discovered that T'ai Chi and QiGong were highly effective stress-reducing exercises, these powerful mind/body health tools were used in more and more hospitals and prescribed by more and more doctors.

Studies show that reaction to stress can damage the entire body. It causes chronic hypertension (high blood pressure), which can cause the arteries to harden, and causes kidney damage and enlargement of the heart. Stress also has been shown to impair our ability to think and actually shrinks the hypothalamus and the hippocampus parts of the brain. Yikes!

> **A T'AI CHI PUNCH LINE**
>
> TCM sees the body and mind intertwined. A rigid body can cause us to think rigidly as well. Or perhaps more accurately, a rigid mind can cause us to have a rigid body.

T'ai Chi and QiGong are proven stress busters. An article in *Occupational Therapy Week* explains that T'ai Chi's emphasis on posture (see *Sinking Your Qi and Locating Your Dan Tien and Vertical Axis* in Chapter 2's Web Video Support for proper posture examples) and diaphragmatic breathing (breathing from your diaphragm, see *QiGong Breathing Tutorial*) accounts for a practitioner's reduction in muscular tension and the stress it causes. Patients using T'ai Chi report a greater ability to cope with fear and anxiety, as that physical relaxation is reflected in their mental attitude.

Bellevue Psychiatric Hospital in New York City provided T'ai Chi to both staff and patients. Its activity therapy supervisor said, "T'ai Chi is a natural and safe vehicle to *neutralize* rather than resist the stress in our personal lives, an ability which we greatly need to nurture in our modern, fast-paced society." View Chapter 2's *T'ai Chi Slows and Calms* on the Web Video Support to see the *resistance-free* model of motion and the *slowing down* of mind and body T'ai Chi promotes. *Research has revealed that just watching the forms being performed can leave you feeling calmer!*

T'ai Chi Is Your Heart, Head, and Body's Best Friend

Harvard Medical School's *Women's Health Watch Journal* reported that "T'ai Chi has *salubrious* effects" and that "practicing T'ai Chi regularly may delay the decline of cardiopulmonary function in older adults … T'ai Chi was found to be as effective as meditation in reducing stress hormones."

A Duke University study revealed that managing stress controls heart disease even more effectively than exercise. Because T'ai Chi provides both powerful stress management and gentle exercise, T'ai Chi is your heart's very best friend.

Studies on mental benefits of these practices include one cited in the *Journal of Psychosomatic Research* reporting that their T'ai Chi study subjects reported less tension, depression, anger, fatigue, confusion, and anxiety. They felt more vigorous and in general had less total mood disturbance.

The *Journal of Black Psychology* states that many African Americans suffer from chronic high blood pressure. The article explains that hypertension is a physical result of psychological stress and proposes T'ai Chi as a holistic way of treating psychosomatic illnesses, or those illnesses caused by stress.

T'ai Chi may also help us think better. Research has shown that stress can limit the development of the hippocampus, the part of the brain that deals with learning and memory. T'ai Chi's ability to reduce stress responses may actually enhance our ability to learn and remember. Sitting QiGong meditation is designed to actually teach you how to un-clench and relax the tissue of the mind, taking pressure off the pineal and pituitary glands as well.

> **SAGE SIFU SAYS**
>
> With all these T'ai Chi and QiGong facts swimming through your mind, now is a good time to practice QiGong's mind-clearing tools. Take a deep breath from your abdomen to your chest, and on the sighing exhale, let your shoulders relax away from your neck as they sink toward the floor. Repeat this several times and, as you release each breath, imagine that every one of the fifty-trillion cells that make you up are absolutely letting go of everything they've been holding on to. Ironically, you will find that the more your mind lets go of trying to hold on to facts, the more easily it can absorb information.

The lowering of "body stress" T'ai Chi and QiGong workouts promote are a huge reason these arts are the fastest-growing fitness endeavors in America (Fitness Manufacturers Association report). In an article on T'ai Chi, *Working Woman* magazine noted that "increasingly mind/body workouts are replacing high-impact aerobics, and other body punishing exercises … These mind/body workouts are kinder to the joints and muscles and can reduce the tension that often contributes to the development of disease, which makes them especially appropriate for high-powered, stressed-out baby boomers."

T'ai Chi is an exercise few doctors will ever tell patients to *stop* practicing. It provides perhaps the lowest-impact weight-bearing exercise there is. We all need weight-bearing exercise to help build bone mass and connective tissue, but for those with rheumatoid arthritis or some other conditions, weight-bearing exercise is a problem. For these people, weight-bearing exercise can aggravate joints, causing tenderness or swelling.

However, a study cited in the *American Journal of Physical Medicine and Rehabilitation* wanted to see if T'ai Chi would harm rheumatoid arthritis patients. To the researchers' pleasant surprise, T'ai Chi did no damage whatsoever and provided the study participants with the safe weight-bearing exercise they seriously needed. The forms were modified for these patients, and everyone with arthritis or knee problems should be sure they do only forms that feel good to them, but this T'ai Chi discovery is good news for all of us because it gives us all a weight-bearing exercise that is safe even into old age.

A Boost to Your Immune System

Prevention Magazine reported a study on T'ai Chi's effects on the immune system, supporting an idea the Chinese call *bu qi, bu xue*. It found that regular T'ai Chi practice may increase the body's production of T-cells. These T-cells are T-lymphocytes. "Lympho-whats?" you might ask. It doesn't matter. What matters is that these little T-cells help the immune system destroy bacteria and possibly even tumor cells. If T'ai Chi can make more of these little buggers, what are we waiting for? Let's T'ai Chi one on!

KNOW YOUR CHINESE

T'ai Chi and QiGong have long been known to boost the immune system. Ancient Chinese medicine understood the concept of the immune system, which the Chinese called *bu qi, bu xue,* meaning "tonify the Qi and blood." When Qi and blood are strengthened, we are better able to fight off infection and disease.

In China, QiGong is commonly prescribed as an adjunct to chemotherapy and radiation. Studies indicate that when QiGong is combined with standard cancer treatments, favorable results are obtained, treating virtually all forms and stages of cancer. Part of the reason for this success is that QiGong helps patients feel less helpless. Studies show that feelings of self-empowerment can have powerful healing benefits on the course of almost any disease, including cancer.

A T'AI CHI PUNCH LINE

I was once studying T'ai Chi and QiGong in Hong Kong. Because of the time difference, I was waking up at 3 A.M. with nothing else to do, so I became a particularly diligent student and practiced Gathering Qi or Standing Post for nearly an hour and a half each morning. After about a week of this, I began to visually see the Qi flowing around people, especially their heads. I noticed that those who seemed to be enjoying the day had large pluming expanses of energy around them, while those appearing driven and stressed had tiny, restricted energy emanating from them.

How Does T'ai Chi Fight for the Immune System?

American QiGong master Kenneth S. Cohen has dubbed a hormone called DHEA the Health Hormone. In his *brilliant* book *The Way of QiGong: The Art and Science of Chinese Energy Healing,* Mr. Cohen explains that this hormone is believed to be linked to Qi.

DHEA is short for dehydroepiandrosterone. Yeah, I know, *forget about it.* But don't forget that DHEA is related to youthfulness, less disease, and a more functional immune system. According to Cohen, low DHEA levels have been directly linked to cancer, diabetes, obesity, hypertension, allergies, heart disease, and most autoimmune diseases.

When we are under a lot of stress, our body exhausts itself of this important hormone. Therefore, by practicing T'ai Chi, we can increase DHEA levels, thereby increasing our immune system's ability to fight whatever steps in the ring with it. Let's rumble!

T'ai Chi does two wonderful things to help us age healthfully: it maximizes the body's full potential to regenerate healthy cells, which actually slows the aging process. And it promotes a deep self-acceptance and self-awareness so that as our body goes through the challenges of aging, we are much better able to handle and adjust to those changes, both physically and emotionally.

DHEA and T'ai Chi

T'ai Chi helps us increase DHEA levels and slow aging (*fan lao huan tong,* as the Chinese say). DHEA is also involved in the aging process. Levels of DHEA tend to decline with age, but the decline is much worse when you're under chronic stress. Add natural aging and chronic stress, and you have an express train to an old body. Once again our old friend T'ai Chi comes to the rescue. T'ai Chi's gentle movements and breathing techniques promote the serenity that can keep DHEA from being depleted.

KNOW YOUR CHINESE

Fan lao huan tong means "reverse old age and return to youthfulness." This is what the Chinese believe T'ai Chi and QiGong offer, and, of course, Western scientific methods are beginning to tell us how and why that happens. East meets West.

Of course, the increased circulation of blood and Qi also fully oxygenates the skin, which provides nourishment to your outer beauty. The Zang Fu system's being balanced by T'ai Chi's stimulation of acupressure points and massage of the internal organs also moves the liquids and oils of the body to the tissues that need them, further adding to your external beauty and internal health.

Reducing Free Radical Damage to Age More Slowly

There's a pesky little free radical atom in your body called superoxide that causes the body to age. Not only does it cause wrinkles and age spots, but it can also weaken cartilage and joints. In fact, this superoxide may even induce cancer or other immune system disorders. Obnoxious little thing, isn't it?

T'AI SCI

Free radicals are atoms with an extra electron that bounce around wreaking havoc throughout the body. We see this with our eyes as aging. The calming effects of T'ai Chi and QiGong not only affect the mind, but can also reduce the damage done by free radicals, thereby slowing the aging process.

Regular T'ai Chi and QiGong practice can protect your body from these pesky free radicals by activating an enzyme called superoxide dismutase (or SOD). SOD is our cellular superman and defends our cells from the ornery superoxides that break down our health systems.

A study of those who practiced QiGong for a half-hour a day for one year showed that their levels of SOD increased dramatically compared to people not doing QiGong. Another study showed a large increase in SOD after only two months of QiGong practice.

Maximizing Bone Health

The National Institute of Mental Health (NIMH) released a study showing that women under chronic stress with depression had weaker bones than those in normal emotional states. In fact, the stressed/depressed women had the bones of 70-year-old women, even though they were only 40 years old.

T'ai Chi lessens the incidence of depression and the body's stress responses and is a gentle, weight-bearing exercise. These qualities might make T'ai Chi the best thing you can do to keep your bones healthy, even into old age, as indicated by Harvard Medical School's health publication that reported, "A review of six controlled studies by … Harvard research indicates that T'ai Chi may be a safe and effective way to maintain bone density in postmenopausal women."

You Can Dramatically Improve Your Balance!

For aging Americans, the simple act of stumbling and falling can often be fatal. The sixth-largest cause of death for older Americans is complications from falling injuries. This costs our country about $10 billion a year and causes tremendous suffering for older people as well as their families. We are all paying for our nation's poor balance in human suffering and in higher healthcare and health insurance costs.

T'ai Chi was part of a balance study by Harvard, Yale, the Centers for Disease Control and Prevention, Washington University School of Medicine, and Emory University. T'ai Chi practitioners fell and injured themselves only half as much as those practicing other balance training. This is an amazing finding that can change the lives of older Americans.

Although you may not be in the age group likely to suffer serious injury from falling, we can all benefit greatly by having better balance. Better balance puts much less stress on the body throughout the workday, and as T'ai Chi practice improves your balance, you will find that you have much more energy.

Compared to the best balance training in the world, T'ai Chi is about twice as effective. Some of the other balance exercises studied in an Ivy League study on balance were very expensive computer models that required participants to go into a lab and practice. The simple exercises of T'ai Chi are not only much more effective than the other exercises, but they are very cheap!

T'ai Chi & QiGong: Healthcare of the Future

Most Chinese hospitals have long integrated Western crisis medicine with TCM. This is now happening in the United States as well. The American Medical Association recently recognized acupuncture as a valid treatment, which is also causing medical universities to incorporate T'ai Chi and QiGong into their educational curriculums.

Growing numbers of neurologists, cardiologists, general practitioners, physical therapists, hypertension specialists, and psychologists are already prescribing T'ai Chi and/or QiGong as treatment or supplemental treatment for many conditions. (See Part 6 for examples of T'ai Chi prescribed for specific conditions.)

As more Western scientific research is completed on the benefits of T'ai Chi and QiGong, this trend will expand. The result will be lower healthcare costs for all of us.

Access the Healing Power of the Mind

When you first hear of the benefits of T'ai Chi and QiGong, effective for helping treat *all things* on *all levels*, it may sound like snake oil. "How can it do that?" you might ask. It's simple: it does this by connecting us to the most powerful healing tool there is—the healing power of the mind. The power of the mind is at the heart of our healing.

It is estimated that placebos can positively treat about 60 percent of our health problems. Placebos are sugar pills (or fake treatments) doctors sometimes give to fool patients into curing themselves. This gets the mind/body to trigger the electrical signals and chemical releases that comprise its internal healing processes, by the mind simply telling itself it's okay for the body to heal. This indicates that the body has a tremendous potential to *self*-heal, if we *believe* in the cure.

T'ai Chi and QiGong are not placebos. They are powerful health tools that can help to unclog the tremendous natural healing power of the body, the power *behind* the placebo. Their healing benefits are extensive and well documented, and new research is emerging all the time. Again, it's important for you to understand just how powerful these tools are so your mind will relax into allowing them to do their magic.

A T'AI CHI PUNCH LINE

Studies have shown that if patients believe something can cure them, the possibility that it actually will is much higher. Cynicism is found to be one of the single-most hazardous behaviors for our health. If I have a choice between being smart enough to realize I'm incurable, or stupid enough to fool myself into curing myself—I'll be the fool any day.

The Least You Need to Know

- T'ai Chi facilitates the flow of Qi and health to your cells.
- Narrow thinking squeezes off life energy.
- T'ai Chi integrates the mind, body, and emotions.
- By toning your Qi, you tone all your healing systems.
- Only T'ai Chi provides an acupressure treatment and organ massage while promoting circulation and centeredness.
- You don't have to memorize how T'ai Chi and QiGong work. Just relax and do it!

Expanding Your Mind and Lightening Your Heart

In This Chapter

- Discovering the power of calm and peace
- Knowing you can be as powerful as you want to be
- Accepting that you are perfect
- Flexing your imagination muscle
- Web Video Support: *T'ai Chi's unfrazzling, internal-awareness quality*

Before moving to the nuts-and-bolts instruction, read on to slip your mind into the T'ai Chi gear. You'll get more out of the instructional chapters by doing so.

The demands of the day-to-day rat race ravage our mental and emotional well-being. The same way T'ai Chi's engineering adjustments show us how our physical efforts can be more efficient, and thereby more effortless and powerful, T'ai Chi also reveals that *life does not have to be that hard.* The simple ways T'ai Chi and QiGong look at movement and life can be powerful self-improvement tools, as well as a soothing balm to frazzled nerves. As you view the T'ai Chi exhibition sections on the Chapter 3's Web Video Support, *Watching T'ai Chi Unfrazzles* (www.idiotsguides.com/taichi), you'll likely feel yourself *unfrazzling,* just by watching.

Leave the Rat Race Behind

Chinese masters constantly repeat "Soong Yi-Dien" ("loosen up"). The goal of T'ai Chi is to weave silken threads of calm into our lives, soothing us as we face the daily rat race. The calmer we are, the calmer our workplace and our home are.

However, at first, rather than bringing T'ai Chi's calm to the rat race, students often unconsciously bring the rat race into the T'ai Chi class or into their home T'ai Chi practice. They do this because they want to "efficiently" learn T'ai Chi. Our work, lives, and technology are all geared toward making things happen faster and faster. So we naturally want to "hurry up and relax." This can't happen.

We have to let go of urgency and efficiency to truly and deeply experience what T'ai Chi offers. T'ai Chi helps us become less urgent, while surprisingly becoming more efficient. Here's how.

Frantic Action vs. Efficiency

T'ai Chi's ability to calm, energize, heal, strengthen, and tone the mind and body in a short, half-hour workout is unequaled. However, if you try to do T'ai Chi efficiently, it doesn't work as well. It's when you relax, and *don't try*, that T'ai Chi works its magic.

The idea that we can get something very worthwhile done without having high anxiety to hurry up and do it is a new concept for most of us. When you're viewing T'ai Chi exhibitions on this book's Web Video Support, notice how *unhurried* and how powerful the movements look.

T'ai Chi Is Smelling the Roses

Our heart and mind seem to be in a constant state of turmoil. With the tidal wave of data the Information Age has swept into our lives, it's easy to always feel two steps behind the pack. We struggle to understand the latest technology, knowing full well that a newer version will be out before we master the one that just came out. We forget to breathe and enjoy the *learning* in life, which, when you get down to it, is pretty much all there is to life. We are not and never will be done learning. So we might as well smell the roses on the way.

Learning to "love the learning" of T'ai Chi is one of the most important lessons T'ai Chi offers our frantic lives. Students sometimes come to T'ai Chi classes gung-ho to learn one set of forms and then move on. The concept that T'ai Chi is a lifelong process comes as a big shock. Students think they can hurry in, get fixed, get calmed, get healthy, and then get going. They want to hurry up and *finish* so they can hurry up to finish the next thing they want to hurry up and do. But by living this way, our lives just become a lot of hurrying. There is no finish in T'ai Chi or in life.

> **OUCH!**
>
> Many Western students feel hopeless upon learning that T'ai Chi is a lifelong process. We in the West are conditioned to expect immediate, short-term results. Don't be discouraged. T'ai Chi is a lifelong process that gives immediate results. Even if you just took one T'ai Chi class and practiced what you learned, you would get great benefit. It just gets better and better for the rest of your life.

T'ai Chi's calming effects can be felt immediately the very first day of practice, but not if you hurry up to feel them. You have to let go of the outcome and let the nice feelings be a pleasant surprise rather than an urgent demand. See Web Video Support's *QiGong Breathing Is About Letting Go*, to get a sense of this release of urgency.

T'ai Chi's movements flow one into the other, just as life's events do. By learning how to breathe and relax the body while moving through these events, we become an island of soothing calm even when we're in the center of the rat race. Our habit of letting go of the frantic demands of the day that fill our minds becomes easier and easier as we practice T'ai Chi.

Remember to Breathe (Everything Else Takes Care of Itself)

As a student in a T'ai Chi class (or at home), the very first thing you should do is close your eyes and breathe. Take deep breaths all the way into the bottom of your lungs and then let go of your breath, your muscles, and your day. Let go of everything you've done before getting here and everything you plan to do later. Just be here and now, breathing. Enjoy the *QiGong Breathing Tutorial* at Chapter 3's Web Video Support.

As your mind fills with remembering to breathe through your T'ai Chi movements, and gravity forces you to focus on your balance, you must let go of the worries of the day. You cannot do T'ai Chi without letting go of thoughts about what to defrost for dinner or the laundry that needs to be done.

T'ai Chi does not advocate starvation or wearing dirty clothes. It does, however, advocate being 100 percent in the moment, whether you're doing T'ai Chi or washing clothes. This is what is called *mindfulness*, or being here and now. You'll find that the more you can let go of the dinner and the laundry to feel your breath, your muscles releasing, and the silken flow of your T'ai Chi movements, the more you'll enjoy doing the laundry or cooking dinner when you do get to it. The T'ai Chi practice of being here and now will seep into your daily life by reminding you to breathe as you move. While making dinner, you'll relax and breathe, enabling you to truly smell the fragrance of dinner.

We don't have to race if we are always where we like being. Then we never have to fear looking in the mirror and seeing a racing rat.

SAGE SIFU SAYS

As T'ai Chi helps us "feel good" on a regular basis, we want more of that feeling. You might spend more time with people who nurture you and less time with those who put you down. This is a powerfully healthful, transformative part of doing T'ai Chi. As the movements in T'ai Chi teach you to ease around areas of discomfort in the body so as to expand mobility without injury, this echoes out into your life. You begin to find nurturing ways to move and live socially.

Lose Your Grip on Reality: The Power of Effortlessness

In our fast-paced, dog-eat-dog world, it's hard to believe that we can be more powerful when we are not straining. However, that is exactly when we are most powerful, not only mentally and emotionally, *but also physically.*

I am always encouraging my students to "lose their grip" on life—to breathe, to untangle, and to let go of *everything*. Have you ever noticed how society uses the phrase "he's losing his grip"? This idea that we must constantly keep a GRIP on reality tells you something about society that needs to change.

T'ai Chi and QiGong's practice of increasing effortlessness will show you that you do not have to *grip* reality in your cells, mind, and heart. Truth and reality exist without our clutching hearts or minds *keeping it all in order.* Another negative in our vernacular is, "she's out of control." These arts are all about learning to, or remembering how to, *let go of control.* We were pretty good at it as kids; we just forgot how when our mortgage payments, student loans, and credit card debt began squeezing down on us. T'ai Chi and QiGong are about not only allowing yourself to be out of control, but celebrating it. A new you cannot expand through you if you continually grip onto what you think you are, or what you think the world is. We are evolutionary beings, continually evolving into more, and the less we grip onto control, the more easily we will be flowed toward the expanding future of what our lives are becoming. If you haven't enjoyed the *Sitting QiGong* exercise today, now's a good time to do so at Chapter 3's Web Video Support. This *Sitting QiGong* experience isn't a "been there, done that" kind of experience. As you progress through the mental concepts and insights of this book, each time you go back to do the Sitting QiGong, you'll notice a deeper, more expansive experience. Also, research shows its good to meditate every day of our lives, so bookmark that exercise, and enjoy it daily.

However, because we are so conditioned to be mentally and emotionally straining all the time, many students feel "guilty" for taking quiet, still time to heal their minds and emotions from the strains of the day. Those students need a real and stark physical example of how we function more effectively when relaxed— which is best shown by the Unbendable Arm technique.

The Unbendable Arm

The Unbendable Arm exercise is a terrific physical example of the concept of "effortless action" and how powerful that kind of action is. In the West, we tend to think of big, straining muscles and huge forehead veins whenever we think of power.

T'ai Chi can rescue us from that sweaty, head-pounding delusion. In T'ai Chi, our goal is to move and stand with as little effort as possible. Ancient *Taoist* poets tried to explain in words the seemingly limitless power found in living a life of effortlessness with a calm mind and quiet heart. However, the concept of effortless power is so strange to Westerners that the following demonstration of the Unbendable Arm is worth a thousand words. (*Note:* If you have any arm or shoulder injuries, you may not want to do the Unbendable Arm exercise. Also, if you have difficulty performing this exercise, you may want to practice the Sitting QiGong exercise in Part 3 and then try again.)

> **T'AI SCI**
>
> Many Western psychotherapists use Taoist philosophy as they encourage patients to let go of obsessing on the outcome and rather enjoy the "process" of life. In fact, T'ai Chi exercises are recommended as an active model to achieve these healing ends.

The Unbendable Arm is a powerful physical example of the principle of effortless power. In my class demonstrations, I ask the largest, most powerful-looking student to try to bend my arm. Resisting with all my muscular strength, they nevertheless eventually bend my arm. However, when I completely relax my mind and body, thinking of an empty flow, or of airy relaxation pouring through my head, shoulder, arm, and on out my fingers through the walls of the building, they can't bend it. The students strain to bend my relaxed arm, yet they cannot.

KNOW YOUR CHINESE

The focus of the ancient Chinese **Taoist** (pronounced *dowist*) philosophy is the invisible force of nature's laws. Its premise is that life flows through all living things the way ocean currents flow through the ocean. The Tao nurtures life and cannot be defined because it applies to all things. When we are calm and still in our hearts, minds, and bodies, we can feel or sense the subtle direction of Tao. Living the Tao is the most effortless, meaningful way to live, flowing with the Tao, the way a surfer rides the waves, while adding our own flair and best intentions to its currents. In the West, we may call the sense of the Tao a hunch or an intuition, or what feels right. Renowned physicist Brian Greene refers to a "sense of elegance" when choosing a direction in research. I think that aptly describes sensing the Tao.

Here's how to experience the Unbendable Arm yourself. Prepare to be totally amazed!

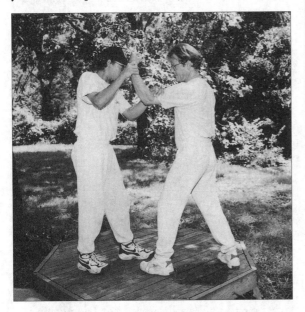

Notice that the person is able to bend my arm even as I use all my muscular strength to resist.

First of all, if you have any arm or shoulder injuries, I don't advise trying this at all. Also, if you do try this, do it with someone you trust to do it gently. He'll push hard, but he won't jerk and wrench your arm; he'll just apply steady pressure.

Step 1:

1. Stand with your feet apart, holding your arm out fairly straight to the side.

2. Have a friend stand to your side, grab your wrist with his right hand, and place his left hand on the top of your upper arm, as in the figure.

3. Tighten your fist and your arm to keep your friend from being able to bend your arm, using all your muscular strength to resist. Your friend will push up on your wrist, while pushing down on your upper arm, so your elbow will be the fulcrum point. If your friend doesn't push down on your upper arm as he pushes your wrist up, your whole arm will just go up in the air. The goal is for your friend to bend your arm at the elbow as you resist. Again, warn your friend to apply steady increasing pressure, rather than trying to quickly wrench your arm into bending. The goal isn't to hurt you, but to illuminate you to your effortless power.

4. If your friend is as strong as you, you'll likely feel your elbow begin to bend as seen in the figure. If you don't, ask your friend to put his shoulder into it as he pushes up on your wrist (see figure).

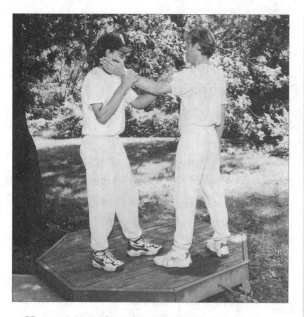

However, notice here that my arm is relaxed, yet the other person cannot bend it.

Step 2:

1. Okay, now that you've felt your arm being bent as you resisted with all your muscular strength, have your friend keep his hands in the same placement on your extended arm, but now just close your eyes and relax.

2. Take a few cleansing breaths, and let your body relax, including your shoulder and extended arm.

3. Think of a down-pouring shower of lightness flowing down through your head, body, and out through your extended arm, hand, and fingers as if that flow continues on through the wall, and all the walls in the surrounding community.

4. When you get a sense of this, a feeling of an airy lightness flowing down and out through your shoulder and arm, as if it were a hollow reed, then ask your friend to try bending your arm again.

5. He won't be able to bend it this time, no matter how hard he tries. In fact, you will think that he isn't really trying this time, to make you feel better or something.

You may feel this, and then think to yourself "Wow, I'm doing it!" and that'll cause you to lose your focus and he'll bend it. It's like when you're typing fast, and you think, "Wow! I'm typing fast!" and then clunk, you lose your focus and your fingers don't work right. As you practice this, you'll get very adept at it if you aren't already.

Note, if this didn't work out for you *at all*, realize that you *will* have an intention not to bend your arm as your friend applies slow steady pressure, you won't let it go completely limp like a wet noodle, but also you will be very relaxed, not straining with your muscles. Your friend should feel your arm as very relaxed even as she strains to bend it. So now try it again after reading this paragraph.

You should be pretty amazed at the power of effortless intent at this point. But, again, if that didn't work out, don't give up. You should go back to the Web Video Support's *Sitting QiGong* meditation to experience the flow of Qi or life energy pouring through your body again. After that 17-minute experience, come back to this and try it again. In my classes, 99 percent of my students are able to perform the Unbendable Arm quite effectively immediately after doing the Sitting QiGong meditation. And even the 1 percent eventually do get it. You'll get it, and when you do, you'll have a great party trick to impress your friends with, but again, warn them not to "wrench" your arm, but to apply steady pressure only.

Our Flexibility Is Our Strength

This Taoist principle of effortless power is even more meaningful in our mental and emotional lives.

I use the Unbendable Arm not to demonstrate the physical power of effortless motion (although it does demonstrate that), but to dispel the myth that our straining is equivalent to productivity. When we breathe and relax while typing at the keyboard or answering the phone, we are so much more effective and real. We have time for the people in our lives instead of always rushing past them to get to the next urgent task.

Learning to See Patterns in the Chaos of Life

T'ai Chi helps our bodies be more effective by relaxing our muscles. This allows a more ordered pattern of muscle use so our muscles aren't fighting other muscles. However, T'ai Chi also has the same effect on the mind. By quieting the mind of all the daily "noise," our mind can open to more orderly patterns of thought. The Web Video Support's *QiGong and T'ai Chi Bring the Mind … Inside the Body* shows the exhibitioners' awareness seems to be "inside themselves" on the process of effortless motion, not elsewhere, wrapped up in life's problems.

Calming the Chaos Within Changes Our World

Similar to the way the body fights itself physically with muscle tension, the mind also keeps itself in needless chaos with noisy thoughts spinning around in it. T'ai Chi and QiGong can end this internal battle and enhance the power of the mind and imagination. The slow, deliberate motions of T'ai Chi that calm the body and get the muscles to work together more powerfully (as demonstrated by the Unbendable Arm) organizes the mind, too, and ultimately the world around us.

A T'AI CHI PUNCH LINE

When studying T'ai Chi in Hong Kong as a young man, I was intrigued by the construction workers there. At the time I was in great shape, being a karate enthusiast who trained very hard. However, I was humbled by the much smaller, thinner Chinese construction workers who hauled enormously heavy bags of cement up bamboo scaffolds on their thin shoulders. They showed barely any exertion. Whether the workers practiced T'ai Chi or not, they had obviously absorbed some of its principles.

Phil Jackson, former head coach of the World Champion Chicago Bulls, is a Zen practitioner, and he introduced the entire Chicago Bulls basketball team to Zen exercises. T'ai Chi and QiGong exercises are from the same roots as Zen exercises and are often indistinguishable from them.

A T'AI CHI PUNCH LINE

The Chinese character for Qi, or life energy, and the Latin root *spir*, as in *spirit*, mean "the air we breathe." Both ancient cultures obviously saw how our breath connects us to the life force. When considering that each of us has breathed an atom of oxygen that was breathed by Jesus, Buddha, and Mohammed, the Taoist claim that we are all connected becomes a very real concept.

The year the Bulls were introduced to Zen practices was the year they became the winningest team in the history of the NBA. This is no coincidence. The choreography the

Bulls displayed that year was mind-boggling; the team often resembled one living entity rather than five separate players. As Zen exercise enables the mind to clear itself of its daily chatter or rubble, it also clarifies the communication between people. So just as the Bulls players began to quiet and clarify their own internal function by relaxing muscles and quieting thoughts they didn't need, they simultaneously clarified their player-to-player communication. This clarity is what we saw in the incredible plays the Bulls made that year.

This was no easy feat, as those as old as me may remember that the Chicago Bulls dynasty was a cast of very diverse personalities, from the flamboyant and controversial Dennis Rodman, to the more reserved and serious Michael Jordan. It could have been easy for these diverse personalities to spend energy in internal ego and turf battles as so often happens with such large personalities. The way Phil Jackson, the "Zen Master," used Zen meditation to relax these potential conflicts, and enable this team of superstars to complement one another instead of conflicting with each other, is exactly how the Unbendable Arm exercise works—teaching the muscles in the arm and body to let go of fighting against one another, so that their effort becomes a super effort that looks effortless.

This same clarity we cultivate through our daily T'ai Chi or QiGong exercises can help us clarify our relationships with others at work or home. Most social breakdowns are rooted in a lack of clarity, for if we aren't clear on what we want and need, we can never expect others to support our efforts. Whether it's our love life, our family, our work, or our social relationships, T'ai Chi's soothing way of moving through life will make relationships more healing and effortless.

People around us become easier to deal with when we are easier to deal with. T'ai Chi shows us how much of the external world reflects what goes on in our own heart and mind. I was once invited to do a T'ai Chi presentation for a horseback rider society, to improve their relationships with their horses. This happened after *Dressage*, the national magazine for the Olympic horseback riding style, promoted T'ai Chi as perhaps the most effective exercise a rider could perform to enhance riding skills. The article pointed out that a horse picks up on the rider's mental and emotional stress levels. Therefore if the rider does T'ai Chi before mounting his horse, the horse gives a smoother and quicker ride.

Imagine how much your unconscious mental and emotional turmoil affects those around you at home or work. Then think of how much your life would change if you did T'ai Chi before riding into work or home from your day.

> **SAGE SIFU SAYS**
>
> The life force is clarity and simplicity and holds no need to compete. By letting go of desires, utmost calm is realized, and all the world arrives at effortless peace.

Releasing Old Patterns Enables Our Evolution

This is what T'ai Chi and QiGong can do. T'ai Chi's physical model of moving with the muscles relaxing off the bones is a model for letting go of mental and emotional obsessions. T'ai Chi enables us to let go of the chaos of life and let our mind lift and observe, unattached to outcomes, grudges, or obsessive desires. It enables us to see more clearly the patterns that cause us to bump our head into the same old walls again and again.

Letting go of attachments or stepping out of the game from time to time gives us a fresh perspective. Fresh perspective is what allows us to exercise our "imagination muscle." It's the most effortless thing you can do. However, it's not always easy because it requires you to let go of all your thoughts, plans, and regrets. Creating space or breathing room in your busy days with T'ai Chi and QiGong helps your mind let go of old patterns. This enables your mind to open to the pure inspiration that wants to bubble up inside it, so you can evolve into the new person you could become.

T'ai Chi Dispels the Idea of Wrongness

Many readers or teachers who read my books often rush past this point, but this is perhaps the most profound benefit I got from my T'ai Chi journey. The most mentally and emotionally healing concept T'ai Chi has to offer our hypercritical world is that T'ai Chi dispels the idea of "wrongness." When you practice T'ai Chi, you never, ever do it "wrong." You just do it. Each time you do it, you relax a little more, you breathe a little easier, and your T'ai Chi gets a little better. On the Web Video Support's *T'ai Chi Slows and Calms*, you'll notice the practitioner's reveling in the simple pleasure of relaxed motion.

OUCH!

If the T'ai Chi instructor you study with is hypercritical, you may want to find another one who has more fun with T'ai Chi. However, be aware that if you are hypercritical of yourself by nature, you may unconsciously project that onto the instructor. Relax and enjoy yourself when in T'ai Chi class and when practicing at home. This will help your instructor relax, too.

T'ai Chi Is a Model for Life

T'ai Chi helps us realize that we are always "perfect," that our lives are ever-evolving perfection. When we learn things about T'ai Chi that we can improve, it is much easier to adopt the new ways if the old ways don't have to be "wrong." This is one of the ways T'ai Chi makes a terrific model for life in general. Again, this realization, this self-acceptance, even in the face of learning the challenging complexity of T'ai Chi movements, was one of the most powerful benefits I got from my 30 year T'ai Chi journey.

Our culture's concepts of wrongness constipate the ability to let go of old ways and move into new ways more easily. If something must be *wrong* before it can be discarded, we judge ourselves as wrong for having done it that way. If we see things in an ever-evolving state of improvement, then nothing is wrong and there are always better ways. Then we can see that we were right for having done it the old way, drop the self-judgment, and proceed smoothly and happily into newer and even "righter" ways of approaching life.

The only wrong thing you can do in T'ai Chi is to tell yourself you're wrong.

T'ai Chi's way of seeing exercise (and life) as a process leaves us always content with where we are, while always taking us past our old limits. When we obsess over getting things "right," whether we know it or not, we limit ourselves by thinking we are "done" when we get it "right." By giving up that myth, we begin to feel a limitlessness to life. T'ai Chi helps us feel bigger, dream bigger, and love bigger.

Each time you do T'ai Chi, you relax a little more deeply and become both a little more self-aware and a little more self-accepting, enabling you to continually improve your T'ai Chi.

When we stick with T'ai Chi long enough, we realize that our T'ai Chi improves each time we do it. More important, it helps us see that we never did T'ai Chi "wrong," for T'ai Chi is not a destination where a fixed level of perfection exists. Like our lives, T'ai Chi is an unfolding rose of improvement that blooms endlessly, more perfectly, and more beautifully each new day we practice it. An 80-year-old T'ai Chi master was being interviewed about his 60 years of T'ai Chi practice. The interviewer asked him, "At what point did you feel you mastered T'ai Chi?" The old master replied with a mischievous wink, "I'll let you know as soon as I do."

SAGE SIFU SAYS

When problems arise, use your energy to fix the problem rather than wasting energy fixing the blame. Fix the problem, not the blame. This concept goes right to the heart of what T'ai Chi offers our harried lives.

T'ai Chi Enhances Life

Does T'ai Chi make life perfect? No, not more perfect than it already is. And it is always perfect, although sometimes it may seem perfectly miserable. T'ai Chi encourages you to let go of outcomes and simply pour your energy into whatever nourishes life—your life and all life. The flow of Qi through the body is like water through the roots of a plant. It doesn't try to fix anything in particular; it just enhances life at all levels. As the Taoist philosopher Lao Tzu put it, "The best people are like water. Water nurtures all things and never is in competition with them." See Web Video Support's *Images of Flowing Qi Enable Us to Un-Grip and Open to Possibility.*

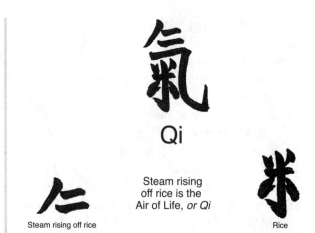

Qi

Steam rising off rice

Steam rising off rice is the Air of Life, *or Qi*

Rice

Notice that the Qi character is a combination of steam or air (the top half) and rice (the lower half). The character for Qi (pronounced chee) represents steam rising from rice, meaning "the air of life," a symbol for effortless sustenance.

T'ai Chi and QiGong Expand Imagination

Sitting QiGong is a motionless exercise. So if the slowness of T'ai Chi makes it seem ineffective to many Westerners, the stillness of QiGong may seem like a colossal waste of time. However, this could not be further from the truth.

These slow, mindful exercises bring the brain into a very calm state known by scientists as the *alpha state.* This is a highly creative state of mind. In fact, three of the great discoverers of our time had their greatest insights while in alpha states. Albert Einstein, Thomas Edison, and Nikolai Tesla all claimed to get their greatest discoveries while in a state of mind that Einstein called "wakeful rest."

KNOW YOUR CHINESE

The **alpha state** is a frequency of brain waves that occurs during a state of relaxed concentration. It is one of four brain-wave frequencies: delta is the slowest, prevalent during infancy or in adults during sleep; theta is present in drowsy, barely conscious states; alpha is during QiGong relaxation exercises; and beta is common when the mind is busy or restless.

Why is the alpha state such a creative state of mind? For one thing, when our mind is filled with normal daily worries, plans, and television/radio noise, there's no room left for creative thought. Also, there may be a deeper knowledge within our minds that we can't access when our minds are busy with daily problem-solving. Psychologist Carl Jung said there is a "collective unconscious" that holds great knowledge, and that we all have access to it. But when our mind is busy with balancing the checkbook or worrying about our next raise, we can't open to that great knowledge. This collective unconscious is the ocean of information our minds get ideas from. It's like all the information on the internet, and our minds are like a computer that can download that information.

A T'AI CHI PUNCH LINE

Bet ya your brain's in beta! The stress we feel in our busy lives is partly because our mind spends too much time in beta brain waves, or "busy brain waves." QiGong can help you drop into a calm state even when you're in line at the supermarket.

When we are tense, our minds are tight and closed to new ideas. This resembles the problem with the internet. The internet has loads of great information, but most computers seem to take forever to access it. This is because information bottlenecks when it passes through the

system's modems because these modems have a limited bandwidth. If your brain is like your computer and ideas are like the internet, then QiGong and T'ai Chi are a way to increase the bandwidth to allow much more access to information.

You've experienced this, whether you know it or not. Have you ever faced a really tough problem you couldn't solve? No matter how hard you tried, you couldn't see the solution. Then when you gave up and went for a walk, or sat on the back porch, or went for a drive, the answer came to you. You saw a pattern you missed when your mind was too busy trying to put the pieces together. Then when you gave up, your mind put the pieces together very easily and very effectively.

T'AI SCI

Every now and then go away, have a little relaxation, for when you come back to your work your judgment will be surer. Go some distance away because then the work appears smaller and more of it can be taken in at a glance and a lack of harmony and proportion is more readily seen.

—Leonardo da Vinci

This is what T'ai Chi and QiGong help us learn to do more often and more easily. They open our mental bandwidth by allowing the mind to let go of its clutter. Things get clearer. As you can see, the stillness and nonaction T'ai Chi and QiGong cultivate are far from a waste of time.

When you utilize the Sitting QiGong experience, your brain waves will go through different vibratory levels, moving from beta to the alpha state. You won't work this out mentally; it'll be an effortless "letting-go" process, a surrendering of your grip on everything again and again with each releasing breath. As your head and heart let go, again and again, permeated by the silken effortlessness of Qi, you will become both more open-minded and more open-hearted. You will become more vulnerable, more empty of yourself. An empty vessel is the only vessel that can be filled with life's adventure and possibility.

The Least You Need to Know

- T'ai Chi heals your mind and heart.
- Real power comes from peace of mind.
- T'ai Chi teaches that life is limitless.
- Stress closes the mind, but QiGong opens it.
- Effortlessness is key to tapping into real emotional, mental, and physical power.

Finding Your Center—*Feeling* Your Center

In This Chapter

- Being here and now
- Letting go of the fight-or-flight response
- Understanding T'ai Chi mastery and discovering the master in you
- Using T'ai Chi to change your world
- Web Video Support: the *centering, internal-scan,* and *block-loosening* qualities of T'ai Chi and QiGong

Usually we don't think about being in or out of "center" until life is completely out of hand. Then we know we are out of it, but we're still not sure what it is we're out of. We often think we are just out of our minds.

Being in center reduces the melodrama in your life so you can focus more attention on the big stuff. Standing in the center means aligning your physical, emotional, mental, and spiritual selves so you function at your very best, using everything you've got in everything you do.

T'ai Chi Walking: Practice *Feeling* Centered

Enjoy the following "T'ai Chi Walking" exercise, to understand the many intricate layers of the letting go, and sinking into here and now that permeates all T'ai Chi and QiGong forms regardless of which style they are.

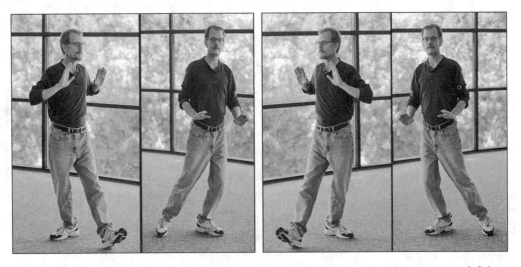

Notice T'ai Chi Walking involves moving across the room, beginning with sinking into your left leg, then right, and so on.

Initial layer of T'ai Chi Walking:

1. Before beginning, think of your head being drawn up toward the sky, and your tailbone relaxing down, causing your spine to elongate. This will align your posture, because as the top of your head lifts up, it brings your chin in, so your head and posture is stacked up above the foot your weight is on. Too often we are leaning forward, always in a hurry to get somewhere else.

   Take a deep breath in, and on the sighing exhale, allow the weight of your body to relax down through your right leg into the earth below. Breathe in again, and as you exhale, let every cell of your being surrender, letting your shoulders sink down away from your neck. Enjoy the sense of being "right here and right now," with nowhere to rush to.

2. Relax your body open to a deep, full breath, as you place your left heel out at a 45° angle (as in the first figure).

3. Now, as you exhale, let your weight sink downward into the left leg (second figure) as your pelvis and your upper body sink forward over the left leg and foot. Relax into this weight shift. Notice how your body remains stacked up above your foot, not leaning forward, aligned and loose. Repeat this process with your right foot out (third and fourth figures), and keep repeating across the floor.

Second layer of T'ai Chi Walking:

As you sink your weight forward onto the foot you are filling or moving over, feel the pads of the foot you are moving onto touch the floor or inner surface of your shoe. Notice how as you shift onto that foot, the pads of the toes, heel, and then entire foot spread as that foot is filled with the weight of your relaxed body.

Also, notice the opposite happening in the foot you are emptying or moving your weight off of. Don't work at this, but just enjoy the sensations. Let the pleasure of sensation, breath, and motion expand through you.

Another layer of T'ai Chi Walking:

Feel how your movements are more effortless when your head stays posturally aligned over your pelvis or dan tien (more on this in Chapter 11). Feel your body deeply relaxing as you shift, or sink, forward into each foot (not leaning forward with your upper body, but letting your pelvis carry you over that foot as your body relaxes onto that leg). Enjoy the sensations of the body in motion.

As you practice breathing, relaxing, and staying aligned in your movements, not leaning forward, you'll discover it will center and slow down your mind over time, and you will find yourself more "in the moment" enjoying the world within and around you. Leaning forward physically is an indication of the mind rushing forward to some other task, appointment, fear, or worry. Most of us will catch ourselves leaning forward a lot in our busy lives.

Always breathe with the tip of the tongue lightly touching the gums just behind the upper-front teeth, allowing your body to relax open to a full inhalation as you pick up your back foot and place the heel in front of you, and then exhaling as you relax your body and its weight onto that leg as you shift forward onto it. This is effortless, so don't try; just enjoy the loosening of the body as it shifts from one leg to the other.

You will discover many other layers of inner awareness as you play with T'ai Chi or Zen Walking meditations over coming days, months, and years.

KNOW YOUR CHINESE

The word **Zen** is a Japanese translation of the Chinese word *ch'an*. Both are translations of the original Sanskrit word *dhyana* (pronounced *jyana*). They describe an art often called "just sitting," or *zazen*. While one sits in Zen meditation, the mind does not calculate or figure, but is still and calm within, like a glass of muddy water slowly becoming clear as it sits still.

Take a few moments to view a video of T'ai Chi Walking in action at the Web Video Support's *T'ai Chi Walking*. Note that the video is of T'ai Chi movements, so when Zen Walking your arms will just hang relaxed by your sides, not in motion as in the T'ai Chi forms. But the foot, leg, and body's weight shifting is exactly the same as in these video excerpts.

This centering capability of T'ai Chi may seem spiritual, but it's really a kind of science that understands that our mind, body, emotions, and spirit are all intertwined, and that if we integrate them through T'ai Chi practice, we become more powerful. If our body and mind work together to nurture our emotional and spiritual well-being rather than against each other, as they sometimes do, life may be less dramatic, but it will be much more fulfilling.

This chapter can make you an expert on what the center is. The Web Video Support's *Breath and Release Centers You* also gives you an example of what is meant by centering here and now and letting go of out there. Then practicing the QiGong exercises in Part 3 and the T'ai Chi in Part 4 will further expand your awareness of "feeling" just how good being centered is.

T'ai Chi is a form of Zen meditation. A wonderful American interpretation of Zen philosophy is, "No matter where you go, there you are." All the toys, trips, and movies in the world cannot take you away from yourself. T'ai Chi is about being right in the center of where you are right now rather than running from it.

T'ai Chi helps us stand right in the center of our lives by focusing our mind and body to release stress that blocks awareness of our spiritual nature and needs. When viewing the *T'ai Chi Loosens Blocks* on the Web Video Support, notice that the practitioners seem to be wholly immersed in loosening any rigid blocks their bodies may have accumulated throughout the day.

Often it seems that life is a merry-go-round, and we're hanging on by our last fingernail as the demands of life pull at us with everything they've got. This is what being "out of center" refers to. When we are out there on the edge just trying to survive, we are not very creative. In fact, we often complicate our lives even more with various coping behaviors. Some people cope by overcharging their credit cards on compulsive spending. Others smoke compulsively or turn to alcohol or drugs. Still others become adrenaline junkies who can't slow down and have to be doing something all the time. All these behaviors have one thing in common: they all distract us from the turmoil going on inside our own minds and hearts. T'ai Chi is like a Zen exercise. Zen is an art of being still, not running from problems but being here and now.

T'ai Chi slows us down inside and out. As our body begins to move more slowly, our breathing slows down. As we hear our breathing slow, our mind begins to ride on the rhythm of that relaxed breath, letting go bit by bit of the storming thoughts of the day. As the mind calms, it has a resonant effect on the heartbeat, the blood pressure, and the body's healing systems. On some level, we begin to realize we are not in a state of mortal danger after all, which is a state that our ancient fight-or-flight response produces in us. It is this response more than the world around us that makes life seem like it is spinning way out of control. Notice on the Web Video Support's *T'ai Chi Breathing Slows the World* the practitioners' look of calm centeredness, as though life's rushing tendencies and storms are beyond them. T'ai Chi promotes that ability to refocus, to disengage, to give the mind and body opportunities to heal so they can tackle real-life problems.

A T'AI CHI PUNCH LINE

Lao Tzu (pronounced *low* [as in "OW!"] *dzuh* in Mandarin, or *lo tzee* in Cantonese) wrote, "In doing nothing, all things are done." He wasn't advocating laziness. He meant that by breathing, relaxing, and enjoying whatever it is we do, all things get done yet seem so effortless that we feel like we did nothing.

T'ai Chi Deprograms Antiquated Cellular Programming

We have all experienced feeling panicked by life much more often than we probably want to think about. This feeling is a product of the fight-or-flight reflex response. This reflex response is like an old memory held in the cells of our body, a cellular memory from our caveman and cavewoman days, when we were the grade-A prime rib for carnivorous creatures. We automatically respond to stress by breathing shallowly and tightening every muscle in our bodies so as not to be heard and to be ready to run like heck or bash the head of our would-be diner.

SAGE SIFU SAYS

The natural breathing T'ai Chi and QiGong promote is a powerful antidote to the fight-or-flight response. Just remembering to breathe when crisis hits can significantly improve your ability to handle it.

How T'ai Chi Frees Us from Ancient Patterns

Our modern cells still think they live in a prehistoric world where mortal danger is everywhere. Our outdated response to stress often leaves us in a minor (or not-so-minor) panic at every red light, supermarket line, or computer glitch we encounter.

This response worked well back in the caveperson days because we really didn't have many options. It does not, however, serve us very well today. Although sometimes the thought of either attacking the source of our anxiety or running away from it seems mighty appealing, it doesn't bode well for our next job performance review:

> **Room for improvement:** Bill should attempt to attack fewer co-workers this quarter, and an emphasis on not fleeing from customers is highly recommended.

T'ai Chi Enables Us to Function Effectively in the Modern World

On a cellular level, the fight-or-flight response is just as inappropriate. When we go into that mode, our heart pounds, blood pressure elevates, oxygen consumption increases, and blood lactate levels (anxiety levels) increase. If it happens often enough, it can actually cause our brain to shrink.

When we enter this state, the energy flowing through our body becomes very erratic, like a stormy sea. When we practice T'ai Chi and things begin to calm and center, our energy begins to flow more smoothly and evenly. The Chinese call this "smooth Qi." Smooth Qi is a healthful state produced by doing T'ai Chi. It soothes our body and begins to soothe our mind as well. Some would say T'ai Chi actually starts calming the mind and then the body becomes calm. Either way, it's a pretty helpful thing to be able to do. So these techniques actually de-program our cell memory so we can adapt to our modern world's needs.

As you view the Web Video Support's *T'ai Chi's Physical Smoothness Reflects Emotional and Mental Grace*, you will feel a sense of progress with your T'ai Chi and Qigong learning and practice. It is difficult to describe, but watching it can help.

Adrenaline Withdrawal

Many of us have actually become addicted to the feeling of anxiety, just like a cigarette smoker gets addicted to the energy level nicotine doses provide. So at first T'ai Chi or QiGong may cause you to feel drained.

If this happens to you, hang in there. You are going through an adrenaline withdrawal. As you continue to practice T'ai Chi and QiGong, you will eventually break through that wall of drowsiness and boredom. You will discover that you can have the best of both worlds. You will experience the relaxed energy that T'ai Chi unleashes within you as you find your center.

As the flow of Qi opens throughout your mind and body, you will have limitless energy, but without the edge. You will run with plenty of juice, but you will be attuned to when it's time to rest, and you will be able to rest when it's time. You'll feel less and less need to be endlessly busy all the time, but you'll have limitless energy for the truly important things in your life. Furthermore, the calmness that T'ai Chi fosters will grant you the wisdom to know which activities are important and which are not.

Today is a good day to get off adrenaline and get to the real juice. Breathe, breathe some more, and do T'ai Chi.

> **T'AI SCI**
>
> Studies show that about 80 percent of illness is due to stress, and that the six leading causes of death are stress related. Most stress-related damage is caused by adrenaline addiction. According to these studies, most of our illnesses are self-inflicted, which means we're creating our own healthcare crisis. T'ai Chi could help us break our adrenaline addiction, while also helping dramatically lower healthcare and insurance costs in the long run.

Demystifying What Makes a T'ai Chi Master

T'ai Chi and martial arts abound with myths of superhuman feats performed by masters who defy physical reality. These feats may be true; some masters have been known to break bricks with their heads.

These performances are compelling demonstrations of the power of internal effortlessness and focus. Often, however, these bizarre demonstrations are a distraction from the real point of these wonderful tools. You are as unlikely to be attacked by a brick as by another person. However, what we are all attacked by every day

is stress—often caused by our effort to grip control in a chaotic world.

What T'ai Chi and QiGong offer us is much more miraculous than the ability to break bricks: they help us understand ourselves and how we fit in the world. They make us masters of our own destiny instead of victims of circumstance. Of course, real masters understand that we are never in control, but merely co-pilots of our destiny. However, a co-pilot is preferable to and more powerful than being an unwitting passenger on this first-class ride we call life.

Overcoming Unconscious Issues Affecting Conscious Actions

Does it seem like life is one surprise after another? Look again. Our physical bodies are the manifest part of who we are. Our thoughts are the unmanifest part of us that creates our body. So our bodies are like reflections of our mind. Our thoughts are energy that triggers feelings or emotions, and that actually changes our physical body. These emotions turn the energy of thoughts into physical responses, just as chronic worry can create ulcers.

Thoughts change our bodies through the communication of emotions. Put simply, our mind in some ways creates our body.

> **T'AI SCI**
>
> Centuries ago, Chinese Taoist philosophers wrote that all things are formed from the same field of potential energy. As modern physics explains it, all atomic particles emerge from the same energy field, meaning that all things in the universe are made of the same essential energy. We are all, therefore, connected to everything else, to each other, and to the universe.

One of the fascinating things QiGong shows us is that the thoughts we are aware of are actually just reflections of what goes on inside us on even deeper levels. Most of our consciousness is subconscious, or below the surface of our awareness. Our thoughts and emotions, and our physical bodies, are results or reflections of an even deeper part of us. That deeper part is the unmanifest part of ourselves. QiGong and T'ai Chi's ability to connect us to that deeper, unmanifest part of ourselves is a potent self-improvement tool.

Imagine that our lives are like a big, clear glass of sparkling water. If you stand up and look down into it, you see only the bubbles bursting up into the air from the surface. This represents the manifest, or obvious, part of life. From this angle, you don't see the deep liquid below that formed these bubbles.

As we experience events in our lives, we are seeing only the bubbles popping up from the surface, not what formed them. These emerging bubbles may take the form of successes or recurring problems. Perhaps we go from one bad relationship to another or constantly fight with our kids.

However, T'ai Chi meditation, and especially QiGong meditation, lets us sit down and look at the water in the "glass of life" from the side, enabling us to see the source of the bubbles. From that angle, we can see that those bubbles, or events of our lives, actually form way down below the surface. This is the unmanifest, or unconscious, part of life.

So our quiet meditations place us sitting on the side, observing the true depth of life. Here we see that experiences are really end results rather than big surprises. Events in our lives are actually results of patterns or habits we have below the level of what we usually see and feel. We set ourselves up for success or failure by how

we think of ourselves every day. If we think of ourselves as valuable human beings capable of success, then we're much more likely to form bubbles that pop on the surface of our lives in the form of success stories.

Likewise, if we continually think of ourselves as bad or worthless, we will probably create bubbles to reflect that worthlessness in the form of relationship problems. If on some deep, unconscious level we believe that we are unworthy of support, we will attract people into our lives who will reinforce that reality. Pop, pop, pop. Seeing only the pops makes us feel like victims of life. (See the Web Video Support's *Sitting QiGong* exercise for a personal experience of this deeper awareness. Appendix C describes other effective Sitting QiGong techniques available.)

Becoming a Master Entails Not Being a Victim

Being a T'ai Chi or QiGong master means we are no longer content to remain ignorant of the unmanifest part of life. However, it's not enough just to know that our responses and actions in life have deeper roots. We have to find ways to change the patterns that form those bubbles way down below the surface of our lives. T'ai Chi and QiGong can help us do this. By quieting our minds and bodies, they can enable us to feel inside where we hurt or hate. By feeling the source inside, we can begin to let it go. For example, if we have a grudge or unresolved hatred in our hearts, we may walk around with a chip on our shoulders. The world will quickly give us confirmation of that grudge or hatred because people we meet will seem cold to us as we greet everyone with the chip on our shoulders, which makes us seem cold to them.

By being more aware of the dynamics of our lives, we feel less like victims. We can begin to affect our world more clearly.

As our lives become less cluttered with bubbles of discord, there is more room for a limitless flow of life energy or Qi to course through us. We become a geyser, watering and nurturing everyone and everything lucky enough to be around us.

T'ai Chi and QiGong's daily pattern of reminding us that we can change with ease, and feel safe in the world without constant muscle-tensing apprehension, is a powerful tool. Sometimes it seems as though the body literally squeezes past burdens within each and every cell. T'ai Chi's ability to allow the body to release those burdens held from the past so each cell can fill with and be nurtured by life energy is a powerful way to affirm that we are worthy of success and love. On levels deeper than we can ever understand, T'ai Chi's easy and pleasant tools help create bubbles in the deepest part of our hearts and minds that burst outward and upward in lives that reflect our very best potential. Cheers, Master! Yeah, that's you.

OUCH!

Modern psychology says we are bombarded on many levels by information and stress that we never consciously perceive. Therefore, trying to attach mental reasons to feelings of being out of control, frightened, or stressed is often a futile exercise. T'ai Chi helps us let go of stress on deep levels that we will never even notice.

Overcome Nature with Nurture

As discussed earlier, the six leading causes of death are stress related. Because stress is something we can control by practicing T'ai Chi and QiGong, using these tools means we can powerfully affect our future in a positive way.

We all are born with genetic tendencies to a certain height or weight, or for some, diabetes or heart disease. Our genes give us those tendencies. However, we can play a big role in how those genes play out. If we drink or smoke heavily and ignore a healthful diet, we can help increase the possibility of the onset of diabetes and heart disease, while likely stunting our growth and expanding our waistline.

On the other hand, we have been lucky enough to live in an age when T'ai Chi and QiGong are available to nurture us to perhaps avoid some of what nature has planted in our cellular structure. We have the ability to put an eternal ace up our sleeve, which heavily stacks the odds in our favor to live long, healthful, productive lives.

My T'ai Chi classes for children always began with one simple question: "Can you feel the inside of your bodies?" With little hands pressing into tiny rib cages, their puzzled faces usually answered no. My next question was, "Have you ever felt a stomachache or a headache?" Obviously, they all had.

T'ai Chi and QiGong are about moving the body, but they are also about feeling the body from the inside. We can feel pain inside, so we can also feel pleasure. Awareness of these feelings enables us to detect normal or abnormal function at a very early stage. By becoming attuned to our internal function, by quieting down, moving slowly, and listening to the signals inside our body, we tune our T'ai Chi antennae. We become conscious of our heartbeat and our respiration rate. The T'ai Chi players in the T'ai Chi exhibitions on the Web Video Support are obviously enjoying the sensations of effortless movement, which provides the added benefit of an internal scan throughout their bodies, alerting them to problem areas long before they would be if they were sedentary, and perhaps before they would be with more stressful exertion exercises.

> **OUCH!**
>
> Dr. Andrew Weil, the Harvard-educated medical doctor who now promotes traditional Chinese medical tools as part of his medical practice, claims that shallow breathing is the main threat to our health. By becoming more conscious of our breath and breathing more fully, we may avoid the health problems many of our shallow-breathing peers seem condemned to.

What amazes most people is that we can affect our heart rate and respiration rate by using some simple QiGong methods to become aware of them. But this is only the beginning. In my children's T'ai Chi classes, I asked children how it felt when they got nervous in school or were in trouble. They described feelings of "tight shoulders," "tight hearts," "tight chests," "hard to breathe," and so on. I asked them to make themselves feel that way, having them clench their shoulders and tighten their chests. Then I asked them to take in a deep breath and to let their chest and shoulders relax like a cloud floating in the sky on the exhale. I asked them to close their eyes and repeat this until they could feel their shoulders and chest relaxing and expanding from the inside.

Try it. Pull your shoulders way up by your ears until your shoulders are very tight and you can feel that tension. Tighten all your head muscles as well, and feel that tension. Now take a deep breath, close your eyes, and let go of everything as you release the breath; feel every cell of your body releasing that breath—absolute

effortlessness, absolute letting go on a cellular level. Feel how good that release feels in your shoulder and back muscles, and how with every breath you let out, they relax a little more. Enjoy the tingling as blood and Qi flow back into those areas.

Our body is a playground of sensation. T'ai Chi exercises and QiGong methods are games we can play in that playground. It's fun, and it makes us healthy. What a deal!

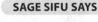

> **SAGE SIFU SAYS**
>
> The Kuang Ping Yang Style of T'ai Chi is a series of 64 integrated postures, one always changing into the other. The 64 postures symbolize the 64 possibilities of change represented in the *I Ching* (pronounced *ee ching*), or *The Book of Changes,* an ancient Chinese book of divination used to tell fortunes or advise people on life decisions. The essence of the *I Ching* is that life is a constant flow of changing circumstances. Its lesson is that we cannot find security by holding on to any one thing or way of being, but by learning to change easily and smoothly as life dictates.

T'ai Chi Can Affect the World Around Us

As you practice T'ai Chi daily, you begin to find that it has an effect on the world around you, not just the world inside your body. Shao Lin folklore spoke of T'ai Chi masters being invisible. That may have referred to the way their nonabrasive personalities enabled them to blend in unnoticed. For example, if two men walk into the same bar, one pushy and ill-tempered and the other very unassuming, the bar will be more dangerous for the ill-tempered man.

T'ai Chi and QiGong can help us focus our view of the world. Look out your window. Do you see a tree, the sky, traffic, smog? Move your chair until all you see is the most pleasing aspect of what your window offers you. Each time you take a break from your work, resume this position and enjoy the view.

Our lives are our minds looking through a window at the world. At any given time, we can see the best our world can be or the worst it can be. In fact, the state of our world has as much or perhaps even more to do with where we are as it does with where the world is. Two people can look at the same situation and see two entirely different things. For example, one person could look at a family and see a miracle she is blessed to be a part of, while another might look at the same situation and view it as a burden on her life, a prison she is sentenced to. In fact, the same person may see her life as either of those things on any given day.

After seeing our world from space, astronauts have experienced a dramatic change in the way they viewed life. They spoke of how precious life on Earth seemed from out there; even the things we think of as annoying—the arguments, the traffic—seemed so precious from outer space.

T'ai Chi and QiGong give us a view adjustment. We begin to notice that the irritating things our children or co-workers do are often irritating because of the way we look at them. With T'ai Chi and QiGong, we get to pull back and remember how precious each moment is. What could be more helpful? This doesn't mean life is a bowl of cherries and that we don't ever have to enact changes to get our needs met. But you'll discover that as these tools help you become calmer and clearer, those conflicts that do arise can be handled more fruitfully and more often in ways that can benefit everyone involved.

The Least You Need to Know

- T'ai Chi puts you in the center, right here and right now.
- T'ai Chi helps you cope with the stressors of modern life.
- T'ai Chi helps you think creatively.
- T'ai Chi masters are aware that they are not victims.
- T'ai Chi changes the world by changing your view of it.

Suiting Up and Setting Out

In This Part

Part 2 prepares you for your first T'ai Chi class, fashion-wise and otherwise. However, for those with T'ai Chi experience, it may also provide valuable insights on how to make your ongoing T'ai Chi experience even more meaningful, both internally and externally.

Knowing when and where to do T'ai Chi can enrich your T'ai Chi experience and can even help treat certain health conditions. You will also learn the ins and outs of T'ai Chi etiquette and how to get the most out of T'ai Chi by becoming aware of the different ways it is taught.

Even advanced T'ai Chi students can benefit from this part's explanation of some of the mental and emotional challenges T'ai Chi practitioners encounter. If you're an advanced student, this part will validate your own experiences. If you're a beginner, these insights will prepare you for those same challenges so you can ride them out and hang in there for the long, beautiful haul with T'ai Chi. If you're a teacher, this part will help you and your student through those rough spots.

Planning Ahead: Where and When to Practice T'ai Chi

In This Chapter

- Finding the best place for T'ai Chi
- Getting the most for your T'ai Chi buck
- Making time for T'ai Chi
- Web Video Support: *Example of What Class Instruction May Look Like*

This chapter explains where and when to do T'ai Chi, as well as what to wear. As you read, you will discover that these questions not only are a matter of etiquette or convenience, but they can also affect the health benefits you get from T'ai Chi.

You also will discover the advantages of a large class versus private instruction and video/book instruction versus (or in addition to) live classes. You'll also find tips on how to make time for whatever T'ai Chi program you choose.

Home Practice vs. Class Study

Although practicing at home by yourself on a regular basis is how you realize T'ai Chi's maximum benefits, studying with a qualified instructor—in class or at home via video, if classes don't work for you—is an essential part of the success of your home practice. No matter how many years you study T'ai Chi, you can still benefit from studying in classes. T'ai Chi, like life, is an endless growth process.

Most of us in the modern world want fast answers. We like to take classes or workshops and move on. And sometimes our educational motivation has more to do with getting our hands on a piece of paper that says we know something than with personally being changed by the knowledge.

Therefore, most people rush through a T'ai Chi course to learn a few moves and then think they're done. Of course, you do get some benefit from any exposure to T'ai Chi. Things you learn on the first day can benefit the rest of your life. But why stop there? T'ai Chi can offer you a deep ocean of experience. After 30 years of T'ai Chi practice, I still study with my instructor and enjoy class, book, and video instruction by other teachers. And even though my very first class was beneficial and wonderful, I still find benefits that carry into my home practice in each and every new lesson. Also, as a teacher, I often get new insights into T'ai Chi by learning from other teachers' classes, books, and videos, even those of different styles.

T'ai Chi provides lifelong benefits and should be practiced for the rest of our lives. However, this isn't a marriage contract. Don't feel smothered by this. Drop in and out of T'ai Chi as often as you like. T'ai Chi will always be patiently waiting for you when you come back, like a touchstone or a port in a storm. Eventually, you will do T'ai Chi simply because you feel pretty spectacular when you do.

Besides finding classes enjoyable, you will discover that T'ai Chi attracts interesting people, and the social aspect will draw you as well. I was among a handful of national T'ai Chi experts commissioned by the National Council on the Aging to create a T'ai Chi for Seniors Efficacy Guide for aging professionals seeking to begin T'ai Chi classes for their clients. All of the attending T'ai Chi experts agreed the "social aspect" of T'ai Chi was a very important benefit of the practice.

If self-confidence is an issue, you'll find that most T'ai Chi classes are friendly and low key. However, you can also boost your confidence by learning T'ai Chi from a video program, to help you feel more comfortable beginning live T'ai Chi classes, even a different style.

The basics of T'ai Chi often transcend styles. Bottom line is this: do *whatever it takes* for you to enjoy T'ai Chi and QiGong!

SAGE SIFU SAYS

If you get frustrated by a class and drop out, don't make it a life sentence. Keep coming back to T'ai Chi. Each class will make you more confident. Repeat the beginner class as many times as you like; there are no deadlines or expectations in T'ai Chi. Relax. Take your time. Play.

Making the Most of Learning T'ai Chi by Book

T'ai Chi books are great for helping you understand the philosophy, art, and science of T'ai Chi, and as supplements to classes, or video instruction if classes don't work for you right now. However, a book cannot replace a live instructor or the other benefits of a class or the verbal/visuals of video lessons.

It's difficult to explain body movements in books because books are dependent on still photographs. This book, however, includes a vast library of T'ai Chi and QiGong video exhibitions in the Web Support Video to provide you an unequaled, and profoundly deeper, T'ai Chi book experience. But, beyond reading this book, the ability to see an instructor move and to ask for clarification or hear other students' questions is invaluable. Also, it's easier for instructors to explain things in person in stages while you relax; when using a book, you have to remember facts because the instructor isn't there to remind you.

But, again, this unique book's voluminous Web Video Support will greatly enhance the book's text and illustrated instruction with information that can benefit you no matter what style you study.

Making the Most of Video/DVD T'ai Chi

If you don't have access to T'ai Chi classes or simply can't work them into your life yet, a video or DVD is the next best way to learn. You can use books to supplement your understanding of what videos teach, too. Using books and videos together can help maximize the benefit of your T'ai Chi practice. As the videos teach visually and audibly, enabling your mind to relax, the books round out your intellectual understanding of the movements and exercises.

Consider that the average 8-week introductory T'ai Chi class entails at least 12 hours of instruction. The average T'ai Chi video is one hour. As you can see, it's difficult for an instructor to explain a 2,000-year-old art and science that's so rich in benefits in a one-hour video. However, some videos are done in multi-volume, several-hour sets, which is the best way to go if you don't have access to or time for live T'ai Chi classes yet. Don't be intimidated by this. You won't work out for hours, but you will use lesson segments of the DVD, progressing through the multi-hour instructional over a period of weeks or months.

DVDs' video instruction can also be used in conjunction with a live class, enabling you to remember what you may have not noticed in class, or to help you practice more between classes. Some instructors have their own videos, or can refer you to one (See Appendix C on DVDs).

SAGE SIFU SAYS

Videos can be great supplements to your ongoing T'ai Chi class, especially if your instructor has produced one or approves one for the class. Be aware, however, that even if a video covers the same style you are studying, it might look different.

Understanding TCM's Horary Clock

TCM, or Traditional Chinese Medicine's, acupuncture, Chinese herbal medicine, and T'ai Chi understand that the body has natural rhythms that align with certain organs and functions. You can actually use this "horary" (hourly) clock to treat problems. Each organ has certain hours, called peak hours, that are generally the best for treating that organ:

11 A.M. to 1 P.M.	Heart
1 P.M. to 3 P.M.	Small intestine
3 P.M. to 5 P.M.	Bladder
5 P.M. to 7 P.M.	Kidney
7 P.M. to 9 P.M.	Pericardium
9 P.M. to 11 P.M.	Triple burner
11 P.M. to 1 A.M.	Gallbladder
1 A.M. to 3 A.M.	Liver
3 A.M. to 5 A.M.	Lung
5 A.M. to 7 A.M.	Large intestine
7 A.M. to 9 A.M.	Stomach
9 A.M. to 11 A.M.	Spleen

In Part 3, I introduce some QiGong exercises for specific organs. However, T'ai Chi can generally *tonify* all the aspects of the body and every organ. Therefore, T'ai Chi practice at a peak hour could provide a good therapy. Yet if your peak hour is in the middle of the night, you may prefer a Sitting or Lying QiGong exercise to focus Qi into the desired organ. The Sitting QiGong exercise in Part 3 gives you a great technique to use in peak hours. To clarify, you'll find great benefit from T'ai Chi and QiGong practice even if you don't observe the horary clock. Generally speaking, most instructors agree that morning is the optimum time for T'ai Chi practice.

Outdoor vs. Indoor Practice

The single most important thing about practicing T'ai Chi is that you actually *do* practice it. Where you practice is secondary. Don't construe the following recommendation to do T'ai Chi outdoors to mean that you should not practice inside. If you can do T'ai Chi outdoors, do so. However, if you don't feel comfortable doing it outside because of where you live or the weather, then by all means do it inside.

The Benefits of Practicing Outdoors

The purpose of T'ai Chi and other QiGong exercises is to promote the flow of Qi. Qi's life energy flows through us and all living things. Therefore, the Chinese have always advocated performing T'ai Chi outdoors, where you can enjoy and benefit from the Qi of other living things. In fact, TCM teaches that when we do T'ai Chi, our relaxed body and mind benefit from nature's healing energy even more.

Just being in nature has a soothing quality, so if T'ai Chi can magnify this benefit, all the better. German physician Dr. Franz Mesmer, from whom we get the word *mesmerize*, worked with patients suffering from psychotic episodes.

Reportedly, Dr. Mesmer would instruct his patients to sit with their backs against a tree whenever they felt an episode coming on. His patients were said to benefit greatly from this "nature therapy." As you practice T'ai Chi in your backyard, the park, or even next to the plants in your house, you may experience the benefits of this therapy for yourself.

Choosing a Surface to Practice On

T'ai Chi should be practiced on a level, predictable surface, especially when you are beginning. As you play over the years, you may experiment with more uneven and challenging surfaces. You can perform T'ai Chi on grass, sand, dirt, or pavement. It's good to practice on varying types of surfaces because this gives your mind/body communication even more information for improving your balance.

Try to choose a flat area out of direct sunlight. Soft morning sunlight or evening light is all right, but do not practice in direct sunlight during the hot part of the day. You will discover that practicing T'ai Chi in different light is challenging as well. Doing T'ai Chi in the dimming light of sunset challenges you to use more internal and less external balance references.

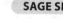

Practicing Indoors

The benefits of doing T'ai Chi indoors are pretty obvious if it's freezing or smoldering hot, or the mosquito population is in full production. Although outdoors is optimum, you can experience the benefits of T'ai Chi anywhere and at any time. When you're having a tough day at the office, it's great to slip off to the restroom or the supply room to drift into a T'ai Chi getaway. If you practice T'ai Chi at home before work or in the evening, it's often just more convenient to practice inside.

One problem students encounter indoors is space. As you move through your T'ai Chi repertoire, you often will cover more ground than your living room provides. If the next step takes you smack into a wall, just remember where you are, move back a couple steps, and pick up where you left off. Eventually, you won't even think about it. T'ai Chi pours into your living room, just like it easily and naturally flows into your life. Just as T'ai Chi encourages an almost liquid relaxation of mind and body, its use and benefits can seem to pour into every nook and cranny of our lives with much benefit.

Last but not least, when you're doing T'ai Chi indoors, minimize noise around you by turning off the TV and stereo. However, don't let noises *beyond your control* be an issue. Noise is in the ear of the beholder.

Large Class vs. Private Class

Surprisingly, learning in a large class has several advantages over more expensive private lessons, although both have their own strengths, depending on your needs and budget.

The Pros and Cons of Large Classes

If an instructor is in great demand, his or her classes will inevitably be larger. Therefore, you will get less personal attention but will benefit from the quality of instruction. On the other hand, you might find instructors with smaller classes who can provide you with more personal instruction. Decide what your priorities are, and choose a class size that meets your needs.

You can learn very effectively in a large class setting. In fact, being in a large class has distinct advantages. As fellow classmates ask questions for clarification, you can benefit by their inquiries. Also, you will discover that T'ai Chi classes have a *group energy*. Just as plants emit life energy, so do other people, and as your classmates practice T'ai Chi, you can bask in the glow of their presence—and they in yours.

Usually, an accomplished T'ai Chi instructor will have numerous advanced students who will help as assistants. In a larger class, you can benefit from the expertise these students have to offer. Note that advanced students probably are less than perfect, but so is the instructor. You will learn T'ai Chi in layers, and the advanced students can give you a layer of instruction that the instructor can add to or polish over the months and years.

T'ai Chi or QiGong classes will benefit you even if you take them for a short time, providing you with tools you can use for the rest of your life. However, it's best to take classes for a lifetime. It is fun, beneficial, and a great way to meet interesting people, so why not? Relax. Enjoy your classes as playtime. You have no deadline or rush to progress at a certain speed. If you practice for a few minutes every day, you will likely learn the forms quite easily.

However, if you need to repeat the beginning class again—and again—that's no problem.

> **OUCH!**
>
> Do not assume the instructor is aware of a problem you have with a movement or the class program. Ask questions during class to clarify instruction. However, if you have concerns about the program, discuss it with the instructor after class. Before you stop attending a T'ai Chi class in frustration, discuss your concerns with the instructor. Most instructors want to help you get it—that's why they're there.

If you're in a large class, you may have to move around a bit to see what the instructor is doing. Move to wherever you need to be to see. T'ai Chi is very informal. Usually, in a very large class advanced students will position themselves in various locations so you can follow them if you cannot see the instructor clearly. If you're not sure what's being taught, raise your hand and ask for clarification. Don't be shy about this. The best T'ai Chi classes are ones in which students interact and ask questions. The least productive classes are those in which the teacher does all the talking.

The Pros and Cons of Private Lessons

Very few people get private lessons. Part of the reason is that they can be very expensive. A good T'ai Chi instructor usually will begin at about $75 per hour and can go up significantly from there.

However, some people, such as emergency room physicians, have erratic, demanding schedules and are forced to take private lessons. This is a highly effective way to learn the T'ai Chi forms in a very short period of time, because the instructor's entire focus is on you.

Private lessons can also be beneficial to those learning to be instructors, thereby enabling them to learn minute details and background on movements and their purpose.

> **T'AI SCI**
>
> Any malady should be discussed with a physician. However, in addition to your medical doctor, you might want to discuss your condition with a certified doctor of TCM. Using T'ai Chi and QiGong on your own can be a powerful adjunct therapy for a condition you may be treating; however, if used under the direction of a TCM practitioner, they may be even more effective.

How Often Should I Practice?

To maximize your T'ai Chi benefits, it's best to spend about 20 minutes in the morning doing T'ai Chi or a Sitting QiGong meditation exercise. Then spend another 20 minutes in the evening doing whichever one you didn't do in the morning.

Usually the first response to this suggestion is, "I don't have an extra 40 minutes a day!" If that is your response, ask yourself the following questions:

Do I spend 40 minutes a day watching TV?

Do I spend my morning and afternoon breaks drinking soda or coffee and chatting?

Do I ever spend time eagerly waiting for my computer to access the internet, or to print a document, or do I ever spend time just waiting for dinner to bake in the oven?

For most of us, the answer to at least one of these questions is yes. If you look, you probably do have an extra 40 minutes a day. So the main difficulty in doing T'ai Chi isn't really having the time, but *deciding* to do it. When we decide to do it, we find that we will make time. Beginning new life habits is one of the single-most difficult things people attempt. But T'ai Chi is worth it. Also, remember that if you practice T'ai Chi or QiGong two or three times a week for a few minutes, that's much better than not doing it at all! Enjoy! Lighten up!

SAGE SIFU SAYS

Because T'ai Chi practice calms us and clears our minds, it actually provides us extra time in a sense. When we are calmer and clearer, we tend to be more efficient, we are easier to live with, and we find it easier to relax and sleep. So the 40 or 50 minutes we spend on T'ai Chi and QiGong can save us hours in effort and frustration.

T'ai Chi Is a Model for Easing Life Changes

T'ai Chi is new for you. You will find that it will take time to get used to doing it every day. Don't punish or scold yourself when you forget. Just enjoy it when you do it. The following example will help you see just how difficult it is to change life habits so you can go easy on yourself as you begin to adapt to a new life with T'ai Chi:

A study of cardiac recovery patients shows just how difficult it is to change. Patients were given a choice of two therapies to follow after their heart attacks. The first was only to take medication and be released within days. Unfortunately, that first choice carried

a prognosis of another possible major heart attack within a few months. The second choice involved staying in the hospital for a much longer period to learn stress-management techniques and new dietary changes, and it offered a much rosier forecast of the patients likely going several years before another coronary. Amazingly, nearly all the patients opted to leave immediately, even though it increased the likelihood of a premature death.

What is ironic about T'ai Chi is that even though it may be difficult to incorporate into your life at first, it will make all other healthful life changes much easier. T'ai Chi is a technology designed to help us change with less effort and stress. Therefore, the longer we practice T'ai Chi, the easier it is for us to change. So if you decide to go on a more healthful diet, or start getting out in nature more, the effort you make to learn T'ai Chi will make all those other efforts to change more effortless.

Let Go of Your Grip on Expectations or Results

Studies show that when we change for positive reasons, we are much more likely to change our habits. Therefore, rather than do T'ai Chi because your blood pressure is high or your stress levels are unbearable, do T'ai Chi because it feels good. Don't rush through your T'ai Chi, but make it a little oasis in your busy day. Slow down enough to feel the pleasure of the movement and the stretches. Enjoy how good it feels to breathe deeply and let the whole body relax. This will condition you, day by day, to love the feeling T'ai Chi gives you, causing you to look forward to it and miss it when you don't do it.

Make a Calendar

If you want help remembering to do T'ai Chi, create a T'ai Chi calendar and place it on your refrigerator door. Every time you do your T'ai Chi or QiGong, mark a big X on that day's square. As you begin to get a few days in a row, you'll want to keep that string going. You'll also begin to notice that the more X's you have on the calendar, the better you feel. Your awareness becomes more subtle and pleasant, which will help you make the transition from doing T'ai Chi for the calendar accomplishment to doing it for how it makes you feel.

OUCH!

When you forget to do T'ai Chi, don't scold yourself. Your mind plays funny games to keep from growing and changing. Making ourselves "bad" for not immediately adopting new life habits is one of those games. If you forgot to do T'ai Chi yesterday, just relax and do it now—no big deal. Breathe and enjoy.

The Value of T'ai Chi's Social Aspect

T'ai Chi clubs are increasingly popular in the United States (and worldwide)—as they have been for centuries in China—because even though T'ai Chi is a terrific personal exercise and is thoroughly enjoyable alone, it can also be a terrific social event. T'ai Chi clubs offer a group energy that can heighten the pleasure T'ai Chi provides. When I was commissioned by the National Council on Aging to join a group of other top T'ai Chi experts from around the country to create an *efficacy guide*

for T'ai Chi for aging population classes, we all agreed that the "social component" of getting together with your T'ai Chi group is a very beneficial aspect of T'ai Chi study.

T'ai Chi clubs also are very supportive and encourage T'ai Chi players to practice on their own. When we have a class or a club to get together with, we are much more likely to practice on our own at home. We want to improve our T'ai Chi so we can play more complex T'ai Chi games using mirror-image forms and other games involving several players. Continuing with a T'ai Chi class or club for the rest of your life is a great way to stick with T'ai Chi for the long haul. Social T'ai Chi is also terrific because T'ai Chi practice can extend your life substantially; if you outlive all your peers, you won't be lonely because you'll still have your T'ai Chi club to hang out with.

The Least You Need to Know

- If you don't have access to, or just can't make it to, live T'ai Chi classes, then videos (see Appendix C) and books can be very useful.

- Treat certain organs by using T'ai Chi and the "horary" clock.

- Although outdoor T'ai Chi is optimum, indoor T'ai Chi is great, too.

- Large classes can be great if you ask questions. If you use video or DVD instruction, find a presenter who'll respond to questions.

- Use a T'ai Chi calendar to get used to practicing. Eventually, T'ai Chi will become an integral part of your life.

Be Prepared: Your First Day of Class

In This Chapter

- Dressing for T'ai Chi
- Preparing mentally and physically for class
- Knowing what is expected of you
- Learning T'ai Chi lingo
- Web Video Support: *What Live T'ai Chi Class Instruction May Look Like*

In this chapter, you learn what to wear to do T'ai Chi. Yet beyond fashion concerns, this chapter prepares you mentally, emotionally, and physically for your first day of class. Even those currently involved in T'ai Chi will find these mental and emotional insights into T'ai Chi challenges helpful.

This chapter also provides you with many ways to get the most out of T'ai Chi training by describing class structure, explaining what is expected of you, and clarifying terms you may encounter in class.

Choosing Your T'ai Chi Wardrobe

Ultimately, you can do T'ai Chi in any kind of clothing, but certain clothing *is* suggested for class. Typically, T'ai Chi students wear anything they want, but wear something loose enough to move freely in. The rest is often up to you. The most common T'ai Chi suit is a T-shirt and sweat pants. Spandex or body suits, although not prohibited, are not typically worn in T'ai Chi.

If you practice T'ai Chi at the office, know that longer dresses can make it more difficult for an instructor to see your posture or leg placement, but don't skip class just because you have a longer dress on that day. Also, even though everyone will likely be wearing office clothes, they should kick off their heels. If you go from the office to a studio or community class, or if your company holds classes in an exercise area, bring some sweats and tennis shoes to change into.

Some studios, especially martial arts studios, may require more formal attire. If so, they will direct you to a martial arts supply store that sells the appropriate garb, or the studio may provide it.

What footwear you wear depends on the location. Tennis shoes are fine for most T'ai Chi classes. However, some studios that offer T'ai Chi, such as martial arts or yoga studios, require bare feet. It's not advisable to wear only socks in these studios because socks can be slippery. If you need arch support and attend a class in these locations, you may be able to wear tennis shoes that have never been used on the street or Chinese kung fu shoes. These nonstreet shoes will not damage the floor, but check with the instructor before purchasing them.

OUCH!

Some Chinese masters caution against practicing T'ai Chi barefoot because it opens the feet to "pernicious influences." This sounds sinister, but it may only mean that you could chill if the ground is cold or pick up an infection if the ground is dirty. Conversely, others say it is good to practice barefoot because it connects you to the earth, whereas your rubber shoes electrically isolate you from it.

The only hard-and-fast rule all instructors follow on footwear is that you cannot wear heeled shoes. Heels are hard on your back, make balance difficult, and change the way your whole body moves. If you're doing T'ai Chi at the office, just kick off your heels or bring tennis shoes if they feel more comfortable, and the best tennis shoes are the ones with lower heels.

Class Rules and Internal/External Hygiene

T'ai Chi has very few external hygiene rules, but internally, it's good to prepare yourself mentally and emotionally by letting go of some myths about yourself and exercise classes.

External Hygiene and Class Rules

Unlike most other martial arts, T'ai Chi usually requires no contact between participants. Therefore, hygiene rules are pretty much like those for daily life.

However, it is important not to wear heavy cologne or perfume into class because it might be overwhelming to others during the deep breathing you do in T'ai Chi. Also, leave jewelry at home, especially jangly jewelry.

The last and most important rule is a combination of external and internal hygiene. Cell phones must be turned off! This is very important, because in most T'ai chi or QiGong classes you'll experience calming meditative states that will come in layers of deepening. Each external distraction will lift you, and all your classmates, backward out of this deeper state of mind, thereby erasing progress and causing the teacher to have to go back and regain that depth.

My teacher extolled us to think of our T'ai Chi or QiGong class and personal practice as a "sacred space" where we don't allow the world's rat race to intrude. This creating a "sacred space" in our consciousness is a powerful part of both T'ai Chi and QiGong, and as you nurture this space, like a garden it will grow out into all aspects of your daily life, making all aspects of your world more sacred places. After 30 years of personal exploration using T'ai Chi, QiGong, Yoga, and other mind-body arts, I have begun to realize that each sliver of each moment is sacred. This life is the only game in town, and it's here for us to play with and enjoy. The Chinese call T'ai Chi a return to childlikeness. Children are mesmerized by life experiences. We can be, too, but we have to leave the rat race outside our classes and home practice.

The only time I saw my teacher get angry in all the years I studied with her, was when I took a cell phone call during a class. In my classes now, I tell *my* students, "You can only leave your cell phone turned on during class if you are expecting an organ transplant; otherwise, they must be turned off." You want this time in group or class to be a special time, a time to let yourself completely unplug from the world.

Internal Hygiene—A State of Mind

Cleansing the clutter from your mind, heart, and body is the *most* important thing you should do before attending your first—or one hundredth—T'ai Chi class.

In the long run, T'ai Chi will help relieve allergy problems, but if you have serious allergies and are heavily medicated, it may be helpful to lighten up on the medications before T'ai Chi if your medications make your balance more difficult or make it harder to focus. However, never adjust your prescription medication without your doctor's approval.

If you haven't tried acupuncture for your allergies, now might be a good time to try it. It can be a terrific nonpharmaceutical way to alleviate allergy symptoms with great results.

Acupuncture treatments cannot harm you, but they can enhance your clarity or balance. There are also some proven dietary approaches to allergy issues. More on TCM's diet tips later.

T'ai Chi and Massage Therapy

T'ai Chi is like an internal self-massage, as it is meant to loosen the mind and body and increase internal awareness (see preview of Chapter 11's *Moving QiGong Warm Ups Excerpt* on the Web Video Support's *Moving Qigong Is Internal Massage* for more on internal awareness www.idiotsguides.com/taichi). Tension disconnects the mind from the body. But, in addition to T'ai Chi and QiGong, you may find it very complementary to begin massage therapy and to continue it for the rest of your life as well. Most good T'ai Chi teachers will advocate massage therapy as part of your T'ai Chi training, just as many good massage therapists will recommend T'ai Chi to their clients. You also might find that massage therapy is helpful in relieving chronic problems such as allergies. T'ai Chi and QiGong work from the inside out, as massage works from the outside in, to expedite and deepen your internal looseness.

SAGE SIFU SAYS

As T'ai Chi teaches the body to move and change more easily and effortlessly, it provides a model for the mind and heart to change more easily. As you continue with T'ai Chi, you may discover you eat more healthfully, drink more water and less soda, get better rest, adopt habits such as regular massage therapy, and spend more time with people who make you feel good about yourself.

Resistance to Change Tempts You to Drop Out

T'ai Chi helps us change. Our minds and bodies get accustomed to the way we have always done things, even things that are not really good for us. Therefore, on a subconscious level, parts of us resist good changes that T'ai Chi fosters because we don't want to let go of the way we've always been. Part of us likes to be a "couch potato" and doesn't like the way T'ai Chi is getting us more involved in an active life. Resistance to change may manifest itself in many ways and may …

- Cause you to scold yourself, to tell yourself you are too clumsy, too uncoordinated, too slow, or too tired to do T'ai Chi.

- Tell you T'ai Chi is for other people who are better, smarter, stronger, or more coordinated than you are.

- Have you think the teacher doesn't like you or T'ai Chi is dumb and useless.

- Have you believe it would be much more fun to watch TV and eat potato chips tonight than going all the way out to your T'ai Chi class.

- Tell you, "You're already too far behind; don't go back there," if you miss a class.

If you hang in there long enough, however, you will discover that after nearly every T'ai Chi class, you will feel much better than you did before going. If you become conscious of the voices of "resistance" and see them as the debilitating illusions they are, you will be more likely to stick with T'ai Chi.

"Wrongness" Is Our Culture's "Resistance"

Your T'ai Chi progress will be held back by something that affects our entire culture. If you understand this, it will take a great deal of pressure off you and your instructor. Most Western students are obsessed with learning the T'ai Chi movements "perfectly," and this causes them stress, which slows their ability to learn and enjoy T'ai Chi. In fact, we often convince ourselves that our attempts to learn are so "imperfect" that it is pointless to continue with our study.

What you will discover is the judgmental voice or thought that plays inside your head, the one that negatively judges your skill or actions, is an energy knot or tangle in your energy body, psyche, and heart. As you progress through your T'ai Chi or Qigong journey, this knot will flare up from time to time and cause you to doubt yourself, or to doubt the value of your practice, or often to doubt the value of your teacher.

My teacher warned us this would happen, and it did, and trust me, it does. She called it "resistance." I described this in detail earlier in this chapter, but it bears repeating. It is the mind and body's tendency to resist change. As T'ai Chi and Qigong expand your world, a part of your consciousness will want to recoil back to older, more unconscious ways of living and behaving. It will try to get you to give up this mind-expanding journey you have embarked upon. Just by recognizing this dynamic, it will help you to not only stick with T'ai Chi and Qigong, but to smooth out these tangles of thought we are often unconsciously manipulated by that hold back our evolution on many levels and in many areas of our life. See Web Video Support's *Qi Is About Letting Go.*

OUCH!

Students often obsess on remembering each detail the instructor tells them; some even bring a pad and pencil to class. Don't do that. Relax. Good instructors will repeat important things over and over. Let yourself enjoy the class. Don't make T'ai Chi class another "important," "serious" thing in your life. Let it be playtime.

T'ai Chi will show you on a very basic level that you are never "wrong." You are growing and learning how to do things better and better each and every day of your life. T'ai Chi is simple enough to use the very first day of practice, but its richness is so subtle that you can refine your T'ai Chi movements for the rest of your life. Therefore, you don't need to "perfect" the first movement before learning the second. You learn a layer of the movements, and learning that layer changes who you are and how you function. Your new and improved self can then learn the movements at yet a deeper, subtler level, and so on for years and years. T'ai Chi leaves you in an endlessly blooming state of perfection.

Attending Your First Class

When entering your first class, you probably aren't sure what it will look like, how to treat the instructor, or what is expected of you. So let's look at these expectations one at a time.

Mainly, you will be expected to relax and enjoy yourself. You will also have a little homework, but as you'll see, this could be the best homework you ever had.

How to Address Your Instructor

You have several possible options for addressing your instructor. The safest way to find out what is right for the class you enroll in is to simply ask the teacher how he or she would like to be addressed. The formal Chinese term for T'ai Chi teacher is *Sifu* (pronounced *see-foo*), meaning "master of an art or skill." However, many T'ai Chi classes in the West are very informal. Most instructors simply go by their first name.

If a Chinese teacher asks you to call him Sifu, this is not because of an inflated ego. Actually, this is a great compliment. This means he considers you a worthy student, and that is an honor.

Class Structure

T'ai Chi is informal, and each class is different. Some classes begin with a Sitting QiGong exercise, using chairs forming a circle. For this relaxation exercise, the instructor will likely lead the group through an imagery exercise as she sits quietly with her eyes closed. Other classes will not use chairs and may begin with a standing relaxation exercise, also with the students' eyes closed. Still other instructors may begin the class by leading students in warm-up exercises without first practicing a QiGong or relaxation exercise.

OUCH!

Your main goal in T'ai Chi class should be to relax and breathe. By not trying too hard, you learn more easily. Students who frustrate themselves by mentally repeating that they "can't get it" usually prove themselves right. If you really can't learn the movement, just follow the other students as you breathe and relax. You'll feel good after class, and you can repeat the session again—and you'll be the expert in class the second time around.

Once relaxation exercises are done, the physical class structure will probably have students staggered throughout the room, facing the instructor. The instructor usually faces the class, which forms lines throughout the room, giving each student enough space to swing his or her arms without striking another student. However, smaller, more informal classes may form a circle. An instructor may alternate facing the class or demonstrating the moves with his back to the class. He might also move around the room to give students different angles to see from.

If you're in a class that's formed in lines facing the instructor, find a place where you can see what he is doing. Many large classes will have advanced students to help, and you can watch them if you can't see the instructor. If you can't see what's going on, ask questions or change places. Be clear about your needs. The teacher wants to help you understand the movements, but in a larger class, he may not know you need further explanation. Don't be afraid to speak up.

The following list gives you an idea of the process a T'ai Chi class might go through; however, each instructor has her own format:

- Sitting or Standing Relaxation Exercise (if your class performs this).

- T'ai Chi warm-up exercises—gentle, repetitive movements that prepare you physically and mentally for T'ai Chi (many warm-ups are moving QiGong exercises and are discussed in detail in Part 3).

- After warm-ups, the instructor may teach individual movements to practice, or if she teaches by exhibition, she will begin performing the entire T'ai Chi set and you will be expected to follow along.

- Your homework is the movements themselves, although it is highly recommended to begin using the QiGong relaxation exercises at home for your own health and pleasure.

T'ai Chi usually does not require anyone to sit or lie on the floor; however, some instructors may have warm-up or cool-down exercises that require it. If you are unable to do so because of an injury or physical limitation, discuss alternatives with the instructor.

SAGE SIFU SAYS

You can get all the benefits from T'ai Chi without straining. You don't have to memorize all the terms, do the movements exactly like your teacher does, or read any certain books. T'ai Chi's amazing benefits will come to you by simply breathing deeply, relaxing your mind, and playing T'ai Chi in class and every day at home. Play T'ai Chi every day, and everything else will take care of itself. See Web Video Support's *Willingness to Let Go*.

How Are T'ai Chi Movements Taught?

T'ai Chi forms involve a series of choreographed martial arts poses that flow together like a slow-motion dance. How these movements are taught can vary. Some classes are taught by example, meaning the instructor will lead the group all the way through the entire T'ai Chi form and the students mimic until, over time, they remember all the movements.

However, many classes are taught for different levels. In these classes, the movements are broken down into one or two movements per class. If you are an average learner, these classes are preferable. It's much easier to learn one movement at a time and practice it all week than it is to try to assimilate an entire T'ai Chi form. It's easier to memorize movements in smaller bites. Realize your learning will be much easier if you don't miss classes, because for each class you'd miss, that would make the learning bites get larger. View the Web Video Support's *What Live T'ai Chi Class Instruction May Look Like* to get a feel for how movements may be broken down in classes.

To help you get the most out of your classes, review the following points on how T'ai Chi is taught or might be studied:

- Warm-ups and relaxation techniques are usually repeated weekly, but you will benefit if you practice these every day on your own.

- You must learn and practice the actual T'ai Chi movement of the week on your own that week.

- Each week a new T'ai Chi movement will be added to your growing form or repertoire.

- The form will get longer and longer each week until you learn the entire form.

- Long forms of 20 minutes take between 6 and 8 months to learn.

- Short forms of 10 minutes may take 2 to 6 months to learn, depending on the instructor and the form.

- Advanced students often repeat beginning or intermediate classes for years to refine their performance of the T'ai Chi forms.

- Advanced students may serve as assistant instructors in class.

In addition to the preceding points, also understand that in most classes T'ai Chi is taught in three stages:

1. The movements are learned.

2. The breath is incorporated into the regimen by learning an inhalation or exhalation that's connected to each movement.

3. A relaxation element or awareness of the flow of energy through the body is learned. Although the first step offers many benefits from the first day, the benefits get richer and deeper with each level you learn. This last element involving an expanding internal awareness will deepen within you for years and years.

Advanced students may be asked to assist new students learning the forms for the first time. T'ai Chi, like all martial arts, is based on a mentoring system. Assistants will usually teach the first of the three stages of T'ai Chi instruction.

SAGE SIFU SAYS

Normal T'ai Chi exercises can be easily adjusted to conform to your living room's size. Also, the more advanced Sword or Fan forms some styles teach, although more challenging, can easily be done indoors, too. For example, you can use retractable swords and leave them retracted when you're practicing indoors. The bottom line is, you can always practice T'ai Chi, no matter what style it is or where you are.

Yes, There Is Homework Involved

T'ai Chi class exposes you to the movements, but then you must practice those movements at home. There are two ways to look at this: either as another burden on your life's full plate or as a chance to take a break and let all the weight of the world roll right off your shoulders.

The very first movement you learn on the very first day of class is a fantastic QiGong relaxation exercise that, if you do it in the right frame of mind, can help you begin to dump stress. If you do the T'ai Chi movement only to prepare for the next T'ai Chi class, it won't be that relaxing. However, if you breathe deeply and let every muscle of your body relax, allowing the burdens of the week to roll off your shoulders each time you practice the movement, it'll feel great! Refer to the *T'ai Chi Learning Can Be a Relaxing Qigong Experience* on the Web Video Support to see how the first movement can be used as a *relaxation therapy*, even as you learn it, by including deep, full breaths. Learning in this spirit can make all the movements become relaxation therapies even as you learn them (more on deep breaths in the Web Video Support's *Let Breath Flow Your Movements*).

> **OUCH!**
>
> At first it will be difficult to discipline yourself to practice daily. If you fall behind in class, just play along and repeat the multi-week session again. There are no deadlines. You'll get it eventually. Don't sabotage yourself into thinking you just can't get it. Regular attendance and daily practice make T'ai Chi effortless and fruitful. Although some instructors may help you individually to catch up if you miss class, you can't expect it.

To learn T'ai Chi, you will need to practice at home. But we learn T'ai Chi because it feels good, so why wouldn't we want to practice something that makes us feel good?

T'ai Chi Etiquette

Most instructors are happy to get questions during class. The rest of the class, or at least some of them, are probably facing the same uncertainties or challenges you are. A good instructor has been studying many years and may not remember all the challenges new students have, so your inquiries help him *help you* as well as the other students in class.

If your questions are criticisms of the format or structure, it would be best to offer them to the instructor personally after class. The instructor may not be able to fix it, but he may explain why it is done the way it is.

The Least You Need to Know

- Before your first T'ai Chi class, ask the class instructor what you should wear.
- T'ai Chi can encourage healthful lifestyle changes, such as massages or drug-free treatments for health problems.
- Practicing T'ai Chi makes life changes easier.
- In a T'ai Chi class, your instructors will tell you what is expected of you.
- Practice T'ai Chi not only to learn and remember the movements, but also because it feels good!

Horse Stance and Other Terms

In This Chapter

- Understanding the importance of T'ai Chi posture
- Learning how T'ai Chi protects your joints
- Discovering how T'ai Chi's moves teach effortless living
- Knowing that breath is the beginning of everything
- Web Video Support: *Locating Your Dan Tien and Vertical Axis; Sinking into the Horse Stance; and Your Rotating Dan Tien Massage Your Organs*

This chapter explains the core concepts that will ensure a rich T'ai Chi experience for you, whether you are beginning classes or a video instruction program. You will discover the basic concepts of T'ai Chi, how its movements are to be performed, why they are performed that way, and how to breathe when performing them. By understanding that T'ai Chi is very different from Western exertion exercises, you won't make it harder than it is, and by relaxing into it, you unlock its full, effortless potential.

T'ai Chi Posture Is Power!

I introduced the dan tien in Chapter 1. See *Locating Your Dan Tien and Vertical Axis* in Web Video Support: www.idiotsguides.com/taichi. In T'ai Chi, we move from the dan tien by first sinking into the Horse Stance. This is how we sink our Qi, which makes us more solid, more balanced, and more down to earth physically, emotionally, and mentally.

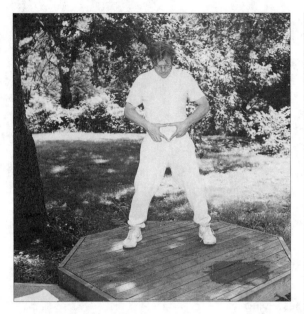

Make a triangle with your thumbs over your navel and with your forefingers extending downward. Your fingertips will meet at the level of your dan tien. Refer to the Web Video Support's Locating Your Dan Tien and Vertical Axis sections.

Where Is the Dan Tien?

Where the dan tien is located on the outside of the body only tells its height, for the dan tien is actually inside the body. Here's how to find your dan tien inside:

1. With your fingers forming a triangle as described in the previous figure, point your fingers as if they could extend inside your body.

2. Your fingers are now pointing toward your dan tien; however, the dan tien is near the center of your body, so it only can be felt on the inside.

3. Now tighten your sphincter muscles, as if you were pulling up your internal organs from within, and then immediately relax. Repeat this over and over until you experience a subtle tugging sensation inside, just beyond where

your fingers are pointing to your upper pelvis or lower abdomen.

4. The place where you feel that subtle tugging feeling is where your dan tien is. That isn't your dan tien itself—that was a muscle tugging—your dan tien is an energy center.

5. Dan tien only can be experienced as energy, tingling, or other light sensations. This is where all powerful movement or action comes from, and cultivated awareness of the dan tien with T'ai Chi makes any action you take more powerful, with less likelihood of injury.

The Horse Stance and Three Dan Tiens

The dan tien is the basis of the Horse Stance. The Horse Stance is the basic stance for all martial arts, including T'ai Chi. It aligns the three dan tien points, upper or Shang dan tien (associated with the *Yin Tang acupuncture point*), middle or Zhong dan tien (*Shan Zhong point*), and lower or Xia dan tien (*Qi Hai point*), to give you the best posture and most effortless movement. Refer to the Web Video Support for a deeper understanding of the energetic nature of the three dan tiens.

KNOW YOUR CHINESE

Although the *dan tien* usually refers to an energy point below the navel, there are actually three dan tien points, all near the center of the body: one below the navel, **Qi Hai**; the second at heart level, **Shan Zhong**; and the third at eyebrow level, **Yin Tang.** Each dan tien is an energy center where certain energies are focused or supercharged into the system.

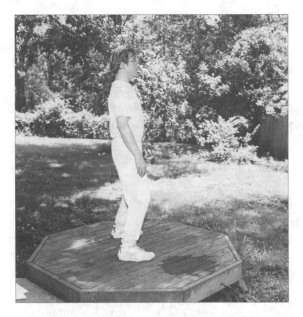

Note that the head is drawn upward toward the sky, as if a string were pulling from the center of the head. The chin is slightly pulled in, and the tailbone or sacrum is dropped down. This has the effect of lengthening the spine.

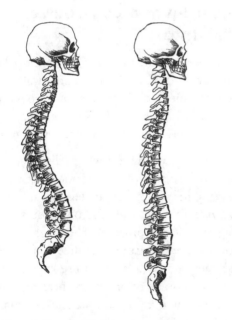

This figure illustrates how the spine is lengthened as you drop into the Horse Stance, although this is an exaggeration.

OUCH!

The lengthening of the spine that occurs as you sink into your Horse Stance is not a "forced" position. Do not "stand at attention"; rather, allow the muscles around the backbone to let go, enabling you to relax into a lengthened posture. Refer to the Web Video Support's *Sinking into the Horse Stance* section for more on the Horse Stance.

The Vertical Axis Aligns Posture

Many lower-back injuries are caused by poor performance posture. T'ai Chi encourages you to maintain good posture and reminds you when you get sloppy. To achieve proper posture, align the three dan tien points over the soles of the feet, with the weight slightly more to the heels than the front.

As you practice T'ai Chi's slow, gentle forms, your back may experience discomfort whenever you forget posture and let your butt creep out too much. However, when done correctly, the slow, gentle, low-impact nature of T'ai Chi will alert you to correct your posture or any other poor physical habits long before real damage occurs. This is what sets T'ai Chi apart from other training. In fact, you often don't become aware of problems in high-impact sports until the doctor is telling you not to play that sport *ever again*.

The vertical axis is not just about posture, but also about giving your body an effortless support to sink its weight onto each time you exhale. Chapter 13's instructional figures show a short line extending from the top of the head out through the bottom of the filled-foot. Your body's weight sinks down through the leg you are filling, down into the earth, to take the load off your body. See *Vertical Axis in Motion* in Web Video Support.

This will seem kind of esoteric at first, but as you again and again *pretend* to let your entire body sink onto the support of the *energy rod* that extends from 12 feet above your head, straight down through the center of your body, and roots down 12 feet into the earth below you, which we refer to as the vertical axis, it will begin to feel very tangible, and will literally hold you up. So, how do we "sink"?

The Sinking

T'ai Chi is about sinking. All teachers of all styles often talk about "the sinking." This isn't like heaviness as in a ship sinking, but more of a weightless release of muscles, allowing the skeleton to effortlessly hold the weight of the body. Let your relaxed shoulders sink away from your neck as you sink into your movements. It's as if you were swimming through an atmosphere of effortlessness as you move through your forms. The Web Video Support's *Sinking into Your Horse Stance* provides a visual support for these instructions. The Sinking is not just physical, for as you know by now, there is a mental and emotional awareness aspect to the physical. When you let your breath and muscles go, your mind and heart are also sinking into a deeper internal awareness, and letting go of their grip on the world. You are sinking into a Zen state of being *here and now*.

A T'AI CHI PUNCH LINE

An advanced T'ai Chi student went to study with a grandmaster in China. The grandmaster told him to stand on one leg and said, "Keep standing; I'll be back." The grandmaster returned 15 minutes later and reached down to squeeze the student's calf muscle on the leg he was standing on. The master scoffed, "Too tight! Why is your leg so tight? Keep standing; I'll come back and check later."

Sinking Your Weight

Each T'ai Chi movement is associated with an inhale and/or an exhale. When you move and exhale, you allow your body to sink into a feeling of effortlessness. As you transfer your weight from one leg to the other, relax the entire weight of the body down into the weight-bearing leg. The Chinese call this "sinking your Qi."

By practicing this in T'ai Chi, you will move more effortlessly and your balance will improve. This also promotes blood and energy circulation through the body and encourages less joint damage by removing chronic tension from your daily movements. Tight muscles make tighter joints. The Web Video Support's *Let Breath Flow Your Movements* provides a visual image of how the breath is related to "sinking" into the movement.

Never Pivot a Leg You've Sunk Into

If you ever watched the TV series *Kung Fu*, you may have seen Kwai Chang Caine walk across the rice paper for his graduation ceremony at the Shao Lin Temple. This looked very mystical, but it was actually a very practical test.

The purpose of the test was to discover whether he was pivoting the foot that was carrying his weight, or the leg that he had just *sunk into*. In most T'ai Chi, once you sink into a leg, you do not pivot on that weight-bearing foot because this can destabilize your balance and, more important, can cause knee damage. Styles that do pivot on weight-bearing legs do so rarely and take certain precautions to prevent injury. These pivots are not recommended for arthritis sufferers, but most styles will make a clear point of not pivoting on a filled leg.

OUCH!

To pivot a weight-bearing foot with no damage to your knee, lift your dan tien at the same time, so as to relieve pressure on your knee. If you have knee problems, I recommend not performing these types of pivots, or else modifying the form to be safe for you.

T'ai Chi movement is a process of "filling" and "emptying" each leg of Qi, or weight. The position of the dan tien over a leg determines that it is full and the other leg is empty. You "fill" the opposite foot by shifting your dan tien over that opposite foot. Then your "empty" foot has no weight on it and can be pivoted with zero damage to the knee. The Web Video Support's *Filling Left Leg to Pivot Empty Right Foot* provides a visual example of how only the emptied foot is pivoted. Chapter 13's *shadowing illustrations* also clearly explains this for all the long form's movements in that chapter.

When you begin doing T'ai Chi, you will benefit from rereading this and the other earlier chapters. You'll notice things you missed this first time through. It doesn't mean you goofed; it means there are multiple layers and dimensions to the motions and to each chapter that you can't comprehend all at once.

Some of the highest level of T'ai Chi and QiGong teachers have read this book several times and reported finding new insights in it each time. This is why, in a few instances, you see Web Video Support titles repeated in more than one chapter. The depth of these ancient teachings, evolved over thousands of years, is so great that you can discover whole new dimensions of each topic as you view it from different perspectives.

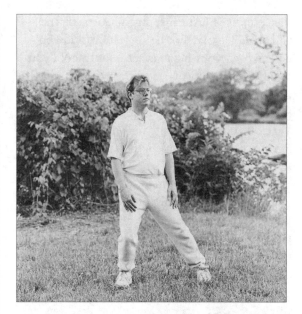

The Vertical Axis of the head and heart dan tien points lines up over the lower dan tien. This axis moving over a leg fills that leg with Qi, or weight. As you let your breath out and relax your body weight onto a leg, you sink your Qi into that leg.

Active Bones Under Soft Muscle

T'ai Chi is unlike any exercise you have ever done because it is done best when it's done easily. T'ai Chi's way will also provide a model for practicing the art of effortlessness in everything you do. When viewing the Web Video Support's T'ai Chi exhibitions in Chapters 13 and 14, notice how *effortlessness* seems to be the T'ai Chi player's goal.

T'ai Chi Is Not Isometrics

Most Western exercises involve some type of force or strain. T'ai Chi does not. The more effortlessly you are moving, the better you're doing it. You may catch yourself subconsciously tightening muscles because we have been taught that exercise must cause strain. Also, at first your balance may not be very solid, and you will tighten your leg muscles a lot to hold you steady. This is normal, and over time you'll find that you can relax your muscles more and more. As you get used to proper posture, using the Vertical Axis alignment you'll need less muscle tension to hold you up. So don't be discouraged if T'ai Chi doesn't feel so "effortless" at first. We are learning how to move effortlessly, by first becoming aware of how tight we are and then using QiGong breathing techniques taught in Part 3. Soon we begin to "let go" of needless effort as we move through T'ai Chi movements *and* life.

OUCH!

Becoming more comfortable with your forms and using proper posture with the Vertical Axis enables you to relax more as you move. At first you will notice yourself losing balance as much as or even more than before you started T'ai Chi. This is not unusual. Before, you probably held your balance by holding your body tightly. Now you are learning to balance while loose, by discovering your center alignment.

When doing T'ai Chi warm-ups, allow your mind to let go of thoughts and center on your effortless breath. Then enjoy the sensations of the muscles loosening as you move. On each breath, think of letting the muscles beneath the muscles let go of each other, as they also let go of the bones beneath. As we relax our muscles, the bones moving beneath provide a deep-tissue massage and the body can cleanse itself of toxins. Also, the relaxed abdominal muscles allow a gentle massage of the internal organs, which tonifies them and improves their function. View the Web Video Support's *Your Rotating Dan Tien Massages Your Organs* for a visual image about relaxed internal massaging of the organs.

Don't force yourself to go as low or deep in your stances as your instructor. You have the rest of your life to get lower. Right now, just focus on breathing, relaxing, and letting the muscles relax on the bones, again by allowing the entire body to relax as you exhale.

SAGE SIFU SAYS

Don't fall into an "all or nothing" trap of self-sabotage. For example, if you have a knee problem that prevents you from rotating your knees the way the instructor does, or if you have asthma that restricts your breathing, that's perfectly fine and natural. Do what you can in a way that feels good to you. Also, just because T'ai Chi and QiGong often help people lessen their reliance on pain or asthma medications doesn't mean you *must* give up your medication. Over time, T'ai Chi and QiGong may reduce your reliance on the very medications that help you feel comfortable enough to move and breathe through T'ai Chi. Talk to your doctor.

Always keep the knees bent in T'ai Chi and QiGong. The depth of that bend depends on what feels good to you. Someone with knee problems may bend his or her knees only slightly at first, whereas someone more athletic may bend more. Don't let competitiveness cause you to go any deeper than what feels good. You won't win a prize, and you'll enjoy the class less because you are straining too much. The relaxed bend of the knees allows the rest of the body to be more loose and flexible, especially the hips.

When It's Easy, It's Correct

As you become more familiar with your T'ai Chi forms, your body will become more adept at sinking into them, as your vertical axis's postural alignment takes pressure off your body. What you'll find is that when your T'ai Chi forms feel "easy" is when you are doing them correctly. Moving with poor posture and muscular tension makes the movements harder. T'ai Chi's slow biofeedback aspect will reveal to you that "easiness" will, over time, become an *internal tutor* that will improve your T'ai Chi forms much more than any teacher can correct from the outside looking in at you. When your movements feel hard, you'll begin to automatically check into your posture, breathing, and tension levels to help the movement become "easier." See Web Video Support's *Internal Tutor for Vertical Alignment* to help get a sense of what this is about.

T'ai Chi is a mind/body exercise that integrates your mental, emotional, and physical aspects. Therefore, as you learn to move more effortlessly, you will notice that emotionally and mentally you find ways to move through life with less and less effort. This doesn't mean you'll get less done. You'll probably get more done because someone with calm emotions and a relaxed mind is much more creative than someone who is in constant mental or emotional turmoil.

T'AI SCI

Some doctors believe our central nervous system is affected by the rhythms of our breath. Because the central nervous system regulates all other organs, a restriction in a freely moving respiratory system could lead to disease. The goal of T'ai Chi is to foster unrestricted breathing. By doing so, T'ai Chi may improve central nervous system function, which may reduce the incidence of disease.

As you study T'ai Chi, be aware of any patterns you have that make learning T'ai Chi more difficult. You may find that you push yourself very hard, straining at every movement. Or you may discover that you are hypercritical of yourself, or perhaps you sabotage your progress by avoiding practice and skipping classes. All these patterns are probably something you do in all aspects of your life, not just in T'ai Chi. By learning how to "play" T'ai Chi in a process of effortless learning, without strain, self-judgment, or self-sabotage, you will discover a new way to learn T'ai Chi and create a new, more effective way to learn in all your life's endeavors. You will become more successful and self-actualizing by becoming clearer and more self-aware of unconscious patterns that inhibit the realization of your dreams.

T'ai Chi Motions Are Round Motions

In Chinese, the word for "round" is roughly equivalent to the American slang word *cool*. The Chinese felt that roundness was calming and comforting, and T'ai Chi is filled with images of roundness. In practicing T'ai Chi, we often move our hands over imaginary orbs or spheres of energy that, over time, become tangible enough to feel. This practice, although at first a little alien, eventually becomes very soothing. It helps us become attuned to our sensations. It is like practicing "feeling." Practice makes perfect, and this is no exception. Refer to the Web Video Support's *Roundness Is Soothing and POWERFUL* for a visual on this idea of *roundness* as part of the T'ai Chi movements.

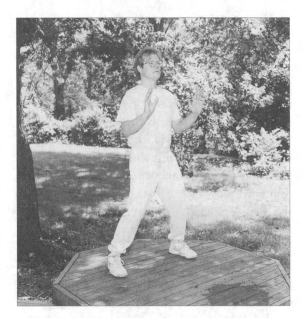

After the hands slide up and over the giant pearl, they descend along the backside until coming to rest in front of your chest, as if you were about to push someone.

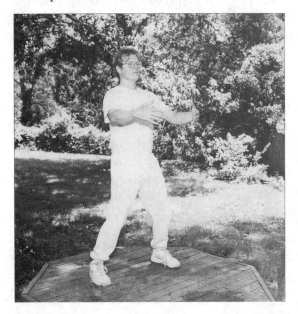

In this Moving QiGong exercise, your hands begin at groin level and circle up as if stroking a huge 3-foot pearl in front of your torso. Move your hands up, over, and down the back of the pearl.

Breath Is the Root of T'ai Chi and QiGong

The essence of T'ai Chi is the breath. While doing T'ai Chi, you inhale or exhale with every movement. There is nothing more effortless in the entire universe than the release of a full breath. Therefore, T'ai Chi's ability to weave exhales with the relaxation of sinking your Qi into your weight shifts creates a powerful habit. This habit of relaxed breathing through everything you do is simple and yet may change the way you live the rest of your life. But again, the reason to do it is because *it feels good*.

Postbirth Breathing

There are many QiGong breathing exercises. In fact, all QiGong exercises are breathing exercises, when you get down to it. However, among all of them there are two main forms of breathing: *postbirth breathing*, which is pretty normal, and *prebirth breathing*, which takes a little more getting used to.

The names of these breathing forms may be based on the fact that we drew breath in through the umbilical cord before birth, and we draw air in through the upper body afterward. This is reflected in the way we draw air into the body during QiGong breathing, depending on which type we are doing.

With postbirth—or normal—breathing, the abdominal muscles expand out a bit as you breathe in to the abdomen; then the chest expands as the tops of the lungs fill. They then relax back in as you exhale, emptying first the chest and then the lower lungs. This is how T'ai Chi and many QiGong exercises are done. However, some QiGong exercises employ prebirth breathing.

OUCH!

Rapid expansion of the chest cavity may not efficiently oxygenate the body. However, QiGong's relaxed abdominal breathing can be highly effective in increasing circulation of blood and Qi.

During postbirth breathing, don't force the breath, but rather allow the body to relax as the breath enters. The following figure illustrates postbirth breathing:

1. Breathe into the lower lungs as the abdomen relaxes slightly outward.

2. Allow the lungs and upper chest to fill as well.

3. As the body relaxes with the exhale of breath, the upper chest deflates first.

4. Then the abdomen relaxes in, completely expelling the air from the lungs.

Repeat this for 10 or 15 minutes if you like, with wonderful results for mind and body. This image is animated in the Web Video Support's *Qigong Breathing Tutorial.*

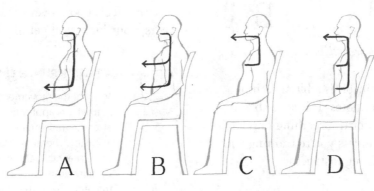

Four-step postbirth breathing.

Prebirth Breathing

Prebirth breathing is just the opposite of postbirth breathing. As you inhale, draw your abdominal muscles in gently, and allow them to relax as you exhale. (Each breathing method has different qualities and is discussed during the moving exercises in Parts 3, 4, and 5.)

In prebirth breathing …

1. Slightly draw in your abdomen, especially your lower abdomen, as you inhale.

2. Then, when you exhale, relax your abdomen back out.

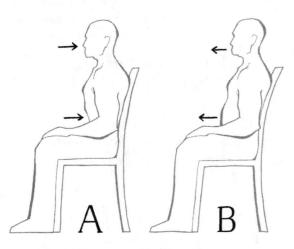

Two-step prebirth breathing.

Prebirth breathing involves a bit of training and some cautionary notes. It is advisable to practice normal postbirth breathing only during your exercises, unless you're training with an experienced QiGong instructor.

A T'AI CHI PUNCH LINE

The Chinese believe that prebirth breathing moves our Qi through the lower dan tien. This energy is associated with cell regeneration and sexual or procreative energy. Therefore, it is believed that prebirth breathing heightens the regenerative ability of our life energy and actually slows the aging process.

Knowing Your Martial Terms for T'ai Chi

Because T'ai Chi was originally a martial art, an introduction to some martial arts terms may be helpful. When you learn T'ai Chi, your instructor may use these or similar terms to describe the T'ai Chi movements.

Understand that any one of these martial arts movements can be done any way that you need to do it for your own comfort. So if you have an injury or condition that limits your movement, do it in a way that feels comfortable to you. Never strain yourself to do something that doesn't feel right; just modify it a bit, kick lower, or reach less. As you play T'ai Chi in a way that feels good, over the days, months, and years, your kicks will get higher and higher.

A T'AI CHI PUNCH LINE

Many of the movements in T'ai Chi have martial arts applications and were patterned after the movements of creatures or images in nature. Therefore, T'ai Chi movements serve practical self-defense purposes and simultaneously are soothing natural motions that encourage the flow of Qi through the body just as Qi flows through all of nature.

Punches

T'ai Chi has punches. They're not hard, grunting punches, but instead soft, relaxing punches. There are generally three types of punches used. Both punches illustrated in the following figures begin with your fist by your hip, with the palm side of the fist turned up toward the sky. The first is a common T'ai Chi punch and begins with the fist at the waist, palm turned in toward the body, with no rotation of the fist as you punch. The other two are slightly more complex and therefore are shown in the following figures. However, then you do a full twist as you send it out to punch in front of you, so the fist ends up with the palm facing down toward the ground.

The second punch is a Half Twist Punch. This begins with the fist near the hip with the palm turned up. When you throw the punch out, the fist rotates only a half turn, leaving the knuckles lined up in a row, top knuckle toward the sky and pinkie knuckle toward the ground.

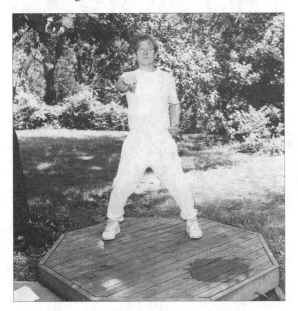

In the Full Fist Turn Punch, the fist ends up palm down.

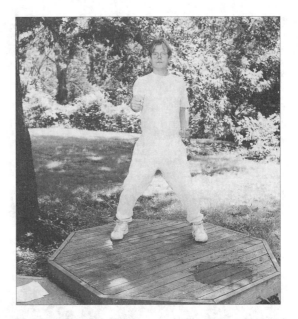

The Half Twist Punch is more common in T'ai Chi, with the knuckles ending up vertical.

Punches are generally not thrown out in big, circular haymaker punches like you've seen in old Westerns (think John Wayne). They come straight out from the hip like a piston, with the elbows tucked in. The elbows *usually* don't extend out from the sides, but stay in near the body.

Because of the many Western movies we've seen, most Westerners also try to punch with the whole upper body, actually leaning into the punch. However, in T'ai Chi and all martial arts, you don't normally lean into the punch. When the punch is complete, your head will still be posturally aligned above your dan tien.

Although there may be exceptions to how punches are thrown in various T'ai Chi forms, usually the rule of not leaning forward is observed. However, there are times when the fist may circle around rather than punch straight out from the hip. Such as in Chapter 13's Movement #46, "Box Opponent's Ears," where you *will* see an example of this rounder punch.

Blocking

There are three types of blocks: In Blocks, Out Blocks, and Up Blocks. Their names explain whether the arm is blocking in toward the center of the body, out away from the center of the body, or up away from the body. One other less-used block is the Down Block, which looks like an Out Block in reverse. An example is seen in Chapter 13's Movement #23, "Wind Blowing Lotus Leaves."

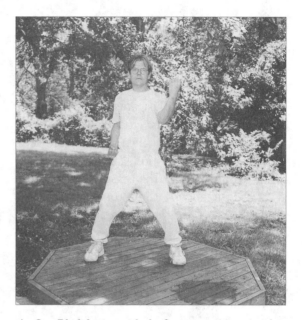

An Out Block begins with the fist near your groin; then your arm is pulled in a circular sweep up across your body to block outward.

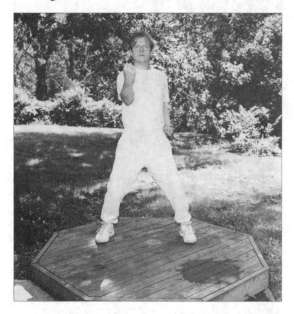

An In Block begins with the fist near your ear; then your arm is pulled in a circular motion across the front of your body.

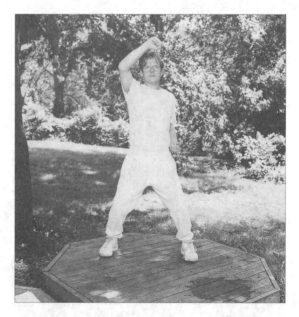

An Up Block begins with the fist palm facing your face; then your palm is twisted away up to the sky, blocking up and away.

Kicks

T'ai Chi generally uses three kicks: Side or Separation Kicks, Crescent Kicks, and Front Kicks. Examples of these kicks can be viewed in Part 4, where the side kick is called "Separation of the Right Foot (and Left Foot)," the Crescent Kick is called "Wave Hand over Water Lily Kick," and the Front Kick is called "Front Kick."

The Least You Need to Know

- Your posture is your power.
- Sinking Qi improves your balance.
- T'ai Chi practice protects your joints.
- Roundness is the image that permeates QiGong and T'ai Chi.
- Proper breathing techniques provide the foundation of your power and health.

Starting Down the QiGong Path to T'ai Chi

In This Part

Part 3 details how QiGong can ease the way for us to fit into a new world evolving around us in these rapidly changing times. Practical exercises for young, old, and everyone in between will help you breathe the breath of life and have some fun doing it.

In this part, you will also learn some QiGong history and see why some QiGong is different from T'ai Chi. Learning QiGong will make your T'ai Chi experience much richer. It is said that medicine cures, but the best medicine prevents. To that end, you'll learn not only about the personal healing powers of QiGong, but also how you can share your Qi, or life energy, with others.

This part also alerts you to some common challenges you may encounter as you begin exploring your inner self with Sitting QiGong. The Sitting QiGong exercise in Chapter 11 will get your Qi overflowing. In fact, it will lead you through an explanation and exercise that may actually change the way you view the universe you live in. Chapter 10 exposes you to the beautiful and wonderful feeling of Moving QiGong exercises, or Dong Gong. There are thousands of them, so in this chapter you will be able to only dip your toe into an ocean of what's out there. The T'ai Chi warm-up exercises in Chapter 11 are QiGong exercises that not only calm the mind, but also prepare the body for T'ai Chi. These exercises alone can have a wonderful impact on your day.

Introducing QiGong

In This Chapter

- Understanding why breathing is so important
- Finding out how QiGong and T'ai Chi differ
- Reading up on the history of QiGong
- Surviving and flourishing through QiGong challenges
- Discovering the healing art of External QiGong
- Web Video Support: *Physical Structure and Breath: The Core of T'ai Chi and QiGong*

The purpose of QiGong is to let go of energy blocks by relaxing the mind, body, and emotions. All the many thousands of QiGong exercises share this goal, including T'ai Chi forms, which most consider to be one of the many forms of QiGong.

QiGong differs from standard meditations but shares many of their healing potentials. QiGong can be used as therapy for specific conditions as well as a general tune-up. Also, we can actually treat another person with the life energy QiGong fills us with.

There are two types of QiGong: active QiGong, or Dong Gong, and passive QiGong, or Jing Gong. Active QiGong involves obvious movement, like T'ai Chi, or other Moving QiGong exercises. With passive QiGong, the external body is still, but the awareness is directed and felt in various areas of the body, by breath, imagery, or both.

We encounter many challenges when beginning QiGong practice. By realizing that these are common, we can begin to move past them and get all the benefits QiGong offers. These challenges to QiGong practice represent challenges we face in all aspects of our lives and personal growth. Therefore, by learning to move through these challenges in QiGong, we begin to untie knots in many other parts of our lives as well.

Let's Do Some Heavy Breathing

Many ancient cultures have recognized the breath as our connection with the life force, or *Qi*. In Chinese, the character for Qi, or life energy, is the same character used for air, as in breath. In Latin, the *spir* of *spir*it or re*spir*ator means "to breathe." Spirit is the *breath of life*, or life energy, which is another word for Qi. So in both the East and West, breath was and is recognized as the key to life's energy. Therefore, if you breathe shallowly, you're cheating yourself out of a lot of life.

KNOW YOUR CHINESE

Literally translated, *Qi* means "air" or "energy," and *gong* means "work." Literally translated, *QiGong* means "breath work" or "energy work."

Many T'ai Chi classes begin with Sitting QiGong exercises that require us to breathe deeply. When we begin, we sometimes might find this difficult because our lungs might have lost capacity from lack of use, or our back and chest muscles are tight with tension. This will change; as your rigid muscles relax, you will soon discover your lungs finding new capacity. The Web Video Support's *Physical Structure and Breath: The Core of T'ai Chi and QiGong* gives visual insight on full abdominal breathing and shows you how to begin to *loosen up* your chest, back, and torso muscles to facilitate breathing. You'll find that Moving QiGong enhances and supports Sitting QiGong, and vice versa, and all will support your coming T'ai Chi experience.

Sometimes we're just embarrassed to let other people hear us breathe. Maybe it's because we think of hearing deep breathing only during sex or other intense feelings, and we're taught not to show our feelings in public. After a few classes, most people get more comfortable with each other and get comfortable with the idea of breathing. Then the tentative group transforms into *a wild adventurous bunch of breathing bohemians!*

If you forget everything about QiGong except to remember to breathe deeply when you're under stress, you will find great benefit. Of course, that's only the beginning—the key to the door of what T'ai Chi has to offer–so don't stop there.

A T'AI CHI PUNCH LINE

A corporate executive arriving promptly for a QiGong class informed the instructor, "My doctor said QiGong would be good for my heart condition, so I want to learn QiGong. But I heard about all that weird breathing you do. I want you to know, I am not into the breathing thing." The instructor responded, "We'd better hurry and get you into it before it's too late, because I don't do CPR."

QiGong first teaches us to feel good about ourselves and to follow what our bodies want and need, like breathing deeply, *even in public*. In fact, QiGong practitioners get to where they can even yawn in public. I know that may seem pretty risqué now, but after learning QiGong, even you will be able to yawn unashamedly in public. And this ability will reflect an even deeper ability to believe in yourself enough to do what your body tells you it needs, whether it's more rest, better foods, regular gentle exercise, or a good, solid yawn, even in the middle of a department meeting.

T'ai Chi vs. QiGong: What's the Difference?

T'ai Chi's goal of relaxing the mind and body to encourage the flow of energy through us makes it QiGong. However, not all QiGong is T'ai Chi (because some QiGong is sitting or lying, and all T'ai Chi is moving and standing). The mental strain of trying to figure out whether you are doing T'ai Chi or QiGong will limit your ability to get the benefits, so forget about it. As you practice T'ai Chi and QiGong exercises, the differences will become obvious. *Doing* is the best way of *seeing*. But let's skip ahead just a bit to see some short video examples of T'ai Chi and various Qigong, so you'll have a rough idea, in the Web Video Support's *Seeing QiGong vs. T'ai Chi in Action*.

Above all, don't sweat it. The following chapters will show you clearly what the difference is, and after Parts 3 and 4, you'll be an expert on the tenets of both T'ai Chi and QiGong. Remember, much of T'ai Chi and QiGong are interchangeable and synonymous anyway. As stated before, the premise of all Traditional Chinese Medicine (TCM), of which T'ai Chi and QiGong are integral parts, is that energy flows through the body, and when that energy flow gets blocked, we are likely to get sick. So QiGong's goal to allow the mind and body to release the past and fears of the future to live a more flowing, healthful life is also the goal of T'ai Chi.

QiGong is a form of meditation; however, it can be more as well. QiGong can actively be used to treat a specific organ or an area of pain and discomfort by directing Qi to that area.

Like other meditations, such as zazen or transcending meditative techniques, QiGong enables the mind to empty of active thought and be passively aware. In zazen, this state of mind is achieved by not thinking about anything, but just letting thoughts drift through the mind without fixing or holding on to them. In transcending meditative techniques, a *mantra* (a verbal utterance used in meditation) or perhaps a *mandala* (a visual meditation tool) is used to take the mind out of the problem-solving mode and into a state of free flow, whereby it "observes" rather than "thinks about" things that flow through the mind.

QiGong combines this passive awareness, or "letting go," with an active healing intention. If we're treating a headache, for example, once we think about the energy filling the muscles in our heads, we have to let that thought go and then just experience how nice it feels as Qi's healing energy, or light, relaxes the head. We observe the healing release in the tight muscles, and in a way, the passive observation of our own healing becomes a mantra or mandala.

A T'AI CHI PUNCH LINE

The ultimate source of Chinese medical knowledge is The Yellow Emperor's *Classic of Internal Medicine* (200 B.C.E.), which prescribed QiGong for curing and preventing illness. According to this ancient book, true medicine cured diseases *before* they developed. T'ai Chi and QiGong can be very effective at doing just that.

A Brief History of QiGong

QiGong is believed to be more than 2,000 years old. Its roots are with ancient Chinese farmers who observed that nature's balance makes things strong. Moderation, flexibility, and constant nurturing filled crops with the life force, or Qi. These ancient observers developed exercises that mimicked that healthful way of cultivating life energy.

Ancient Science Is the Future

What many Western hospitals are now considering as cutting-edge treatments for cancer, for example, can be found in the 800-year-old *Taoist Canon*. At the Simonton Cancer Center, mental imagery exercises are successfully used to help cancer sufferers live nearly twice as long as their peers who don't use imagery techniques. The Taoist Canon wrote of thousands of visualization techniques meant to heal various conditions.

KNOW YOUR CHINESE

The *Taoist Canon* (1145 C.E.) held all the early writing on QiGong, although at that time it was known as *Tao-yin*. (*QiGong* is a fairly modern term.) Taoist philosophy emphasizes being attuned to the invisible laws of nature. QiGong, or Tao-yin, was viewed as a way to connect with that deeper part of ourselves that knows what's best for us.

Is Your Mind Half Full or Half Empty?

Here in the West, we have no trouble understanding and accepting that our mind can make us sick. We know that worry can cause an ulcer or that chronic anxiety can lead to skin rashes or even a heart attack. However, we have a big problem accepting just the opposite: that our mind can also heal us.

So the world has come full circle, and what was ancient treatment in China is now the cutting edge of modern healing in the West. *Welcome back to the future.*

KNOW YOUR CHINESE

QiGong has had other names in the past, such as *tu gu na xin,* "expelling the old energy, absorbing the new," and *tao-yin,* "leading and guiding the energy." Actually, the term *QiGong* is a fairly recent way of saying "energy exercise." Refer to Ken Cohen's brilliant book *The Way of QiGong* for rich explanations of Chinese medical terminology.

It's an "Is the glass half full or half empty?" kind of thing. We know our stress can cause our shoulders to tighten and our breath to get shallow and constricted, leading to hypertension and maybe a headache. But the concept of using our minds to heal us is often thought of as a weird idea. Ponder this: we all know that recalling an argument we had a week ago or even a month ago can cause our muscles to tighten, our breathing to become shallow, and our blood pressure to skyrocket. *Now, that is strange!*

So if something as abstract as a week-old memory can wreak havoc on our health, it makes perfect sense that the mind can have a healing effect on itself today. Unlocking its grip on worry and tension, the mind can allow each cell to bathe in the radiant glow of health.

Bored? It's QiGong Time!

If you're wondering when to do QiGong, the short answer is, anytime you need it. In fact, as you practice energy work more and more, you'll find that, in a way, you *always do it*. As you open more to the feeling of energy flowing rather than being squeezed off by stress, you will automatically sit back and breathe yourself open each time stress begins to close off your flow of Qi.

I always remind students that after learning QiGong, they need never again be bored. Any time you catch yourself getting anxious in a line or in a waiting room, you now can just mentally kick back and practice these wonderful exercises instead of stressing out.

Although you can practice QiGong with great results at any time of the day, TCM has found that the energy flowing through your body is different at different times of the day. Just as Chapter 5 explained how T'ai Chi can be performed at different times of the day for different effects, so can QiGong exercises. (Refer to Chapter 5 to see the times and related organ systems.)

T'AI SCI

Western medical research has discovered that the immune system follows certain rhythms and is weakest at about 1 A.M. and strongest at about 7 A.M. This may partially explain why when you are sick, your cold or flu symptoms keep you from sleeping at night, and then suddenly in the morning you are ready to sleep well. Ancient Chinese doctors were not only aware of this general pattern, but also began to distinguish similar cycles in specific organs.

Mental Healing and QiGong Challenges

QiGong helps heal us mentally, emotionally, and physically, but the beginning of healing entails *becoming more aware*. This can present challenges for the novice because when we become more aware of our mental, emotional, and physical discomforts, we often think this means T'ai Chi and/or QiGong doesn't work. Many of us think a mind/body exercise such as T'ai Chi means "instant and permanent nirvana," and when we discover that we have to feel discomfort such as tension before we know to let it go, we may mistakenly think the tools don't work.

Remember, this new self-awareness is part of a healing process, and you will get enormous benefits from your practice if you stick with it. Over time, you will find those little tight spots you tried to avoid feeling so you could pretend they weren't there will become little "pleasure nuggets" you will enjoy discovering in yourself. Nothing feels as exquisite as discovering a tight spot that hasn't seen much action in a while, getting the deep tissue massage your relaxed T'ai Chi or QiGong movements will become.

Bliss vs. Discomfort

T'ai Chi, QiGong, and other mind/body fitness exercises are sometimes mistakenly seen as "escapist," whereby we can use them to run away from our problems. Although T'ai Chi and QiGong can sometimes seem like a soothing vacation from our problems, they also help us heal or release the source of those problems.

These mindfulness tools can take us right into the heart of our reality. First they enable us to become more aware so that we might be relaxed and clear enough to effectively change a behavior or situation for the better. By being relaxed and clear we are less likely to be depressed about dysfunctional aspects of ourselves or our society, and more likely to jump in and be part of the solution. Many of my T'ai Chi students are surprised to discover that I have been an environmental and human rights activist over much of the three decades of my T'ai Chi journey. They thought my practice was about transcending the macrocosmic societal issues of life. I explain that the tools have helped me breathe through my fear and trepidation, so that I am a calmer, clearer human being, filled with life energy, feeling more empowered and capable of taking on and untangling those big societal issues rather than being stressed out by them.

A more personal microcosmic example can be seen when doing Sitting QiGong exercises or meditations, where you may feel your shoulders getting very tense. Remember, the exercise is not making you tense. The exercise of sitting mindfulness is helping you become aware of a pattern or habit you have of holding tension in your shoulders. Now that you're aware of it, you can practice the release and relaxation systems presented in Chapter 9 to begin to let that pattern go.

As you practice T'ai Chi and/or QiGong, you may experience tension or even anxiety. Don't let that stop you or make you think you're doing it wrong. The emergence of these feelings is an opportunity to begin releasing them, using your new tools of breath and life energy. Where you feel discomfort or angst within, as you release your deep full breath, think of allowing the light or energy to expand within that restricted area, and then enjoy the sensation as it begins to *lighten up*. Over time, your practice will "smooth out" those tension blocks, and you'll experience the sense of soothing flow as the T'ai Chi players obviously are enjoying

in the Web Video Support's *T'ai Chi Slows and Calms.*

Trying Too Hard to See the Light?

If your QiGong exercises make you feel intensely anxious or tense, it's usually because you are trying too hard to make the tools work. Ironically, the harder we *try* to relax, let go, and *make* light or life energy flow through us, the more we squeeze it off. This isn't just about doing QiGong better, because most of us in the modern world have this tendency of trying way too hard and making life a pressure cooker; you will begin to lighten and release from all aspects of your life as you learn to let QiGong become more effortless.

Life energy flows and expands effortlessly through us when we let the mind and body let go. In fact, Qi, the tingly life energy, is limitless and waiting to radiate through our relaxed being, anytime we're ready to let go of our grip on life. We *are* light/energy. It expands through us, and expands us, when we stop trying, like kids trying to float on our backs at the swimming pool, who find that only by surrendering themselves can they be lifted, lightened, and floated. This is what QiGong teaches us to do. Furthermore, QiGong practice will teach you how to let your conscious mind work with the effortless power of life energy. This will take practice. You'll catch yourself trying too hard to feel life energy or trying too hard to make muscles relax. Always remember that the Qi, or life energy, is completely effortless, and is expanding throughout our being all the time. It's only our tension that is squeezing it off. You don't *make* Qi, you *let* Qi. Your awareness of discomfort will direct your Qi to tense shoulder muscles, but once that thought is directed, you can and must let your mind relax, letting go of the outcome. Let the light or energy do its loosening expanding work, effortlessly, just by breathing and being willing to *let go.* Enjoy this Web Video Support's *Becoming Effortless, Lightened … Lighted,* offering a short preview of next chapter's Sitting Qigong experience.

Allow Healing Qi to Flow Through You

That's right, you are a healer, *master.* After practicing the Sitting QiGong exercise in Chapter 9, you will feel the Qi flowing out of your hands. Medical studies have shown that this energy can help people heal. Many nursing schools in the United States now teach a form of External QiGong (Wai Qi Zhi Liao) called Therapeutic Touch (TT) and are finding great success with everything from anxiety reduction to facilitating healing. If someone you know has a headache, you can usually get some results even if you're a novice. Whether you completely heal the headache or not, the sufferer will likely get some relief, or at the very least, his headache won't last as long as it normally would. View Web Video Support's *Lighting Your Hands* to get a preview of the External QiGong exercise you'll experience in-depth in the next chapter.

KNOW YOUR CHINESE

Wai Qi Zhi Liao is the term for External QiGong. Modern Therapeutic Touch (TT) used in many Western hospitals is a form of External QiGong.

In the following figures, you will see one form of an External QiGong exercise you can begin practicing today. After completing steps 1, 2, and 3 and before proceeding to step 4, ask the recipient to describe to you how she feels. Your experience with these tools is the best teacher of what they offer you and others.

1. As you let your Qi flow through your hands into the receiver's heart, slowly bring your hands over her shoulder and down, keeping her arm between your hands so your Qi can flow into her arm.

2. Bring your hands back up to her heart, and repeat three times.

3. Shake off your hands between each brush down to let go of any stress or heavy energy you might have brushed off on the receiver.

4. Repeat this entire process after moving to the other side so the recipient's left and right side are both brushed down.

Many other healing exercises exist for various purposes. These are general cleansing treatments that will benefit anybody. However, the recipients have to feel comfortable with the process, because if they feel tense, it won't work as well. Many nurses simply place their hands on patients to comfort them and then let their energy flow into the patients without their conscious awareness of it. This enables the patients to relax.

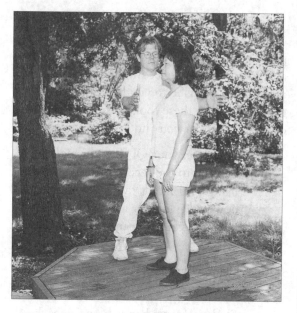

The giver of energy stands to one side of the receiver, with his hands extended over the recipient's heart.

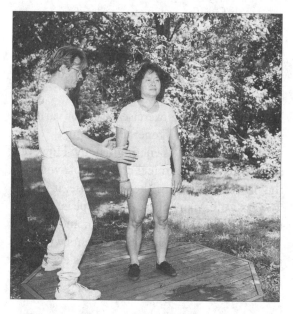

Then he slowly brings his hands over the recipient's shoulder and down her arm to allow the giver's Qi to flow from his hands into the recipient's arm.

Try to do much more of your own Sitting QiGong (Chapter 9) for *self-healing* than you do working with others. Encourage others to learn their own QiGong practice rather than depending on you for relief.

The Least You Need to Know

- If you breathe, the rest is easy—*all of it*.
- T'ai Chi is one form of QiGong, but there are thousands of QiGong exercises that are not T'ai Chi.
- QiGong is an ancient/modern healing art.
- Discomfort is information, not an enemy. Rooting out blocked areas and feeling *dis-ease* helps avoid future disease.
- You are a healer and a master, and understanding this involves letting go of self-imposed limitation.

Sitting QiGong (Jing Gong or Nei Gong)

In This Chapter

- Seeing and feeling Qi
- Remembering that we are made of energy
- Experiencing how Sitting QiGong lights you up
- Web Video Support: *QiGong Facilitates Our Energy Flow*

If you are a T'ai Chi or QiGong teacher, and you haven't enjoyed and incorporated Sitting QiGong meditation into your own practice and your teaching, you are missing out on a huge opportunity to deepen your Qi awareness.

This chapter will enable you to experience a profound Sitting QiGong experience that will give you a good start into dramatically expanding the depth and breadth of your T'ai Chi and QiGong journey or teaching. Your T'ai Chi or QiGong moving forms will deepen to an entirely new level as Sitting QiGong is used to prep you or your students for the moving forms. Someone in the UK emailed me after using my T'ai Chi DVD for about a year. He'd gone directly to the Moving QiGong and T'ai Chi instruction, skipping over the Sitting QiGong for a year. Then one day he decided to try the Sitting QiGong and was stunned by how much deeper his Moving QiGong and T'ai Chi experience was after using the Sitting QiGong technique.

It can help make your T'ai Chi forms a deep QiGong experience. I've included for this chapter a short exhibition of the Long Form of T'ai Chi I teach in Chapter 13, with "breathing techniques" so you can ultimately learn to make your T'ai Chi experience a deeply relaxing internal one that incorporates QiGong's Postbirth Breathing into each form. See *T'ai Chi with QiGong Breathing* in the Web Video Support, www.idiotsguides.com/taichi.

At its core, Sitting QiGong is about tuning into our vibratory rate. As you know by now, we are made of energy. Our thoughts, emotions, and feelings are varying vibratory rates of this energy field that we are, but it may in a way be creating our external reality as well.

An acclaimed book titled *The Hidden Messages in Water* was written by Dr. Masuru Emoto, a Japanese researcher, who discovered that people's thoughts affected the water he was studying. When two exactly alike bottles of water were placed on two different tables, one with a group of people directing hateful thoughts at it, and the other bottle on a table surrounded by people thinking loving thoughts, the water looked much different in analysis. The researcher was photographing the water just as it reached the freezing point and was forming crystals. The "hateful-thought-programmed" water crystals looked like vomit, while the "loving-thought" water had formed beautiful crystalline shapes.

If the vibratory rate of thoughts physically changed the water, and we are made mostly of water, what impact does our thoughts, or in other words the energy vibratory rate of our consciousness, have on our bodies? Conversely, as you enjoy this Sitting QiGong exercise and are immersed in acceptance, safety, and nurturing, then consider how this affects your vibratory rate, and in the end, your cells and body. By using techniques like this again and again, day after day, we re-program our energy field's vibratory rate in a positive way, and this energy field that we are is the most basic part of our existence. Our physical body is built upon the template of that field's state of being, which is influenced by our state of mind.

Once I became extremely ill after a botched dental procedure, and I thought I might not survive. A healthcare professional validated my years of T'ai Chi practice, when she said, "You must have been super healthy to have survived this; most people wouldn't have." During that life challenge Dr. Effie Chow, a great QiGong master from California who'd served on the President's Council for Complementary Medicine in the early 1990s came to my aid,

and reminded me that I *must* let my mind see myself as getting well. She worked with me to shift my consciousness through counseling and QiGong practices. This close call was one of the most powerful QiGong lessons I ever learned. But this programming of the physical with the mind can affect the world beyond our bodies as well.

In Chapter 21 I'll detail our ability to use T'ai Chi to change the world on a practical level, but it's worth mentioning here, because over the 15 years since this book's first edition came out, science has discovered some amazing facts about our connection and ability to affect the world *around us* as well.

Scientific research has revealed that subatomic particles thousands of miles away from one another can affect one another, and that our human energy field extends far beyond the body, and in fact that human consciousness actually *affects* the physical world around us. The Global Consciousness Project's research (that evolved out of original research at Princeton University) has proven this.

So if Dr. Emoto's research proves that our energy vibratory rate can impact things outside our physical body, and other research has proven that the world is physically influenced by our vibratory rate of consciousness, then our energy's condition, when multiplied by 7 billion people, is actually forming the world we see around us in many ways. Mind blowing, isn't it?

But for the purposes of this chapter, let's focus on our *internal* energy field. We can measure the Qi flowing through our bodies in many ways. A common way to see energy flow is through Kirlian photography. This chapter provides some examples of how Kirlian photography captures images of our energy.

QiGong practice isn't about pretending to be energy; it's about feeling what we really are, which is energy. Actually, the entire universe is energy. This chapter ends with an exercise of Sitting QiGong, which will enable you to actually feel the nature of your energy and how life energy, or Qi, feels as it flows through your body. You'll love it!

Energy Medicine and QiGong

Previous chapters explained how Traditional Chinese Medicine (TCM) works by unblocking or directing the energy flowing through the body. QiGong and T'ai Chi also work to balance and unblock that energy. See Web Video *QiGong Facilitates Our Energy Flow*.

However, QiGong is also about realizing that the body isn't a solid entity but, instead, an open, moving wave of energy. QiGong will actually help you realize your energy nature by providing quiet sitting exercises that enable you to feel it. Over time, you'll begin to feel your energy aspect in your T'ai Chi practice as well. Some of the instructional figures in Chapter 13 include notes on energy flow during T'ai Chi, and when you view those *figures/instructional notes* while watching the Web Video Support's *Exhibition of the T'ai Chi Long Form*, you can get a feeling of the T'ai Chi player's loosening flow of Qi as he or she enjoys the T'ai Chi forms, which Sitting QiGong helps prepare you for *internally*.

The Sitting QiGong exercise presented at the end of this chapter enables you to feel the Qi or energy that moves through your body. Before I get to that, however, I'd like to show you how the process works. Then, when you do the exercise, you can let your brain—and skepticism—relax and get out of the way. The energy flows more easily when you are *effortless*. So don't worry about memorizing any of these facts. Rather, sit back and be entertained by the fascinating insights into who you really are.

OUCH!

Some studies identify cynicism as our greatest health risk. Being constantly suspicious of the world around you triggers unhealthful stress responses. Keep an open mind and relaxed body as you learn about your energetic nature.

Kirlian Photography: Seeing Qi Is Believing

There is actually a way to take photographs of the energy aspect of our bodies. (You may have heard this energy referred to as *aura*.) Kirlian photography has been around since the 1950s, but it received a lot more attention as we in the West learned about Qi and QiGong because it seems to be able to take pictures of Qi, or at least aspects of Qi.

When a Kirlian photograph is taken, the person, or leaf, or any living thing rests on a photographic plate, and a mild electrical current is run through it. Then the camera takes an image of the energy or Qi of the plant or person.

The Science of Qi

In China, modern scientific studies over the last three decades have detected that what has been called Qi includes a mixture of electromagnetic field, infrared light, ultraviolet light, and even traces of visible light. However, Kirlian photographic research is what significantly sparked interest in identifying Qi as a scientific reality.

When Kirlian photography was first introduced, skeptics argued that the photography captured nothing more than the electricity running through the plant or person's hand or whatever was photographed. However, this all changed with the discovery of the "phantom effect." The following figure illustrates the phantom effect, seen on a leaf.

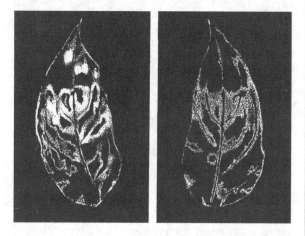

This illustration represents the "phantom effect" as it appears in a common Kirlian photograph of a leaf.

In these front and back images you see a leaf, but what's amazing is that the top part of the leaf you see in the figure *isn't really there!* The top quarter of the leaf was torn off before the photo was taken. So what looks like the top part of the leaf is actually the Qi, or energy aspect, of that missing top. You can see where the leaf was torn but still see the veins and edges going up. This discovery changed not only the way people viewed Kirlian photography, *but also the way science looks at what we are made of.*

Having *Smooth Qi* Means Being in the Zone

Eating right, getting enough rest and exercise, and practicing T'ai Chi and QiGong can positively affect your energy flow, whereas behavior shown to be detrimental to health can

negatively affect Qi flow. The following figure illustrates how our behavior affects our Qi, or energy. This is important for understanding the benefits of the Sitting QiGong exercise we will do later.

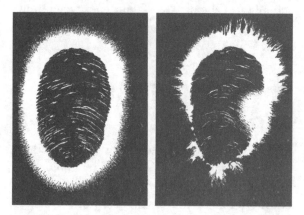

Kirlian photographs illustrate how our behavior affects our Qi, or energy flow, through our body and beyond.

The figure shows a woman's fingertip and the energy flowing through and around it. The image on the left shows this woman's fingertip in a normal state; the Chinese would call that smooth Qi, or a healthful state. However, the image on the right is the same woman after she drank a cup of coffee and smoked her very first cigarette. The energy went wild! In fact, notice that in some places there seems to be no energy.

We all know how smooth Qi feels, as on those days when you wake up and everything just clicks the way it's supposed to. Every paper wad you throw lands right in the center of the trash can. In basketball, it's called being *in the zone.* We all know how it feels when we are there, in the zone, but we might not know how to get there.

T'ai Chi and QiGong offer a way to get into the zone. As we practice our T'ai Chi movements every day, day after day, we find ourselves spending much less time frazzled and wired, like in the second image. And we find ourselves more and more in the calm center of smooth Qi, as depicted in the first image.

T'AI SCI

The Tao of Physics shows how the modern subatomic physicists' view of reality is often very close to the view held by ancient Chinese mystics. By going within themselves in QiGong meditation, these mystics somehow began to understand what modern physicists understand about the energetic nature of reality.

Don't Control Qi, Let Qi Radiate

The following figure is very important in preparing you for the upcoming Sitting QiGong exercise because it illustrates how the mind can direct energy. In this figure, you see two sets of hands; both belong to the same man. In the image on the left, you see his hands in a normal state. However, in the image on the right, you see his hands when he's consciously thinking of *allowing* energy to radiate out from his hands.

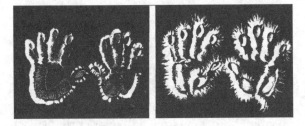

Kirlian photographs illustrate how our energy or Qi flow can be directed by thought.

When the man was thinking of *sending energy* out of his hands, he wasn't grunting and straining. He simply relaxed as he *let it happen.* I mention this before you start the Sitting QiGong to remind you not to "try."

This is an important point because we often think that anything worth doing must be hard.

We want to put our "shoulder to the wheel," our "nose to the grindstone," and "furrow our brow" to get something done. However, the energy work, or QiGong, doesn't work that way. The more you try, the more the muscles tighten up and the less the energy flows through you.

So as the man was sending energy out through his hands, he just thought of it happening and then relaxed and enjoyed the feeling as he let it flow out. You may experience what he felt during the Sitting QiGong exercise, often described as a tingly light feeling.

SAGE SIFU SAYS

Twenty-five years ago, it was nearly impossible for me to sit still for 20 minutes to do Sitting QiGong, because in Sitting QiGong we begin to become conscious of our energy disruption—or tension knots. However, over time, as my energy flowed more smoothly, I found that the pleasure of my renewed energy flow had always been effortless. I had made it hard.

The Sitting QiGong is a very effortless process. When it begins, I'll invoke images, such as a soothing flow of relaxation or light energy pouring over your head and face, relaxing all the muscles. When you read this or hear it on the Web Video Support that follows (you may find it helpful to record the Sitting QiGong in your own voice as well), you will want to imagine the shower of lightness or relaxation pouring over you. But then let go of the image and just enjoy the feeling of effortless relaxation spreading through your head and facial muscles as the lightness spreads through them. Researchers have found that if you think of the image, let go of that mental image, and then let the lightness flow through, you will be more able to feel the pleasure of that flow.

E = MC² Means You Are Only Energy

It's easier to relax and let your Qi flow through you if you know that everything in the universe—*including* you—is only made out of energy. Einstein's famous $E = MC^2$ equation means E (energy) equals M (mass) times C (speed of light) squared. Don't get an algebra attack, though, because all it means is that all things, including you, are made of energy.

Actually, we are mostly just empty space, or energy field. To understand just how spacious we all are, consider the following: if you could take an atom out of anything in the universe, like one of your body's atoms, and blow it up to the size of a football field, the nucleus of that atom would only be the size of a BB in the center of that football field. The electrons that revolve around it would be like dust motes 50 yards away in the end zone. So everything between the BB and the dust mote 50 yards away is energy field, or empty space.

In fact, imagine if you could take all the atoms of *all the human beings on the whole planet* and somehow smush all their atomic particles together, getting rid of the empty space or energy fields we are made of. All the humans on the entire planet's smushed-up atomic particles would add up to just one grain of rice. That is it!

The best image to illustrate that we are mostly open, permeable space is found in something called a "particle chamber." (You might have seen one in your local children's science museum.) A particle chamber is a big glass box filled with ammonia mist. A plaque on the chamber explains that there are cosmic particles falling through space, through the roof of the building, through your skull, your body, your shoes, and right into the earth as you sit here reading this. However, the particles are too small to be seen with your eyes. So the chamber's ammonia mist wraps layers of ammonia around the particles and shines bright flood lights on them, making them big enough to see. When you look inside the particle chamber, you see a blizzard of these particles—the same blizzard that's flowing through us all the time.

I mention all this to set the mood for the Sitting QiGong exercise because it reminds us that we are not a solid, impenetrable mass. We are mostly empty space, and the Qi or life energy can flow through our skulls and brains just as easily as it flows through the air around us.

The only thing that can limit the Qi flow is a thought limitation. So if you invoke an image of a relaxing flow of energy expanding through your head, but then you think, *Hold on there—my head is solid mass,* your muscles will tighten up a bit. This tightening will restrict the flow of energy that flows through you.

QiGong and T'ai Chi don't make energy flow through you. The energy expands and flows through you every moment you are alive. Yet as we age, we often squeeze off the flow of life energy, turning it into a dribble rather than the river of life that flowed through us when we were kids. T'ai Chi and QiGong work by enabling your mind and body to let go of fears, tensions, and grudges that squeeze off your energy flow. This Sitting QiGong exercise is about letting go effortlessly with every breath. The energy flows by itself.

OUCH!

Don't feel as though you have to sit perfectly still while doing the Sitting QiGong exercise. If you need to fidget, roll out your neck or shoulders, scratch an itch, or yawn constantly, let yourself do it. Let your body be as loose and comfortable as possible. However, don't let your mind be distracted by having your eyes open. Close your eyes after reading each point, giving yourself time to experience the effects of each suggestion.

On Sitting QiGong, Jing Gong, or Nei Gong

In this exercise, you will begin to feel your flow of Qi, or life energy. The Qi will be referred to as "light" because the Qi flows right through you, like sunlight seems to soak right into your bones on a nice spring day. Sitting QiGong is also called Nei Gong (pronounced (*nā gong*), which is defined as "allowing the mind to radiate Qi through the meridians, body, and the larger energy field that we are made up of." Jing Gong is another term for it, jing referring to stillness, or spirit.

Remember not to try. You are not *supposed* to see or feel anything. You are just going to have a nice, relaxing experience. So as I offer images, read them and then close your eyes and let yourself feel the result. Qi is waiting to radiate through you, as soon as you begin to lighten up on yourself, which is what this exercise is designed to help you do.

As alluded to earlier, this latest edition of this book includes a new Sitting QiGong video in the Web Video Support (excerpt provided courtesy of *Anthology of QiGong* CD in Appendix C). It will verbally guide you through the following Sitting QiGong exercises, enabling you to sit back with your eyes closed throughout the entire exercise.

SAGE SIFU SAYS

To get better results and enjoy a wonderful experience, complete this exercise from beginning to end all in one sitting. This may take about 20 minutes. To only read this, or only listen to the words of the Web Video Support *Sitting QiGong,* is not enough to understand Sitting QiGong. You must let your mind and body go through the different levels of relaxation to actually "feel" the results. Otherwise, it would be like only reading about water and having never felt water. After reading each instructional byte, sit back and "let" it happen to you, rather than "trying" to "make" it happen.

This exercise is best done sitting upright in a comfortable chair that supports good posture. Your feet should be in solid contact with the floor. Also, if your arms and legs are not crossed, the energy flows easier. When you see spaces between text divided by … (an ellipsis), give yourself a few seconds to assimilate and feel the experience *with your eyes closed* before reading on. The fourth edition's new Web Video Support *Sitting QiGong* video/audio experience enables you to enjoy this experience with your eyes closed.

One last suggestion before you dive in. I used to focus a lot on the idea of energy flowing through my body, and you may experience a sense of this. However, over the years I've realized that this isn't so much about "making" energy do something as it is about us just relaxing out of the way so that this silken effortlessness can expand through us, because, as you now know, when you get down to the little bits we are only made of energy.

Before starting the Web Video's *Sitting QiGong* or this text instruction, I encourage you to review the Web Video Support's *QiGong Breathing Tutorial*. Now, I realize that you've already done the Sitting QiGong video experience in Chapter 1, but you now know a lot more about the energetic nature of your being and effortless nature of T'ai Chi and QiGong, so when you do it this time it will be a new experience.

1. Begin by placing your feet flat on the floor, with your palms flat on your legs. Let your eyes close comfortably and naturally. This exercise is broken into sections, so you can open your eyes to read a section and then close them for a few moments to let yourself experience and feel the responses.

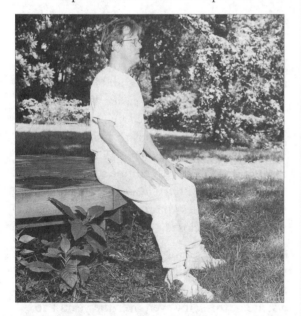

Sit with your feet flat, your palms flat on your thighs, and your back straight but not rigid.

2. All T'ai Chi or QiGong exercises begin by simply becoming aware of the breath. Notice how your lungs fill and empty. Let your chest and back relax so your lungs can fill from the bottom all the way up to the top. Notice how, as you release the breath, your lungs empty from the top, or the chest, and then empty all the way down into the abdomen as the abdominal muscles pull in slightly.

3. Let your mind relax as the muscles in your head, neck, shoulders, chest, and back relax. As the body relaxes, the breaths become not only deeper, but also more effortless. Allow your awareness to relax and ride on the rhythm of that breath, as if the whole body was being breathed by the air. Let the whole body relax as you release each breath.

4. As you feel the body let go of the breath, feel the brain let go of your thoughts and worries of the day. Just as the deep exhales or releasing yawns allow the muscles to let go, the exhaled breath can let go of mental tensions. Likewise, the muscles within and around your heart can hold on to fears or emotions. So as you release each breath, yawn, or sigh, allow the heart to release emotions, the body to release the muscles, and the mind to let go of worries. Each breath is a deep letting go on all levels.

5. Notice that as you let out each breath, it feels as though the atoms of the body are actually expanding away from one another. That's because they are! When we get tense, the body's atoms actually squeeze together, tightening us up. So as we breathe and allow the

body to open, the atoms and cells relax away from one another ... feeling as if the wind could blow right through you.

6. Now think of the sun directly above your head. Just by thinking of an orb of lightness above your head, you may experience a subtle lift or lightening throughout your mind, or your presence. This Qi, light, or subtle energy vibrates at a higher, more silken rate than the body's vibratory rate. Therefore, you may experience a feeling of lightness, or loosening, and a deep letting go throughout your entire being. Good.

7. Let that sun open and release a shower of clear, washing light, or silken energy, to pour over your head and body, and through your feet down into the earth below. Let go of that image and open to the feeling of deep release as you are washed by that silken energy. Like a water hose spraying through a screen door, just let the body open and be washed through, as you release each sighing exhale.

OUCH!

Whenever you notice that your breathing is very shallow or that you are holding your breath, make it a point to breathe deeply. Let the body relax open, allowing air down into the bottom of the abdominal region of the lungs, and let the whole body relax that breath out, as if the breath were breathing you. Do not force—just let.

8. Be aware as a feeling of lightness expands through the tissues of the body. Notice the light spreading through the muscles in the top of your head. As the cranial muscles relax, they release their grip on the skull, allowing that permeating lightness to expand through the scalp. Expanding through the sides and back of the head, the entire scalp is lighted, as light flows out through every follicle and every hair on the head. Feel the scalp relaxing around the root of every hair.

9. Now allow the light to expand into the muscles at the base of the neck, then down and throughout the connected muscles in the shoulders and upper back. As they let go of their grip on the bones, experience the airy lightness permeating between muscles and bones ... a deep letting go.

10. Feel as the energy expands up the back of the head and over the sides, and feel the hinges of the jaw go slack.

11. Now allow this energy to expand over the forehead, over the brow, down the bridge of the nose, and into the temples. Don't try to feel anything or make anything happen; just effortlessly observe as the light expands into the left eye socket ... and then the right. Experience all the tiny optical muscles letting go.

12. Perceive the illumination expanding through all the soft tissues of the face, nose, mouth, and lips.

13. Experience an airy radiance expanding up through the nose into the deepest recesses of the sinus cavity. Feel that opening release as the sinuses fill with light.

14. Now into the ears: feel the deep skeletal muscles in the sides of the head let go as the silken energy expands into the inner ears, allowing a deep letting go in the sides of the head.

15. As the inner ears relax, the Eustachian tubes open, allowing the soothing energy to flow down into the mouth. As the mouth fills with light, the upper palate, upper jaw and gums, and even the teeth seem to lighten, loosen, and let go. And now the lower jaw.

SAGE SIFU SAYS

Don't rush through this. Be sure to close your eyes between each instruction point, allowing yourself to sit back and savor the experience of each image. Don't rush through it. Enjoy. Breathe. Breathe.

16. As you become aware of any saliva gathered in your mouth, swallow it and experience the energy expanding down your throat, through the neck, and into your chest, shoulders, and back.

17. The heart itself can begin to lighten. If you catch yourself trying to feel or make something happen, let all that go. Be willing to feel absolutely nothing as you passively observe the lightness expanding through your heart and chest, permeating all the fibrous tissues of your lungs.

18. This allows every beat of the heart to carry lighted oxygen to all the extremities of the body; in fact, every cell begins to be lighted as the energy moves through the liquid systems of the body. Let the body open to that lightness, even in the tightest places.

19. Allow the light to expand through the abdomen, lighting the stomach ... the liver ... intestinal tract ... kidneys ... and lower back.

20. Now think of the sun above your head again. Think of it opening and releasing an even greater flow of light over and through the body. After you think the thought, let go of it and experience the feeling of expanded release ... as the bones themselves begin to lighten, the deepest skeletal muscles begin to release their grip on the bones.

SAGE SIFU SAYS

The light or Qi heals and lifts without any effort on your part. Let go of those tight head muscles, and enjoy the feeling of release.

21. As the skull becomes permeated with light, the soothing energy expands right into the brain, illuminating the left frontal lobe and then the right frontal lobe, and expanding into the forebrain, above and just behind the eyes, into the midbrain and temporal lobes, and on into the brain stem, or old brain, in back.

22. Experience as all the billions of brain cells open to that silken effortless radiance. It's as if the brain were a muscle we've held clenched very tightly for a long, long time. And now as we allow the light to expand through the brain, we are finally allowing that muscle to let go, to expand open, and to light.

23. Now let the energy expand through the spine to the entire nervous system. Any nervous tension on the frayed nerve endings can now be released into that silken healing lightness now passing through all the nerves to the farthest dendrites in the skin.

24. Experience the light flowing down to the tip of the tailbone and radiating out, filling the pelvic bowl and expanding on down through the legs and feet. Now think of the feet opening to allow this river of cleansing energy to pour right through into the cleansing pull of the earth.

25. Let the whole body open to be washed through as the feet release any loads or heavy tensions down into the earth's cleansing pull.

26. As you allow yourself to be washed through by this radiant cleansing shower, you may become aware of blocks in the flow. Tight spots, tensions, anxiety, feelings of restlessness, or thick drowsiness may appear. Any discomfort you feel is due to a block in the flow of energy. Note where you may feel those blocks or discomforts. Take a deep breath, and as you close your eyes, let the breath out. Think of the light expanding in the center of that tightness or blockage. Experience the opening release.

27. This enables the light to expand in the center of the blockage, allowing that area to open. Release the blockage into the cleansing shower that pours through you to wash away the blockage and release it out through the feet into the earth. Breathe and release yet a bit deeper with every exhale, as if the bones themselves could let go of the load they carry.

28. Sit in this cleansing downpour for a while, enjoying the release. As any thoughts, worries, or tensions surface in your mind or heart, release them into the cleansing shower of washing light. Breathe, release, and enjoy.

29. Now think of the feet closing. Instantly that happens, with no effort. By closing the feet, you may experience a sensation of back-filling energy on the soles of your feet as the light fills the feet and the field around, like a silken cocoon of light, coming up over the feet, ankles, knees, legs, and torso, and spilling over the top of your head to fill the field around you.

> **SAGE SIFU SAYS**
>
> Our thought directs energy, and once directed, it moves there without any effort on our part. Having our eyes closed enables us to experience this within ourselves, to enjoy the cleansing release. This is effortless. The light, or Qi, moves with no effort. After you think the thought, let it go, and sit back and enjoy your responses.

30. With the eyes closed, lift your hands in front of you, as if you were holding a giant beach ball between your palms (see the following figure). Think of the palms and fingers opening, and effortlessly the back-filling energy in your body now flows out through your palms and fingers.

31. Take a few deep-cleansing breaths to release all the muscles in your upper body, even though your hands are raised. It's the letting go that allows the energy to flow through more powerfully.

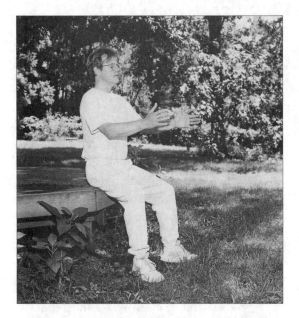

Be sure to let the upper body relax, even though the hands are raised. Slowly move them together and, with eyes closed, open to experience the sensations of Qi in your hands.

32. Slowly begin to move the palms of your hands toward one another, opening them to the experience of the energy you've begun to gather, not only within and around you, but between your palms as well. Move them toward one another until they are almost touching … and experience.

33. Good, now slowly move your hands apart until they are about 3 or 4 feet away from one another, feeling the difference as they move apart. (Repeat moving the hands in and out two more times.)

34. Now gently place your palms back down on your thighs. With each releasing breath, let all that go, relaxing a bit more into your chair with each exhale.

35. As you let go of that experience, reopen yourself to the down-pouring light washing over and through your head

and body. With the feet closed, the body is saturated with light. Allow it to spill over the top of your head, quickly filling the field around you.

36. Soon it will feel as though you are floating within a limitlessly expanding ocean of light. With every exhale, allow yourself to be floating more effortlessly within it. Sit back and enjoy this feeling.

37. In doing so, you can begin to feel any remaining loads or heavy energy squeezed within the muscles or other tissues being magnetically lifted up and out of the body in all directions.

38. You can literally begin to feel burdens being lifted up and off of the shoulders just by breathing and being willing to let go. Any worries and concerns are lifted off the temples or brow, again just by being willing to let go and then observing the release. The deep facial muscles release tensions they've held on to throughout the day.

> **SAGE SIFU SAYS**
>
> After learning and regularly practicing the soothing exercise of Sitting QiGong, you will become very adept at it. So when waiting in line at the supermarket, rather than being bored or anxious, just pretend to be staring at the latest tabloid scandal and open yourself to a soothing flow of life energy as it fills and permeates all the areas where your body is holding on to tension.

39. Now any heaviness or angst around the heart begins to be lifted up and off your chest. As the body continues to release these loads, you become aware of your entire being filling with a limitless, permeable lightness, refreshing and absolutely effortless.

40. This process of release, cleansing, expanding, and enlightening will continue throughout the day. Even when you're not consciously aware of it, the rhythm of breathing and the willingness to let go will enable you to be lifted into the lightness of this ocean of silken energy. Here your stresses and loads can continually be released into the cleansing light, and your cells and surrounding field will be bathed in its effortless healing.

41. Let yourself sit within this ocean of light, assimilating and soaking in the light. Let go. There is no need to hold on to the light, for the more we let go, the more there is.

42. After assimilating the light for a few minutes, very slowly and very gently, when you're ready, open your eyes.

Quite often, the first time you do Sitting QiGong it's quite blissful.

However, if you noticed any discomfort or dis-ease, tension, angst, urgency, etc., during this exercise, you didn't do anything wrong. Whatever you feel is whatever you feel; there is no wrong way to do this. Just don't give up because of encountering any discomfort.

Realize that there is a physical component to all emotions, thoughts, and sensations within us. As you exhale, think of allowing the light to expand within and throughout these physical points of blockage, for beneath this physical sensation or area of discomfort is an energy tangle or knot where we've squeezed onto something mentally or emotionally and unconsciously gripped it in the field of energy that we are. When you think about it, there should be nothing at all stressful or angst producing about sitting in a chair, breathing, for 20 minutes.

So if these issues come up, they are issues you've been gripping for some time, and the space this exercise provides enables this issue to come to the surface of your consciousness—so you can play with the breath and the light to allow those internal tangles to begin to ungrip. I bring this up because as discomforts come up, if and when they do, it is easy to run away from the exercise, thinking erroneously that "Sitting QiGong made me tense or nervous." Again, there is nothing stress or angst producing about sitting in a chair and breathing.

The reason you don't want to just avoid these internal experiences is because trying to stay distracted all the time with TV, etc. seems to help, but it is only putting a band-aid over a cut without cleaning it first. The turmoil that comes up when in meditation is real, and it will stay under the surface until you go deep inside and practice letting go of your grip around it. But don't get all serious about this; look at it like an internal game to play.

How do I know this, you might ask? A growing number of Americans suffer from chronic sleep disorders. These tangles of consciousness we build up in our psyche during the day have no way of being released so long as the mind is occupied. Even watching TV doesn't unload this load because the mind is still busy being stimulated by TV. However, when we lie down and our head hits the pillow, that is the first time during the day when we make space, and so all these collected issues we've been avoiding come swirling in our minds like stranded planes circling above an airport where they've been waiting for a space to land in. By meditating, we create space, and have tools to help the mind, heart, and body ungrip from issues we've unconsciously collected. As you meditate a couple of times per day for a few weeks, you'll notice sleep coming much easier. In fact, you may not even have to wait that long to gain benefit—it could come very quickly—but don't put pressure on it. Let the goals slip off your shoulders and be pleasurably surprised when you look back and remember you used to have sleep problems.

One caution: don't think you have to mentally figure out the solutions to all these circling issues that come up in meditation. Meditation is about letting them come up, sensing where you feel them, how they feel, and then on each releasing breath, thinking of the 50 trillion cells you are exhaling and releasing their grip on whatever your mind starts squeezing onto. Don't expect these things to let go immediately. They may, but don't expect it because that will be a form of hanging on to them. Just exhale and let go, again and again and again. Many of these issues will release in layers, so as you release the breath and allow the silken lightness to expand in the center of where you've squeezed them, let go of outcome and just trust that layer upon layer of these issues are beginning to release.

I think one big thing I got from Sitting QiGong was learning how to "be with" my discomfort and disturbance in this safe place I cultivated by meditating, so these energetic, emotional, physical, and mental knots could have a chance to evaporate. By learning not to judge these internal sensations as "bad" and trying to run away from them by turning away from meditation and toward life's myriad distractions, I was able to learn to play with them, and little by little loosen my grip around them and feel the lightness, centeredness, and flow these tools offer.

As long as you remember to breathe, and let go, everything else will take care of itself. Think of T'ai Chi and Sitting QiGong as a game. Whatever you feel is whatever you feel; there is no right or wrong to this. Just breathe, and let go again, and again, and again, and your tangles will begin to unknot within,

throughout, and all around you as you release them into the *expanding light* that you are, and have always been.

If you stuck with Sitting QiGong long enough, you'd figure all this out on your own. The reason I bring it up here is so that you don't "externalize the blame" for these issues if they come up. They may not come up at all, but after 30 years of teaching, and from my own early experience, I know that it's tempting to blame the issues that come up during Sitting QiGong on the exercise, or the teacher, or on yourself by thinking meditation is not for you and you just can't do it.

You can do it. Lighten up on yourself. You'll get it. Remember T'ai Chi and QiGong are games to play for fun. You play QiGong; you don't work at it. Just like with sports, it's not all easy all the time, and challenges come at you from all angles. But by sticking with this, all aspects of your life will improve, and you'll learn to be much more real and self-accepting, even as you evolve into more and more, deeper and wider.

The Least You Need to Know

- Qi, or life energy, is scientifically observable and measurable.
- QiGong is effortless. It's one of the easiest and most fulfilling things you can do.
- Practice Sitting QiGong every day to supercharge your strength, calm your attitude, and improve your health.
- Use QiGong to program each cell in your body to let go of stress at the earliest indication of blockage.
- QiGong programs your mind and body to radiate health.

Moving QiGong (Dong Gong)

In This Chapter

- Understanding mindful movements and mindless exercise
- Practicing Bone Marrow Cleansing
- Becoming elegant with Mulan Quan
- Learning to make walking a meditation
- Tonifying kidney function with Carry the Moon
- Web Video Support: *Mulan Styles' Montage of Elegance; Tupu Spinning-Stretch*

The Sitting QiGong presented in Chapter 9 is a prerequisite for the simple yet powerful Moving QiGong exercises in this chapter. Remember, "mindfulness" is the act of observing, experiencing, and perhaps enjoying, rather than analyzing the world around us *or within us*. Sitting QiGong's effortless mindfulness of truly experiencing yourself from the inside is a big part of how Moving QiGong works its magic.

In this chapter, you will experience how Moving QiGong can help treat illnesses and organs. QiGong can enhance immune system responses by cleansing the bone marrow of stress.

The following Moving QiGong exercises promote elegance and grace in your movements, while also promoting a calm and peaceful state of mind. The very helpful Web Video Support for this new, fourth edition includes a video exhibition of *Tupu Spinning-Stretch*, an example of Moving QiGong in this chapter.

Mindful Movement vs. Mindless Exercise

Like Sitting QiGong, the goal of Moving QiGong is to let the mind initiate physical, mental, and emotional releases throughout the body. The more we let go, relax, and open, the more easily and healthfully the energy flows through us.

Much exercise is not very thoughtful. We strain and pound our joints and tissue running on pavement or in other high-impact exercises without paying much attention to the toll it can take on the body. Nor do we give much thought to the toll this takes on our mind, as we often listen to loud music or watch the news while scurrying through our exercises. Studies have shown that loud noises and excessive TV watching can actually elevate damaging stress responses. Don't get me wrong, I like TV, so I'm not necessarily urging you to renounce modern life. But taking time to let the world go on a daily basis to let the Qi flow through and untangle you, can make TV much more enjoyable when you do watch it.

Moving QiGong, like T'ai Chi, is different. When you practice these exercises, let yourself take a break from the rat race, the noise, and the endless demands of the day. Practice QiGong in silence, hearing only your breath and the motion of your body. Let your mind be filled with the experience of letting go of *everything*.

Bone Marrow Cleansing

Some Moving QiGong exercises, such as the Bone Marrow Cleansing, have specific purposes. As you go through these gentle motions, the energy is encouraged and allowed to flow through the body, even the bone marrow, to cleanse this tissue of frantic energy. The tissue can function at a higher, clearer level when not burdened by old stress.

I recently got a phone call from someone new to T'ai Chi who'd read this book, and reported that the Bone Marrow Cleansing exercise had been introduced to him as part of his cancer for Leukemia rehabilitation therapy. He'd seen his test numbers improving since he'd begun the exercise, and attributed his success to the Bone Marrow Cleansing. The Australian News reported on a melanoma patient who'd found benefit from practicing QiGong in addition to his vegan, organic, non-GMO (non-genetically modified) dietary changes. In all my T'ai Chi and QiGong classes I now recommend a popular new documentary titled *Forks Over Knives* to my students, which explains how a *whole-foods diet* can further reduce stress on the body. The more stressors we relieve our body from, the more energy we have for immune system and other important tasks inside us. It's simple mathematics.

SAGE SIFU SAYS

Many centuries ago, before modern microscopes, Chinese health professionals understood that blood and bone marrow were associated with the immune system. They studied exercises such as Bone Marrow Cleansing not by viewing another's cells with a microscope, but by practicing the exercise and then observing their own internal health responses.

What follows are the instructions for a Bone Marrow Cleansing QiGong exercise. These instructions are broken into sections. Each section is followed by a photograph that captures a key step in the exercise.

1. Bone Marrow Cleansing begins with the feet about shoulder width apart and the knees slightly bent. Your hands are relaxed at your sides.

2. Bring your hands up in front as if lifting a 1-foot ball to chest level, and then letting the hands come together at the sternum.

3. Lower your hands now back down to your sides and then slowly raise your arms out to the sides.

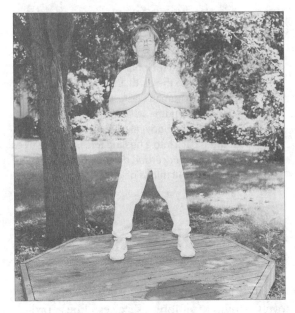

Hands at chest in prayer position.

4. Turn the palms outward. Think of opening the body to absorb the energy of life from the universe. Allow the body and mind to become open and porous.

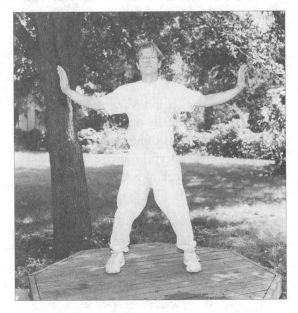

Arms out to sides, palms turned outward to universe.

5. Allow your arms to slowly descend to your sides.

6. One hand now floats up and outward away from the body until eventually it is above your head, with the palm turned down toward the top of your head. Meanwhile, the other hand drifts to settle so the back of your hand is on the small of your back.

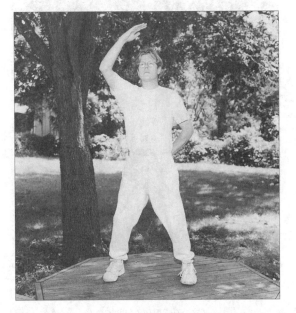

One hand overhead with palm down, and the other hand with back of hand on small of back.

7. As the palm above your head turns palm down, allow the energy to pour over and through the head and body. As the hand descends down in front of the body, the body fills with energy, washing through the bones and bone marrow, cleansing the body of any toxins, which are carried right down into the earth through the feet.

8. Repeat this on the other side, each hand now doing what the other did before. Repeat on both sides three times.

9. Then, with both arms relaxed at your sides, begin lifting both palms up toward the sky.

10. Push your hands up toward the sky above your head, and then turn the palms over to face downward.

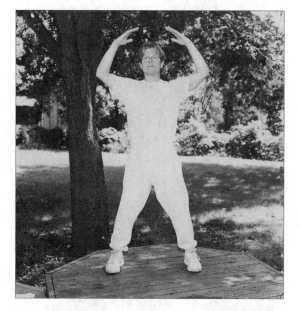

Palms above forehead down, similar to Grand Terminus. See Web Video Support's Grand Terminus excerpt for a wonderful taste of this QiGong breathing and deep stress-cleansing experience.

11. As the palms float down in front of the body, let the energy pour through the bones and other tissues, carrying any impurities or dense energy right out through the feet into the earth.

A T'AI CHI PUNCH LINE

Sometimes in classes, students express their concern for the environmental repercussions of releasing their heavy or toxic energy down into the earth. Look at this like our physical human waste, which becomes fodder or nutrients to the earth. Heavy energy the body releases is transmuted and lifted back into a healing force, just like trees breathe our carbon dioxide to create new oxygen. All things balance.

Mulan Quan Teaches Elegance

Mulan Quan warm-ups incorporate several lovely Moving QiGong exercises. These promote elegance in movement and carriage but have healing effects as well. My teacher told us that elegance, or moving elegantly, isn't about how you look to others, but rather is a state of mind and body that occurs as you nurture a loving and self-accepting relationship with your body, which Mulan is specifically designed to promote. See Web Video Support's *Mulan Styles' Montage of Elegance.*

Spread Wings to Fly

Spread Wings to Fly is a Moving QiGong exercise that specifically helps with upper limb disorders and loosens tightness in the shoulders. This is a wonderful exercise to perform during breaks at work to release job tension.

OUCH!

Although all Moving QiGong is likely an excellent addition to any physical therapy you may be involved in, you should use common sense and not force yourself into positions you are not ready for. Always consult your physician or physical therapist before beginning any new exercise program.

1. Begin with your hands out in front of your chest. Relax your shoulders and breathe naturally, with the tip of the tongue lightly touching the roof of your mouth.

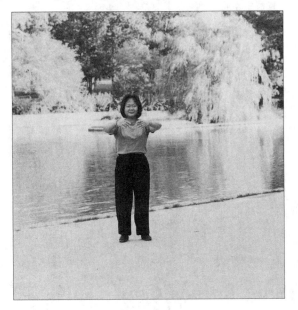

Hands out in front of chest.

2. Begin a long, slow inhalation of breath as you gently pull your arms back around to your sides (as shown in the following figure) until the shoulder blades touch in back, while simultaneously turning your head slowly to the left.

3. Begin exhaling as your arms slowly circle back down and around (rolling out the shoulder sockets) to the start position in front of your chest, while turning your head back to the front.

4. Repeat the entire process, with your head turning to the right this time.

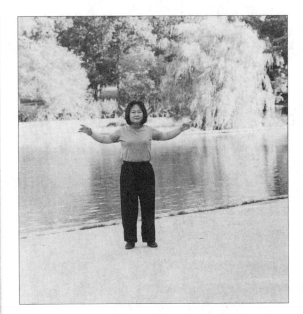

Arms back until shoulder blades touch.

5. Repeat the process, alternately turning your head to the left and then the right until completing eight forms (four with the head turning to the right, and four with the head turning to the left).

Tupu Spinning

Tupu can be therapeutic for movement limitations of the back, buttocks, legs, knees, and ankles. Following are steps for this exercise with more detailed instructions for the Mulan Lesson Example—*Tupu Spinning-Stretch* on the book's Web Video Support.

SAGE SIFU SAYS

If live classes are unavailable to you, detailed DVD lessons are the next best thing.

1. Begin by forming fists held at your waist, with your elbows tucked in and your knees slightly bent. Breathe normally and easily yet fully.

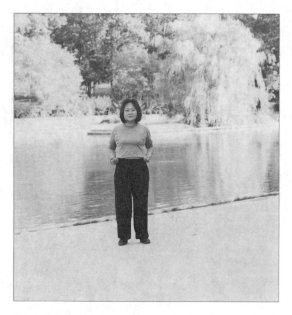

Form fists held at your waist with your elbows tucked in and knees slightly bent.

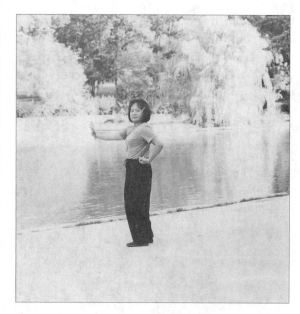

Look left, extend right arm out, left shoulder pulling back.

2. Inhale as you extend the right shoulder forward and as your right hand pushes out in front of your body. Simultaneously, your left shoulder and elbow pull back as you turn your face to look back over your left shoulder. Exhale as you reverse this, pulling your right hand back to square off your shoulders, thereby returning to the start position.

3. Switch, extending your left shoulder out as your left hand pushes, and your right shoulder pulls back as you look back over your right shoulder.

4. Repeat on both sides four times each.

Bring Knee to Chest

This movement not only feels great, it also helps with any pain in the legs and buttocks and is therapy for functional disorders of the leg involving bending and extending.

1. Begin with your hands relaxed at your sides, your knees slightly bent, while breathing easily and naturally.

2. Now begin inhaling as you step forward with your right leg, shifting your weight to the right leg as your arms swing upward and back in great round arcs.

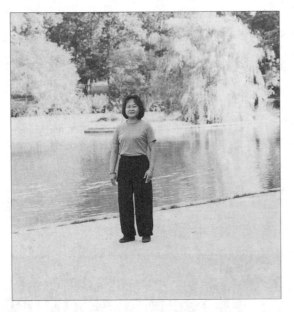

Hands at sides relaxed, knees bent.

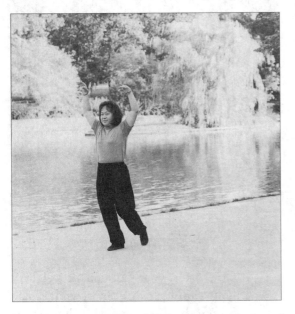

Step forward with your right leg, swing arms backward.

3. As the arms' arcs begin to swing down and toward the front, the left leg begins to lift.

4. Lift your left knee in front, pointing the toes of the left foot down, and wrap your hands around your knee to help it stretch up gently.

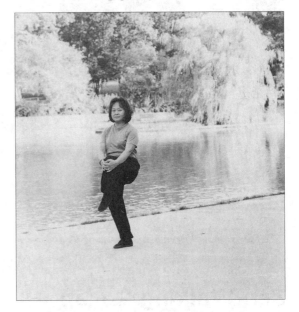

Lift left knee, wrap hands around knee.

5. Now exhale. As the left leg is released, the arms begin to swing down and back.

6. Place your left foot behind you, and shift the weight back onto the left leg as your arms swing from the back over the top toward the front.

7. Allow the right leg to come back even with the left as your hands descend, returning you to the start position.

8. Repeat with the left leg stepping out this time. Repeat the entire process alternating sides (four times on each side).

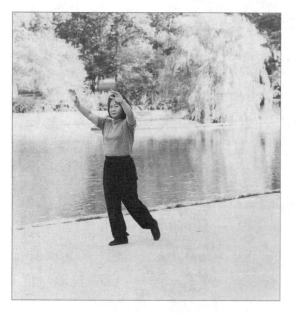

Left leg steps back behind as arms swing up and over.

Zen Walking Recap

Zen meditations involve a mindfulness that simultaneously allows your mind to let go of the worries of the world while attuning yourself to the world in a clear and healing way. Zen walking is a common T'ai Chi exercise. It teaches us how to let our movement fill our minds, while improving our balance and dexterity. Follow these instructions to Zen-walk like the masters, and remember to breathe easily and naturally when Zen walking. Although instructions in Zen or T'ai Chi Walking were given in Chapter 4, here's a recap with a few more details. Revisit the *T'ai Chi Walking* in Web Video Support after reading this.

SAGE SIFU SAYS

Just as Zen walking makes a meditation or relaxation therapy out of simple walking, we can expand this ability throughout our lives. T'ai Chi and QiGong's teaching of mindful awareness of the subtleties of life can help us make anything we do a meditation, whether it's washing dishes or paying bills. In doing so, every moment becomes more healthful, pleasant, and meaningful.

1. Place the heel of one foot outward at a slight angle, while maintaining balance over the back foot.

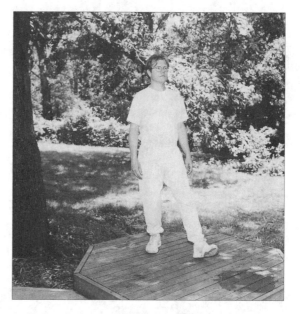

Zen walking is a mindfulness meditation that also improves balance and dexterity.

2. Slowly shift your dan tien, or weight, up toward your front foot, while slowly rolling the foot down onto the ground.

3. The back foot stays flat until your Vertical Axis, or dan tien, is settled over the front foot. Now let your heel lift up, then the foot, and now bring that foot up near your weight-bearing foot before placing it out in front at a slight angle, just like in the beginning.

4. Repeat many times, all the way across your living room or backyard. The goal is to Zen-walk enough that you forget about everything in the world except the soles of your feet, the ground they contact, and the shifting tissue in your body.

Carry the Moon

As discussed in Chapter 2, QiGong can treat specific organs, or systems, in the body. Carry the Moon is great for keeping the spine supple and can also tonify kidney function. It has been said that this may also help reduce premature baldness. This may be because, as with all QiGong and T'ai Chi, it promotes circulation, but in the case of Carry the Moon, especially in the scalp.

OUCH!

Although QiGong may help with premature hair loss, it works best as part of an overall healthful lifestyle. So if you are in a high-pressure job you hate, aren't getting enough sleep, and are smoking too much, the benefits of QiGong will be limited. QiGong practice may help you sleep better, and cut down on or perhaps even eventually help you quit smoking. Therefore, QiGong should be viewed not as a cure-all, but as a stairway to a more healthful lifestyle. Realize that even with a job you hate and not enough sleep, you're still better off doing QiGong than not.

1. Begin by letting your hands and head simply hang loosely over as you bend effortlessly forward. Don't try to strain, as if attempting to touch your toes. Just let yourself hang comfortably, with your hands at about knee level or higher. Breathe naturally and easily, as you enjoy a sense of earth's gravity

pulling the weight of the world out of your hanging upper body.

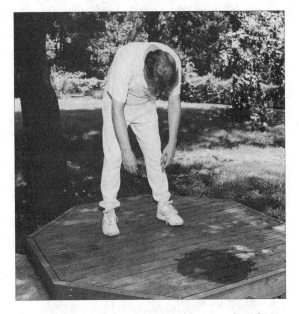

Leaning over with hands hanging down to about knees.

2. Form a circle using the thumbs and forefingers of both hands. As you slowly rise up, the hands ascend above your head.

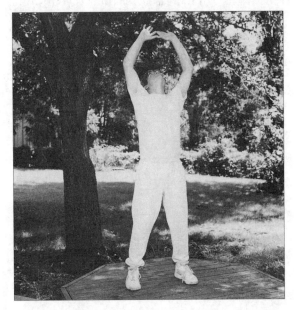

With hands above the head, forming a circle between thumb and forefingers, looking through it.

3. Let the hands go up and slightly back behind as you gently arch your back to look up through the circle your hands form.

4. Hold this position as you breathe effortlessly and naturally for a few moments; then let yourself hang forward again, allowing the earth's magnetic cleansing pull to unload whatever you've been gripping onto. Notice that with each releasing breath, no matter how much you've let go, as you exhale and the lightness expands through your dangling upper body, you'll be able to let go just a little bit deeper and hang just a bit more loosely as the earth draws those loads, surrendering yourself completely into it's pull. Now, begin again, and repeat several times.

QiGong exercises should be repeated as long as they are comfortable, don't push yourself to do it more times than feels good. Your number of repetitions can increase over time as your mind, heart, and body loosen around the movements. Start your journey with short soothing lengths of exercise, and then as your body relaxes into it you'll find you can enjoy longer and longer experiences involving more repetitions.

The Least You Need to Know

- Sitting QiGong prepares you for Moving QiGong.
- Breath and mindfulness are important in QiGong.
- QiGong can improve all organ functions.
- QiGong's circulation promotion may help slow premature hair loss.
- Use QiGong as a launch pad to a healthier you.

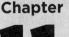
QiGong Warm-Up Exercises

In This Chapter

- Using warm-ups to calm and center
- Loosening the body and the mind
- Healing your joints while perfecting your balance
- Cleansing your tissues and your mind
- Web Video Support: *Shaking Loose the Tension*

T'ai Chi warm-up exercises are meant not only to warm the muscles and other tissues, but also to center the mind. You cannot listen to the radio or watch TV while warming up for T'ai Chi.

Of course, there are exceptions to every rule: when you get to the "Let the Dan Tien Do the Driving"; the "Filling the Sandbags, Sinking the Qi"; and the "Deep-Sinking Your Qi" sections of this chapter, you'll be encouraged to view the related Web Video Support excerpts."

Unlike the way many of us were taught to stretch out our muscles when warming up by using straining stances, T'ai Chi warm-ups start from the very center of our being. We begin by becoming self-aware of that center and then relaxing ourselves from the deep skeletal muscles outward. We prepare ourselves for fluid and effortless movement by allowing our body to relax around our breathing lungs, and then all the muscles relax on top of the moving skeleton.

Each warm-up is a form of QiGong and promotes health and healing on many levels. These warm-ups are a beneficial exercise program even without T'ai Chi, but T'ai Chi offers so much more.

Letting Your Dan Tien Move You

When we start our Sitting QiGong, warm-ups, or T'ai Chi movements, our minds are usually scattered. We are thinking about what we need to do at work, what we need to do to prepare dinner tonight, and so on. So the first task of warm-ups is to center our minds, and the center of our physical being is, as you know, the dan tien. However, the center of our mind and heart is the breath. View *Breathing into Your Center* Web Video Support.

How Breathing Can Center You

There's nothing more calming and centering than hearing and feeling your own breath. Therefore, all T'ai Chi–related exercises begin by simply closing your eyes and feeling the rhythm of your own breathing:

- Let your eyes close easily and naturally as you stand comfortably with your feet fairly close together and knees slightly bent. See Web Video Support's *How to Bend the Knees.*

- Notice how your lungs fill and empty. Think of breathing into the bottom or abdominal part of the lungs and then letting the top or chest area fill.

- As you breathe, allow the muscles in your head and torso to let go. This allows the breaths to become not only deeper, but also more and more effortless, almost as if the breath were beginning to breathe you.

> **SAGE SIFU SAYS**
>
> When doing all T'ai Chi warm-up exercises, let your eyes close so your awareness can relax within. Enjoy the sensations of loosening and breathing. Breathe fully, but don't force yourself. Breathe easily and naturally.

- Let your awareness (or mind) relax, riding on the rhythm of your own breath.

- Now think of breathing down into the dan tien area. You can experience the slight expanse of the upper pelvic and lower abdominal muscles as you breathe in, and notice how those muscles relax in as you release the breath.

- You may experience a feeling of air expanding down into that area. Of course, the lungs don't go down that far, so you are feeling the Qi, or your awareness, expanding through your dan tien area.

Revisit the Web Video Support's *Breathing into Your Center* for a quick video tutorial on abdominal breathing.

Let the Dan Tien Propel Your Movement

The breathing exercises help your awareness expand in the dan tien area, which prepares you to let the dan tien be the movement. This may sound a little odd at first, but after playing the following exercises for a while, it'll be quite natural and will dramatically improve your focus, balance, and movement. The first two T'ai Chi warm-up exercises employing hip rotations help you practice this. See the Web Video Support's *Moving QiGong: Dan Tien Massages the Body* for an exhibition of the first of the following warm-ups and more on *letting the dan tien do the driving.*

> **SAGE SIFU SAYS**
>
> If you are in a wheelchair or have an injury or condition that requires you to sit, let the most inner part of your upper pelvis go into motion and be aware of that motion, allowing the body to relax as much as possible around that motion. If you are paralyzed, let the internal rotation begin in the center of the body at the lowest point your physical awareness begins.

1. With your feet close together, let the dan tien, or hips, begin a counterclockwise rotation, sort of like a hula-hoop motion. If you were looking down at a clock face beneath your feet, you would be going counterclockwise.

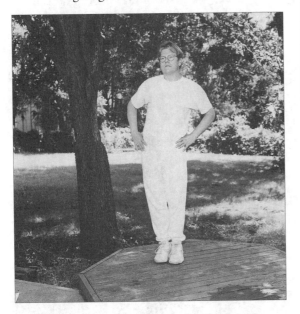

Feet together, rotating hips in hula-hoop fashion.

Notice that the dan tien begins to move effortlessly like a gyroscope in motion, allowing you to let your muscles relax while the dan tien moves the skeleton underneath. The shoulders don't move too much; most of the motion is in the dan tien, or hip area. However, don't be rigid about this. The goal is to get loose.

2. Repeat the counterclockwise hip rotations 32 times, if that feels good to you, and then repeat 32 times in the opposite direction, clockwise.

   Close your eyes as you rotate the dan tien. At first this may challenge your balance, but you'll get better. With your eyes closed, your awareness can

go within. You will notice areas of the body loosening as you rotate and breathe. Think of letting the muscles let go of bones and other tissue, allowing the body to just generally loosen on top of the skeleton. You will notice the lower-back vertebrae loosening as the muscles around them begin to let go. You will also notice this loosening spreading up the back through the lumbar region, up through the dorsal vertebrae between the shoulders, and into the neck and the back of the head. Basically, anywhere you let your light of awareness shine within, your body, mind, or heart can begin to loosen as you breathe effortlessly and move effortlessly in these dan tien rotations.

OUCH!

If your balance is too unstable on the first set of rotations with your feet close together and eyes closed, then open your eyes but soften your focus so your awareness can still go inside. You'll find that when you move to the second exercise of rotations with your feet shoulder-width apart, your balance will be more secure.

3. Now repeat the hip rotations both ways (first counterclockwise and then clockwise), with your feet about shoulder-width apart and knees slightly bent. Relax and enjoy the sensations of movement. With the feet farther apart and eyes closed, you will notice that you can very tangibly feel the top of the femur or hipbone rotating in the hip socket. Slow the rotations, and you will feel the hipbone rotating all the way around the inner rim of the hip socket.

Enjoy the deep-tissue massage the rotating bones give, as the deep hip muscles begin to let go of the tensions built up there. As you breathe and let muscles relax on top of the moving skeleton, you can enjoy this loosening through the back, legs, and the rest of the body.

The enjoyment of this internal loosening helps us almost see inside ourselves. Practicing this pleasant internal vision is a powerful health tool. By becoming aware of how good effortless motion feels inside, we also become aware of tensions or diseases at a very early stage before they actually become diseases.

SAGE SIFU SAYS

We are a very shallow-breathing society. You may catch yourself breathing very shallowly or even holding your breath as you move. Let your lungs fill effortlessly all the way down to the abdominal region and up to the top. Allow the entire body to relax that breath out, as if every cell of the body were letting go at the deepest level with each breath. Each breath lets us practice living effortlessly. There is nothing more effortless than the release of a breath.

Lengthened, Not Stretched

In T'ai Chi warm-ups, we don't strain to stretch out our muscles. We allow ourselves to lengthen until we begin to ease up against strain. The tension we become aware of indicates a block. Then we take a deep breath, and as we exhale, we allow light, or Qi, to fill the area of tension or restriction, which lets the block begin to let go. You can actually feel the lightness or release spread effortlessly through a tight or restraining muscle as you let out the breath. Our mind's awareness of the block directs the Qi, or energy, into the center of

the block as we let the breath relax out of our bodies.

1. With your fingers interlaced, extend your hands up over your head. See Web Video Support's *Moving QiGong: Elongated, Not Stretched*. And do the exercise with this text instruction afterword, because there are details of "letting go" here that go beyond the video.

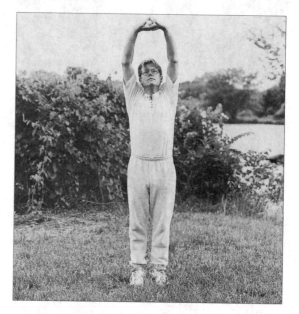

Fingers interlaced, stretching upward.

2. Don't stretch, but allow your body to be effortlessly lengthened, as if the hands were being lifted up toward the sky.

3. As you release each sighing exhale, think of letting the muscles beneath the muscles let go.

4. Enjoy the feeling of effortless release through the back, shoulders, neck, and head, and down into the hips and legs. As you breathe and let go, the entire body gets a bit of a stretch.

5. Now stretch out to either side, but rather than thinking of stretching, think of the hands being drawn out and upward toward the sky, out to the left and then the right. First the hands are drawn outward and up off to the right side of the body, and then easing back upward and over to the left side.

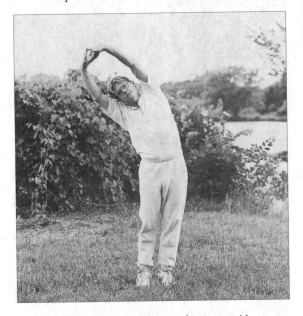

Hands extended, but now stretching over sideways.

6. Go back and forth. Don't stretch so far to the side that you feel a big strain. Rather, go just far enough that you can savor the sensation of the muscles stretching across the back, between the shoulders, and through the neck. Again, as you loosen, the entire body gets a bit of a soothing, effortless stretch.

7. Now lengthen straight up again before stretching out and forward. The back should be fairly straight, bending from the hips and letting the arms just hang down.

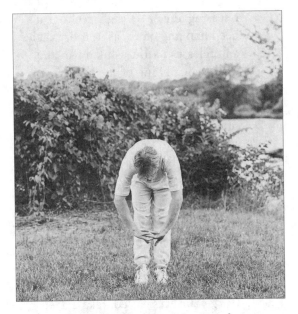

Back bent flat, with hands hanging down.

8. Don't strain to touch your toes. That's not the point. The point is to feel an effortless lengthening through the upper body as you simply let go. As you hang loosely, some of the weight of the world is pulled off and out of you by gravity's gentle cleansing pull. On each exhale, surrender yourself to that unloading. The earth's gravity is like the planet giving you a hug, as with each sighing exhale you surrender yourself into its embrace, allowing it to draw your burdens from you.

9. Enjoy that feeling of effortless elongation through the shoulders, neck, and back of the head. Notice that with each releasing exhale, you can let go even more. With each releasing breath, the muscles in the head can let go even more, showing you that relaxation is not a destination, but an endlessly enriching process of letting go. Think of the heart, just hanging in the chest,

releasing any of the tight feelings it's been hanging on to, as it, too, exhales and releases itself to sink down and out of you. Think of the brain just hanging in the skull, releasing any of the tight thoughts you've unconsciously squeezed in your mind. Feel the scalp actually begin to relax off the skull, as that tingly lightness permeates both skull and scalp.

10. Again, interlace the fingers, and then slowly and gently straighten the lengthened back up to the original position, with hands interlaced high over the head.

11. With your eyes closed, take a deep breath. On the sighing exhale, allow the hands to descend to the sides so slowly that you can feel the air passing between the fingers. As the hands arc down from above the head, out to the sides, and the breath relaxes out, experience the different muscle groups letting go through the head, face, jaw, neck, shoulders, torso, arms, legs—even into the hands and feet. Feel a deep letting go in the field within, throughout, and all around you … releasing *everything*, even down into the earth below.

12. Let each exhale trigger a deeper letting go from the very center of your being, as if the bones themselves could let go. Allow every cell in the body relax those breaths out.

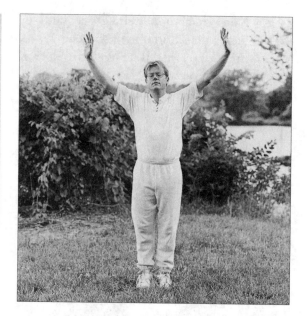

Hands descending to the sides.

13. As you stand with your eyes closed, continue to let go of all the muscles with each breath, and also let go of the heart. Just as the muscles release tensions with each sigh or yawn, the heart can let go of tensions or loads it has squeezed in the heart muscle or muscles around the heart.

14. Think of the brain or mind letting go. Just as the cranial muscles let go of their grip on the skull, the mind can release worries and mental tensions with each releasing breath.

15. Realize that each breath can trigger a deep cleansing on many levels—mental, emotional, and physical. With each exhale, experience a deep letting go. Give yourself a few moments with eyes still closed to marinate in this field of soothing expanding lightness that you are. These exercises don't create this field of lightness, they just help us unload the tension dust, to allow the incredible lightness of being that we are to shine through.

Sinking the Qi Is Like Filling a Sandbag

Settling down into the Horse Stance is sinking your weight down into both feet as if you were sinking down into a saddle on a horse. The tailbone drops as the pelvis tilts slightly up, and the head is drawn upward toward the sky, while the chin is pulled slightly in. This causes the spine to lengthen, which is great for the back, releasing a lot of the pressure daily stress puts on it. Moving from the Horse Stance not only improves posture and balance, but it can also preserve your joints and make you more powerful.

Revisit the Web Video Support's *Sinking into the Horse Stance* for a video supplement of this settling into the Horse Stance instruction.

Moving from the Horse Stance

After you settle in the Horse Stance, let the dan tien flow back and forth from one leg to the other. Picture yourself sitting on an office chair with wheels, rolling from side to side. Or as if you were sitting on the back of a park bench, sliding your bottom from side to side. Notice that the head and shoulder never lead the way, nor do the hips stick out from side to side. The upper body stays stacked above the dan tien as it flows back and forth. View the Web Support Video's *Filling and Emptying* to get a sense of the following, more detailed exercise instructions.

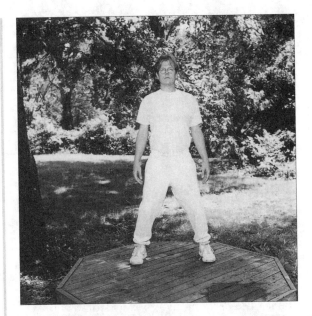

Note that while in Horse Stance, the knees are slightly bent and the upper body is stacked above the dan tien, erect but relaxed and not rigid.

As you become aware of discomfort or tension—the fatigue you may feel in the muscles above the knees, for example—play the following game.

1. Let yourself feel the tension or discomfort, wherever it is in your body.

2. Experience how it feels and where you feel it.

3. Now, as you let the next breath out, think of letting the light, or Qi, expand right in the center of that feeling.

4. Let your awareness sit back and enjoy whatever responses you experience. Often you will experience a lessening of the discomfort or even a pleasure of the expanding lightness.

Sinking the Qi

In T'ai Chi, the upper body does not lean; it stays stacked up above the dan tien, just like in the Horse Stance. The dan tien flowing toward one leg fills that leg with the Qi, or energy (or the weight of your body). Simultaneously, the leg the dan tien moves away from is emptying of Qi, or weight. In T'ai Chi, you rarely ever pivot a leg that has weight on it because it makes your balance precarious. More important, it damages the knees to pivot feet that bear weight. So this Moving from the Dan Tien exercise teaches you to shift your weight from one leg to the other. This simple exercise is the most important T'ai Chi warm-up because this is what T'ai Chi is. All of T'ai Chi's elaborate forms are based on the dan tien moving from one leg to another.

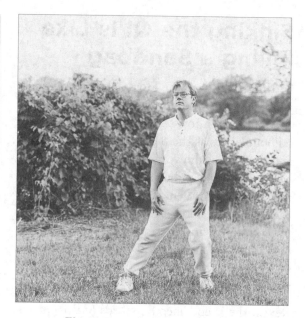

Flowing upper body to the other side.

Deep-Sinking Your Dan Tien

If your mobility permits and you feel adventurous, you can practice a Deep Sinking of the Dan Tien exercise. Also refer to the Web Video Support's *Deeper Filling and Emptying* for a video supplement of the instructions here. Realize that you do not have to do this exercise to get T'ai Chi and QiGong's benefits. This will be too deep for many, so don't feel like you must do this in order to be successful at T'ai Chi or QiGong. However, you may be surprised in a few months or years to find that you can enjoy this because your practice has loosened you and improved your balance so profoundly.

Note that as the dan tien drops deeply down into one leg by bending that knee, the back is not bent over. As always, you don't bend, but you keep the upper body stacked up above the dan tien.

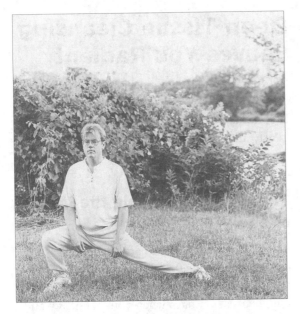

Deep bending of one knee with back straight.

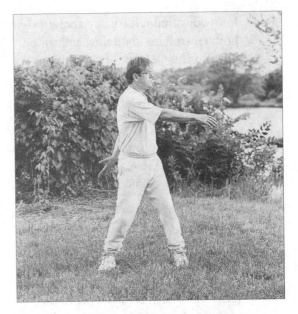

Turning and arm swinging out from body.

The Chinese Drum's Kaleidoscopic Sensations

The Chinese Drum mimics the motion of those little toy drums with the two swinging beads. See Web Video Support's *Chinese Drum Turns.* When the drum is turned from side to side, the beads twist and drum alternately on each side. This is how your relaxed arms and hands will gently strike your body, as you follow these instructions:

1. Stand up with your feet about shoulder-width apart and knees, as always, slightly bent. Gently turn, swinging your arms out. The lead arm swings across the back to strike the flank or lower back, as the trailing arm swings across the front of the body to strike the shoulder.

2. As the hands strike the shoulder and flank in back, close your eyes and enjoy the physical contact. The gentle slapping begins to massage the muscles as you turn back and forth, alternately slapping each flank and shoulder in turn.

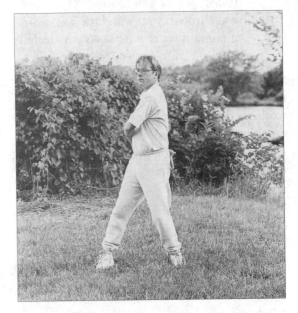

Hands striking body in back and shoulder.

3. Let your mind release any analytical or problem-solving thoughts, and simply open to the pleasure of the motion.

4. With each turn and releasing breath, allow the body to let go even more.

5. Let the mind relax into the pleasure of that letting go, allowing the mind to experience the tens of thousands of sensations throughout the body.

6. With your eyes closed, you can attune yourself to the sensations of the pads of the feet shifting on the floor, the interactions of bones and muscles throughout the body, and the releasing pleasure of each breath. Feel the wind on your skin as you turn through space.

7. Even with your eyes closed, patterns of light and shadow flow across your eyelids, and sounds both internal and external flow over and through you.

8. Don't try to hear, feel, or see. Rather, let your mind relax and allow sensations, images, and sounds to pour over and through your mind the way clear mountain water pours over a waterfall.

Let the mind give up straining to function or reaching out to the world, but rather allow the world to flow to you in a soothing experience of effortlessness. Think of your mind releasing its grip on the dock of logical thought and floating down a river of kaleidoscopic sensation, carried on the beauty of existence, savoring the ability to breathe, flow, and experience sensation … effortlessly.

Deep-Tissue Cleansing Leaves You Radiant

QiGong provides many deep-tissue cleansing exercises, and the following is only one of them. It contains two parts that should be practiced gently and, as always, with awareness of your own mobility range.

Fling Off and Exhale the Weight of the World

Most of the tensions we carry around are energy we've squeezed in our minds, our hearts, and the muscles in the body. You know this is true because on days when you feel heavy and weighted down by the world, if you get on a scale, you don't weigh any more than usual. Therefore, we can simply fling off much of the loads we lug around. See Web Video Support's *Fling Off the Weight of the World*.

1. Begin with your hands above your head and then simply swing them gently outward and downward, flinging off the weight of the world you've held in your body.

2. Think of letting the bone marrow itself exhale and release the loads it's been holding on to, which, of course, it can release.

3. As the hands fling toward the ground, think of the hands and feet opening to release that load to fly out of you into the cleansing earth. As your hands swing out and down, exhale deeply to facilitate the release.

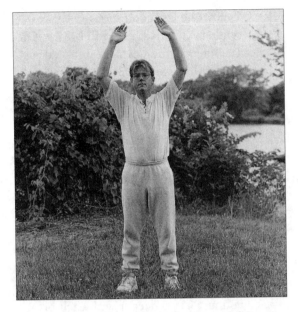

Hands up high, ready to swing out and down.

4. Breathe in as you raise the hands back up over the head, and again release all as you swing the hands out and down again. Repeat several times.

Experience Your Incredible Lightness of Being!

This tissue-cleansing exercise is a fun and soothing jiggling of your entire being that you can practice several times per day to shake the tension dust out of your energetic being. See Web Video Support's *Shaking Loose the Tension* for a visual example of this, and then read through the following text instruction for an even deeper awareness of what you should feel as you do this. A couple of years ago, I caught a news report about a hip new club in New York where people paid a hefty entrance fee to do this very same thing, and they reported that they felt terrific afterward. Enjoy!

1. With your feet about shoulder-width apart, eyes closed, and knees slightly bent, take a deep full breath and then just let your dan tien and skeleton jiggle. Gently let the arms and entire body go liquid and loose. Don't jolt the joints, but allow a liquid wave to ripple through every muscle and joint. It's almost as if the field of energy that you are is vibrating you at the roots of your being, as you just relax out of the way more and more with each releasing breath, as if your entire being could exhale, and let go.

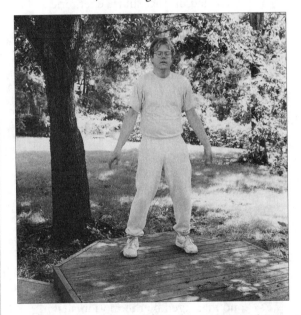

Let yourself go as liquid and limp as you can, with your eyes closed, enjoying a loosening throughout your being.

T'AI SCI

Blood lactates, or lactic acids, accumulate in the deep skeletal muscles during times of anxiety. Studies also show that these acids produce anxiety. Therefore, T'ai Chi and warm-ups like the Elvis Impersonation or Tissue Cleansing allow the body to release these long-held anxieties and to cleanse itself of them.

2. Experience the deep skeletal muscles going liquid on the bones, from the top of the head to the pads of the feet. It's very slight and very subtle, but as those muscles loosen, they begin to cleanse the body of deep toxins. Think of the brain and heart loosening as well, letting worries, angst, and tensions evaporate out of the body with each yawn or sighing exhale. Yawn anytime and every time you feel like it.

3. Even the bones are being shaken and loosened on that subtle energetic level. Think of the bones exhaling and letting go of that bone tiredness they squeeze onto. Feel the tendons, cartilage, and connective tissue all loosening throughout your frame, as all the 50 trillion cells you are made of are gently shaken loose.

4. Notice the rib cage loosening in your torso, and as it exhales you feel it ever more easily jostled inside you.

5. The cranium, cranial muscles, and even the brain are being loosened by this gentle vibration shaking through you. Think of the brain exhaling, and letting go, to be even more loosened and massaged by the motion shaking through your head.

6. Now the spine and spinal fluid, and all the miles and miles of nerves through your body are being shaken out like a dusty sheet in the wind, releasing their static tension loads into the expanding lightness that you are.

7. Enjoy one last good series of shakes while taking in a nice, full breath. On the long, sighing exhale, stop shaking, and with the eyes still closed, just feel the body awakening—the tingly lightness expanding through you—losing that definition of skin, and opening up to this lighter, larger energetic beingness that you are. Notice how every cell expands open with a radiant lightness, clear, clean, and alive. Wherever you notice remaining tension or block, with each releasing breath, think of allowing the light to expand in that area as if the body were expanding endlessly outward. You don't make it happen, you just let go deeper with each breath, releasing any heavy loads to evaporate in that endlessly expanding lightness.

The Least You Need to Know

- The dan tien makes all movement effortless.
- Let warm-ups loosen your entire being and be almost a sensory amusement park.
- Moving from the Horse Stance is the most important warm-up exercise.
- The Chinese Drum cleans your mind and body.
- Doing warm-ups with your eyes closed helps the mind relax within.

Learning a T'ai Chi Long Form

In This Part

Part 4 introduces the Kuang Ping Yang right style's approximately 20-minute long form, augmented by this edition's new Web Video Support, which provides a video exhibition of the entire form, with QiGong breathing, and video-augmenting text and graphic instruction of each individual movement in the long form. Chapter 12 helps you prepare mentally for the physical experience presented in Chapter 13. You will learn how T'ai Chi movements aid certain organs and what T'ai Chi has in common with the ancient Chinese *I Ching*, or *The Book of Changes*. Chapter 13 illustrates the 64 postures of the Kuang Ping Yang style's forms in detailed sketches that help you analyze and study each move individually, as well as see how they flow together. The text accompanying the images further details how movements are performed.

Detailed lessons for a few of the more complicated movements taught in Chapter 13 includes Web Video Support, showing you the very first movement video, overlaid with the instructional illustrations in the book to help you better understand how the illustrated/text instructions in Chapter 13 work. The Web Video gives overviews of several styles. Excerpts from my DVD (Appendix C) bring life to the instructional methods in Chapter 13 in a big way.

Many of these forms can be seen performed in other styles of T'ai Chi as well. So the explanations of the benefits each movement provides and the T'ai Chi principles and insights explained can also benefit those practicing other forms. As you learn and practice T'ai Chi, you will constantly ask yourself one recurring question: *How did I ever get along without this?*

Introducing the Kuang Ping Yang Style

In This Chapter

- Uncovering T'ai Chi's ancient roots
- Learning how T'ai Chi became a philosophy of life
- Absorbing the advantages of the T'ai Chi long form
- Why the Kuang Ping Yang has 64 movements
- How the historical roots of medicine and T'ai Chi intertwine
- Kuang Ping Yang Style is just one of *many* wonderful T'ai Chi styles available

The Kuang Ping Yang style of T'ai Chi has a rich and colorful history, as do all the ancient styles. (See Chapter 1's "Styles of T'ai Chi" for background on the other *wonderful* T'ai Chi styles.) The history of T'ai Chi is a great way to better understand its benefits and why it is so perfect for our modern, harried lives.

This chapter discusses the roots of all T'ai Chi and explains how Kuang Ping Yang and the more extant Yang style became different. You also learn why some styles offer shortened versions and why Chapter 13 offers a long form. Understanding some of T'ai Chi's historical or ancient tenets may actually help you get many more and endlessly richer benefits from its practice. The more your mind believes in your therapy, the more powerfully it heals.

The Origin of T'ai Chi: The Snake and the Crane

According to legend, T'ai Chi was born from an observation of nature. A martial arts master observed how a snake slowly evaded a crane's attack by moving away each time the bird's sharp beak struck. What may have been mortal combat became a gentle exercise that left the exhausted crane flying off for easier prey.

This example of yielding to the brute force of the world has created not only a powerful martial art, but also an extremely healthful philosophy for surviving the stressful onslaught of an accelerating future. If this crane's attacks are compared with today's rapid changes, we may be much smarter to bend, yield, and flow with that change than to dig in our heels and fight it. The snake's yielding was much less stressful than a head-to-head fight with the larger, sharp-beaked crane. See Web Video Support's *Liquid Yielding Nature of T'ai Chi* for a few visual examples of this quality of T'ai Chi (www.idiotsguides.com/taichi).

OUCH!

If the idea of learning a long T'ai Chi form that may take 8 to 12 months to learn is daunting, remember, the journey of a thousand miles begins under one's own feet.

The Shao-Lin Temple: Where It All Began

The Shao-Lin Temple that was featured on the famous television series *Kung Fu* is actually where T'ai Chi began. Around 400 C.E., an 18-movement stretching exercise that eventually grew into T'ai Chi was taught to the monks by a man known as Ta Mo. The purported founder of modern T'ai Chi, however, was a monk named Chang San-feng, who lived about 1000 years later. It was Chang San-feng who is said to have watched the snake yield and avoid the crane's harsh attacks.

From the Temple to the West

The Chen family, founders of the Chen style of T'ai Chi, created one of the earliest family styles. The Chen style was taught to a young martial artist named Yang Lu-chan, who was the founder of today's Yang style.

KNOW YOUR CHINESE

Chinese names begin with the family name. Therefore, Yang Lu-chan, founder of the Yang style, would be called Lu-chan Yang in the West because Yang is his family name.

The Yang family taught a style of T'ai Chi while residing in the city of Kuang Ping. Here, the founding master Yang Lu-chan's eldest son, Yang Pan-hou, was made an offer he couldn't refuse: to teach T'ai Chi at the imperial court and become the emperor's personal teacher. Yang could not refuse the emperor, so he decided to create another version of the family style to teach him, one that was different from the Kuang Ping Yang style. It's worth stating here that *all the various Yang styles* (and other styles) can be powerful health and wellness techniques.

This Kuang Ping Yang style was passed down from Yang Pan-hou to his student Wong Jao-yu, who taught master Kuo Lien Ying. Kuo Lien Ying eventually migrated to the United States and taught this to students, who have since spread this style all across the United States, just as other masters spread the other wonderful styles of T'ai Chi throughout the world.

This can be about as difficult to sort out as the cast of a soap opera, so don't worry about these details. It's just important to remember that the tools you are about to enjoy are the fruits of centuries of study. I include these stories not to confuse, but to acknowledge and to thank these people for making available all that T'ai Chi has to offer in its various forms and styles.

Again, the basic principles are universal to all styles, such as Kuang Ping Style master Henry Look's Seven Important Principles. Master Look was one of Master Kuo's original students, and his Seven Important Principles were: centering; quiet smile; quiet movement;

quiet mind; quiet breathing; coordination; and focus, which can be applied to all styles of T'ai Chi and QiGong.

T'ai Chi Becomes a Philosophy

Around 1500 C.E., the Taoist philosopher Wan Yang-ming began to blend the gentle centering philosophical concepts of Taoism into the equally centering physical concepts of T'ai Chi. This gave practitioners a real way to live a more healing, nonviolent life—not just preaching it or thinking about it, but actually training their mind and body how to live that way through T'ai Chi's gentle mind/body fitness program.

The modern styles now widely practiced—Yang, Chen, Wu, Mulan Quan, Sun, and others—all incorporate the beautiful personal-growth concepts of Taoist philosophy. This book is *not* meant to favor any one style, but to celebrate *all T'ai Chi styles.* As mentioned earlier, when the six grandmasters of the major family styles traveled from China to speak at the International Tai Chi Symposium at Vanderbilt University, all six agreed that *all* styles of T'ai Chi provide similar benefits when practiced correctly.

Taoism is not a religion, but an observation of the dynamics of life and consciousness. Anyone of any religion can enjoy the Taoist aspects of T'ai Chi and QiGong and benefit from them. Taoism is about understanding that we are connected to all of life, and thereby that what nurtures all life in the end nurtures us. Taoism is a philosophy designed to foster compassion, not through intellectual edicts and rules, but rather through immersing ourselves in the field of Qi, or life energy, which permeates all existence. Any T'ai Chi or QiGong player knows that when she lets go of her grip on the world and relaxes open to the Qi or energy field that she is made of, she feels more connected to

the world. When we do this we feel a kinship to the world, and feel more welcome in our world, which thereby makes us more welcoming to those around us.

A T'AI CHI PUNCH LINE

T'ai Chi styles have been created with the same fluidity to the world's demands that T'ai Chi encourages its practitioners to have. For example, the Wu style was created by Wu Quan-yu, a palace guard in the Imperial Court who designed a system of T'ai Chi that could be performed in the restrictive clothing of an imperial palace guard's uniform.

The philosophy of T'ai Chi is based on the idea of the balance of nature, both internally in our health systems and externally in our relationships with the natural world. Therefore, you will see nature imitated in many of the following Kuang Ping Yang T'ai Chi long form names, but also in other styles' form names as well:

- Wave Hands Like Clouds
- Wind Blowing Lotus Leaves
- White Crane Cools Its Wings
- Retreat to Ride the Tiger

See Web Video Support's *Nature's Flow in T'ai Chi*, containing excerpts of "Wave Hands Like Clouds" and "Wind Blowing Lotus Leaves."

The poetic quality of these names does more than just remind us how to perform the movements. On a subliminal level, they make us feel more at home in the natural world, somehow more attuned to our connection to the whole of life.

T'ai Chi movement names can also help us remember our multidimensional nature. We are all physical and mental beings, of course, and

T'ai Chi integrates these aspects of ourselves well, but it connects our minds and bodies with our spirit or energy nature, too. This connection is reflected in movement names:

- Strike Palm to Ask Blessing
- Focus Mind Toward the Temple

T'ai Chi reminds us that we are part of the universe and that, in fact, we are made of the same energy stars and everything else are made of. T'ai Chi is meant to open us to the limitless supply of energy within us, in the earth we walk upon, and from the universe our world hurtles through. That universal connection is also reflected in movement names:

- Step Up to Form Seven Stars
- Grand Terminus

Grand Terminus, the final movement, opens us to the limitless energy of the universe around us. See Web Video Support's *Grand Radiance*, containing an excerpt of Grand Terminus with special effects added to help you visualize the energetic nature of this movement.

Short Forms vs. Long Forms

Today several short versions of the original long forms of T'ai Chi exist. These shortened versions can provide extensive benefits, such as enabling a student to acquire a practice system more quickly. But why stop there, when there is added value in taking the time to eventually learn a 20-minute long form as well?

SAGE SIFU SAYS

Most short forms of T'ai Chi take between 3 and 10 minutes. If you practice a short form, simply loop it so you can exercise for 20 minutes and get more benefit. However, if you ever get an opportunity to learn the long form of your style, do it. The complexity of 20 minutes of different movements keeps your mind in a state of relaxed focus, even more than repetition of the same movements does.

We now know the original ancient forms, which usually took about 20 minutes to complete, were that length for a good reason. In his groundbreaking book *The Relaxation Response*, Dr. Herbert Benson notes that a 20-minute relaxation response exercise seemed to evoke the optimum benefits. Apparently, the mind uses the first few minutes of a relaxation therapy to just wind down; the remaining time truly allows the deep alpha state relaxation these therapies are known for. So it's advisable to take the time to eventually learn a long form of T'ai Chi.

T'AI SCI

Some T'ai Chi movements look very similar to modern physical therapies. For example, Dropping the Duck's Beak, which is an extension of the fingers bending down to touch the thumb, is the same as a Carpal Tunnel prevention exercise used in many corporations. Could it be the therapy for modern repetitive stress disorders had been discovered centuries ago?

Why Sixty-Four Movements?

The more extensive Yang form names 108 movements, and the Kuang Ping Yang style long form claims 64 movements, yet they both average around 20 minutes to perform.

There may be more to the Kuang Ping's 64 movements than just chance. The number 64 has profound philosophical meaning. The Chinese classic *I Ching*, or *The Book of Changes*, is an ancient text of divination and philosophy that attempts to explain how the universal forces of yin and yang ebb and flow, combine and disintegrate, and rise and fall to create the dance of existence. The central premise is that all things are in a constant state of change, including our lives and us. T'ai Chi's goal is to help us flow with the change and not be compulsively attached to the old *or the new*, using what works and discarding what is no longer useful. As if you were a surfer riding the changing waves of life, let go of old waves as they recede, to ease onto the mounting power of the new wave.

The *I Ching* uses Trigrams, or figures with three lines (shown in the following figure) to symbolize the changes in life. When two Trigrams are combined, 64 possible combinations are obtained. These 64 hexagrams are said to represent all possible states of change in the universe. Therefore, Kuang Ping Yang's 64 flowing movements symbolize—and in some ways physically help us to flow through—all the possible changes and challenges of life those changes entail.

OUCH!

It's not important to mentally calculate what movement or direction benefits what system of the body. It's more important to simply allow the mind and body to enjoy the exquisite pleasure of effortless breath and movement as you do T'ai Chi. Rest assured that each aspect of your mind, heart, and body is being nourished and healed by the life energy T'ai Chi practice promotes.

The fact that Kuang Ping Yang-style T'ai Chi forms involve 64 movements may have deeper reasons than we know. The complexity and powerful healing qualities that T'ai Chi offers are only now beginning to be discovered by modern science. Perhaps many other details of how and why T'ai Chi does what it does will be uncovered in years to come.

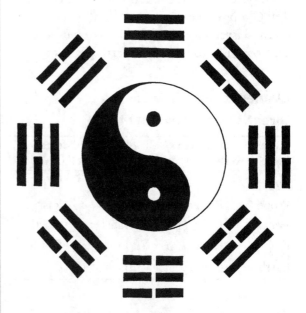

Trigrams are combinations of three lines, which can be broken in half or remain whole, making eight possible combinations.

T'ai Chi and Chinese Medicine

As I discussed in Chapter 2, Traditional Chinese Medicine (TCM) uses the Zang Fu system of understanding how organs interact. Each of these organ systems is represented by one of the five elements of the earth, according to ancient Chinese physics:

Metal	Lungs and large intestines
Wood	Liver and gall bladder

Water	Bladder and kidney
Fire	Heart/pericardium/small intestine/triple warmer
Earth	Spleen and stomach

T'ai Chi movements are described with this same system, and the motion of the body that T'ai Chi promotes may have a healing effect on those systems. The directions of movement each correlate to one of the earth elements:

Elements Correlate to Directions of Movement

Movement Directions Relative to the Body		Movement Directions Relative to Earth	
Metal	Advance	Metal	West
Wood	Retreat	Wood	East
Water	Left	Water	North
Fire	Right	Fire	South
Earth	Center	Earth	Center

The 64 postures of the Kuang Ping Yang style can take anywhere from about 15 to 20 minutes to complete. The movements flow in an unending progression from one to the next until the final movement, the Grand Terminus. The movements move the body outward and backward in all the directions previously described. There is also a meditative quality to that motion that cannot be described or conveyed in print.

Chapter 13 provides detailed sketches of each of the 64 Kuang Ping Yang-style movements, numbered in sequence. It also explains many of the benefits of each movement, complete with pointers, directional arrows, left-leg/right-leg labels, and energy-flow indicators to help you precisely perform them, as well as cautionary

notes to help your T'ai Chi experience be both healthful and profound. There are Web Video Support examples of each of the 64 postures to augment the deeply detailed figure and text instructions.

The Least You Need to Know

- T'ai Chi teaches us to yield when life attacks and to advance when opportunities open.
- Twenty-minute long forms have advantages over short forms.
- The 64 Kuang Ping movements ease the mind and body through changes.
- T'ai Chi movements have healing abilities we've yet to completely understand.
- *All forms* of T'ai Chi can offer profound healing benefits.

T'ai Chi Long Form Instruction

In This Chapter

- Learning the Kuang Ping Yang T'ai Chi long form
- Adjusting T'ai Chi to fit your body
- Breathing through life's challenges
- Using T'ai Chi to help prevent repetitive stress injuries
- Relaxing into "complexity" and tapping into universal, limitless energy
- Web Video Support: *Exhibition of the Entire T'ai Chi Long Form* and detailed lesson excerpts

My 30 years of studying have shown me that even when studying other styles I haven't trained extensively in, I discover much about my own familiar style. So even if you are currently practicing some other form of T'ai Chi, by emptying yourself of your knowledge, you can learn something useful here that will add to your current forms. As in all arts and sciences, there is no one master who knows everything about T'ai Chi. Each teacher brings his or her own unique genius to bear and I've learned much from all the masters and teachers I've played T'ai Chi with.

This book's graphic, illustrated, and Web Video Support instruction will flesh out how and why each movement benefits you, and detail the internal mechanics of posture, weight shift, and Qi flow that is common to *all* T'ai Chi styles, not just this one.

Because T'ai Chi is constant movement, the Web Video Support that complements this new edition gives you visual support for this chapter's already unequaled illustrated and text instructions. Use this chapter's text and illustrated instructions in their proper order for T'ai Chi instruction, *preceding T'ai Chi practice with the warm-ups in Chapter 11.* The Web Video Support for this book provides visual enhancement meant to augment this chapter's text and illustrated instructions—*not* to replace them.

The explanations and instructions you find in this book—now augmented by the new Web Video Support—provide an unparalleled instructional tool that is unequaled in T'ai Chi book instruction. Each movement is broken down into a series of sketches to help you see both external and internal aspects, as the video exhibitions of this *T'ai Chi Long Form* on the Web Video Support bring these illustrated instructions to life.

The video exhibitions supporting each of the 64 postures taught in this chapter are intended to support their corresponding instructional figures, to more effectively familiarize you with the "patterns" of this book's illustrated and text instructional techniques. In this way, you'll be clearer on all the text and graphic movement instructions, which will give you precise details on many levels.

The movement sketches and their accompanying text in this chapter include the following:

- **Directional arrows.** Arrows show how your limbs or body move from the previous "ghost image" position into the current position, taking all the guesswork out of how you get from one pose to another.

- **Markers.** "L" and "R" are marked on the figures so you can see at a glance whether the left or right side of the body is depicted.

- **Shading.** The leg the weight is on, or the *filled leg*, is shaded to a darkness level reflecting just how much weight is shifted onto it. When both legs are shaded, weight is evenly distributed.

- **Posture line.** This is a line indicating your *Vertical Axis* or postural alignment centered over the dan tien.

- **Emphasis.** Occasional *italicized* text explains what *sensations* and *internal awareness*, releases, and benefits you may be experiencing *within* as you go through the motions.

- **"Ghost" images.** Most of the sketches have a ghost image indicating what the previous posture was, helping you see transitions.

Using the very first Chapter 13 Web Video Support link, you'll see how each movement's detailed instructions work *in action*.

Begin by viewing the *Exhibition of the Entire T'ai Chi Long Form* and the first movement's lesson video on the Web Video Support, while viewing the corresponding illustrated drawings in this chapter and reading the associated instructional text in this chapter. This will make all the illustrated instructional cues more tangible as you progress through the instruction for all the 64 movements that follow.

Some of the more complex instructional figures in this chapter have corresponding, intensely detailed Web Video Support, including figures for movements #1, #6 through 8, and #15 through 19, where you'll see "Sage Sifu Says" notations by these figures, indicating they have super-detailed video support.

A few sketches also reflect how the Qi, or life energy, flows outward through the hand or the foot. This is shown only in a few figures because too many graphics would be distracting. As a general rule, when you are physically moving an empty foot to a new location on the floor, you take an *in breath.* When the weight (Vertical Axis) is shifting over/into/onto a leg and foot, *the breath is being exhaled as you sink into the leg,* allowing Qi to flow down through your relaxed "filling" leg and out the extending arms and hands (revisit Web Video Support's *T'ai Chi Walking, Filling and Emptying,* and *The Unbendable Arm*). This illustrates why the practice of Sitting QiGong is such a critical element to a powerful and effective T'ai Chi form (no matter what style you do), as it enables you to practice "feeling the Qi," or relaxation flowing through your arms and body.

The Kuang Ping Yang-style long form takes approximately 20 minutes to complete. Before beginning the movements, to understand why the Vertical Axis and filling illustrations are so important to your T'ai Chi practice, try this simple exercise:

1. Standing comfortably in the Horse Stance, close your eyes and breathe while relaxing the entire body and standing in your proper Vertical Axis with the head stacked up above the lower dan tien.

2. Lean your head forward, noticing how the muscles tighten to hold you up. As the head goes back into Vertical Axis alignment, notice how effortless the stance becomes. The same thing happens when you lean back slightly.

Moving in Vertical Axis posture makes everything more effortless. See the Web Video Support's *Enhanced Internal Tutor for Vertical Alignment.* This will show you that ultimately your greatest T'ai Chi tutor will be *you,* as you learn how to sense the correctness of your own postural alignment by each movement's level of effortlessness. Practicing T'ai Chi with this awareness of effortless versus effortful movement easily and naturally changes the way you move through life as well. T'ai Chi, and life, should be mostly effortless—and strangely, when it is, this is usually when we are getting the most accomplished.

As you go through this exercise, note that the movement names offer two tools: they evoke healthful and soothing mental/sensual images to calm the mind and heart, and they offer visual mental images to help you remember how to move. Part of the calming effect results from T'ai Chi's left brain/right brain integration of feeling and thinking.

Before you dive into learning the movements using the following text and illustrated instructions, again, if you haven't already, view the Web Video Support's *Exhibition of the Entire T'ai Chi Long Form* while flipping through the pages of this chapter to get a general feel for the motion of T'ai Chi movement. Then, view *T'ai Chi Long Form Lesson 1 Excerpt.* Once you've done that, you can begin learning the movements one at a time, following the instructions, and referring to each individual movement's video example when needed.

NOTE: On your computer or smart phone, *bookmark* the web pages www.idiotsguides. com/taichi, and www.idiotsguides.com/taichi13. These will help you quickly find links to each movement's video as you break down each movement individually with this chapter's following instructions, beginning with Movement #1, *Strike Palm to Ask Blessings.* The combination of this chapter and its video support provides an unequaled T'ai Chi book-learning experience.

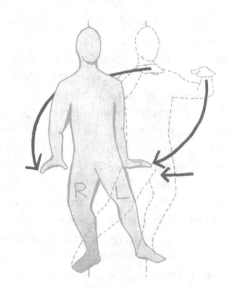

Strike Palm to Ask Blessings, #1

Breathe in deeply and lift your palms as if circling them up in front of you over a large 3-foot ball of energy, shifting your weight toward the left foot as your hands circle up over the ball.

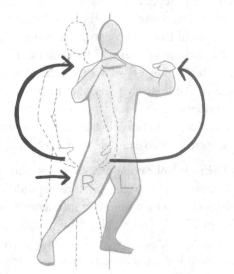

As the palms pull back over, down the back of the sphere, ending up in front of your chest as though you were going to push something away, the weight is shifting back to the right foot, sinking the Qi, or filling the right foot/leg, as palms drop to the sides of the hips.

From palms-down position, palms pull out and behind a bit to gently rotate out the shoulders. As your empty left foot comes out in front, place your left heel lightly on the ground. Continue circling your arms around in front of the body as if hugging a large tree, and the left heel touches just as your palms almost meet. The left palm is lateral as in the sketch, while the right palm is vertical. Although the movement is called Strike Palm, the palms don't actually strike; pretend there is a soft energy sphere the size of a honeydew melon between your relaxed, rounded hands.

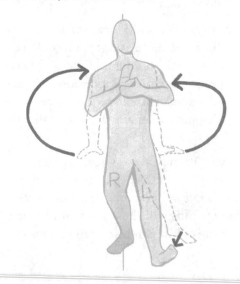

Grasp the Bird's Tail, #2

From completed Strike Palms, reach with your arms up and out to the right as your left toe reaches out to the left and back.

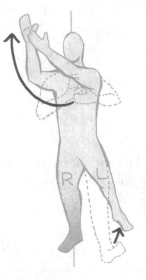

With your right hand palm down on top of your left hand palm up, stroke the bird's tail as your arms pull down and back. Your weight shifts back to the left foot behind.

Your hands stroke down to the groin, releasing the bird's tail. Turn your palms away from your body with your elbows at your sides while your hands continue to circle up in front of your face. Your right foot pulls back, touching your right toe near the left instep.

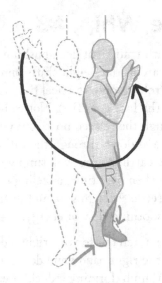

Now turn your dan tien and torso to the right at a 45° angle (front/right), while your arms follow around and in front of your chest, ready to push out diagonally to right.

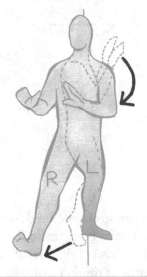

SAGE SIFU SAYS

Strike Palm, Grasp Bird's Tail, and Single Whip are all wonderful for loosening the daily stress from tight shoulders.

Single Whip, #3

Step out with your right heel, pushing your hands forward as the weight shifts onto the right foot (rolling onto the heel first and then the rest of the foot goes flat). Notice how Qi flows through the relaxed body, out your pushing hands, and down through the filling right leg into the earth. At first you simply relax and exhale; then over time, a feeling of "empty flow" will settle through you, and in time you'll perceive a soothing flow of energy.

Your arms stretch out to your right side, as the fingers on the right hand bend down, touching your right thumb (forming a duck's beak).

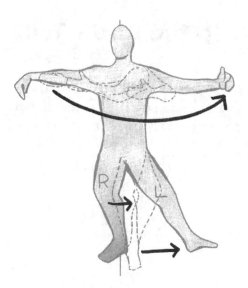

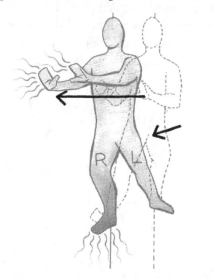

Your left fingers stroke the inside of the right arm. Your left palm pulls across your body in a great half-circle toward the left side as the body follows, turning at the dan tien.

Your left palm continues over to the left side, as if circling a globe on its axis, until your palm is near your shoulder …

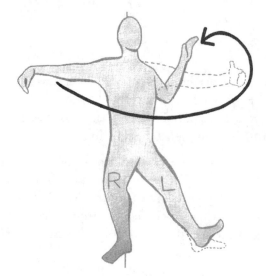

T'AI SCI

T'ai Chi is a uniquely right-brain/left-brain experience. Your analytical mind follows detailed forms, while your sensory mind enjoys a sense of being carried through motions, almost being massaged by the process effortlessly. Book instruction is left brain; video/class is more right brain.

… and then your left hand pushes the imaginary globe away to the left, while the weight sinks onto the left heel and then the rest of the left foot, with about 60 percent of your weight now on the left foot. Again, note how the Qi or life energy flows through the relaxed body, out the body, arm, and hand, and down the left leg and deeply into the earth.

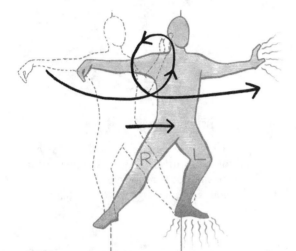

White Crane Cools Its Wings, #4

Your weight shifts to the left leg as the torso turns to the left. The left arm drops down to your side, the palm facing the ground, as the right arm circles from behind up above the head.

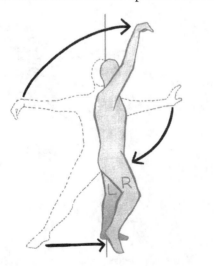

T'AI SCI

Place the tip of the tongue lightly against the roof of the mouth while performing your movements, and fully fill and empty the lungs from bottom to top on each breath, allowing the torso to "relax" around your breathing. Studies show that long, relaxed abdominal breathing oxygenates the body much more effectively than rapidly inflating the chest.

Note that the following two sketches show the same pose, so you can now see it from a front angle as well. The right arm comes straight down as the right foot sticks out a few inches in front.

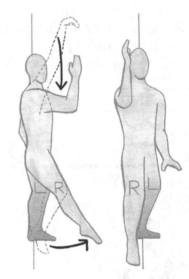

Step out to the right side with your right toe, as the right elbow circles to the left side, to prepare by winding up for upcoming elbow strike. (Both your palms are face down in their respective positions.) See figure on next page.

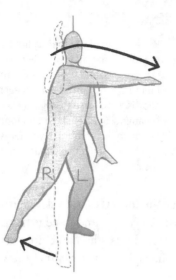

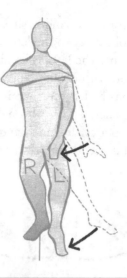

Now shift the weight to the right foot as the right elbow pulls across in an elbow strike, allowing the sinking dan tien to pull the elbow strike across.

SAGE SIFU SAYS

Remember that the "ghost" images in most of the instructional sketches represent the previous posture and are included to help you see *transitions between* positions.

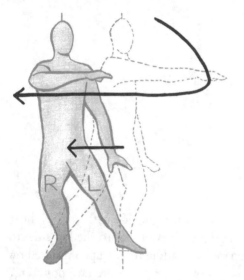

Lift the left foot and place it out in front, as the left hand moves slightly to the front, as shown in the following figure.

Brush Knee Twist Step, #5

The left hand extends out 45° to the left of front, as the left foot steps back behind slightly. The right forearm twists a bit so the "back" of the right hand is facing the chest, and the palm faces out.

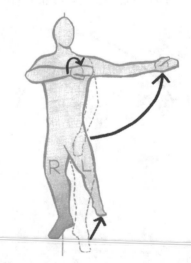

Now the weight sinks back into the left foot as the left arm brushes to the center of the body, as if slapping an imaginary wall in front of you. Exhale and allow the body to relax as the weight, or dan tien, sinks back on each brush motion.

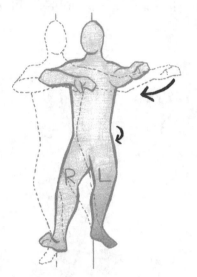

With the weight back on the left foot, the right empty foot steps slightly back as the right hand extends out 45° to the right, and the "back" or left hand is placed in front of your heart.

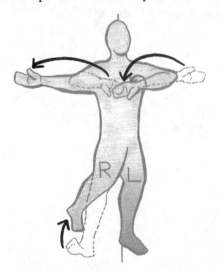

OUCH!

If any of the movement descriptions cause pain, alter them to suit you. For example, if you have a bad knee, share some weight on the empty foot as well.

Just as you did on the left side, now shift your weight back to the right, brushing the right hand toward your center.

Repeat once more on both sides, as in the first four figures of Brush Knee Twist Step (Movement #5). As you finish the last brush, shift to your right foot and brush across your body with your right hand.

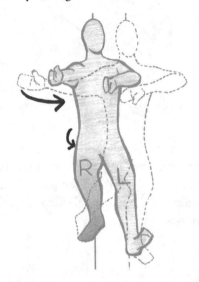

Move the left hand out 45° to the left, but do not move the left foot this time.

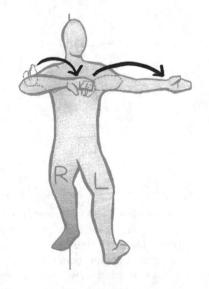

Brush the left hand across the body, and let the left arm circle out in front as the right hand forms a fist by the right hip.

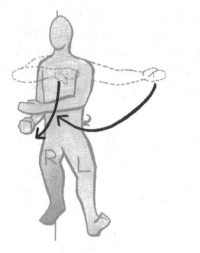

Now shift your weight 60 percent onto the left foot, and throw the right-fisted punch out in front beneath the left arm, circling out in a defensive posture, or parry.

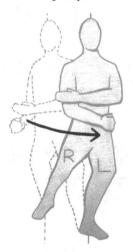

SAGE SIFU SAYS

Look at the figures for movements #6 through #8, and view the *T'ai Chi Long Form Lesson 4 Excerpt* on the Web Video Support. Pay attention to the motion arrows, shading, posture lines, and ghost images on the figures, and relate the video to the book's instructional patterns.

Apparent Closing, #6

From the Parry and Punch position, the palms turn down; then your hands open and come back to the temples as your weight shifts back onto the right leg and the left foot rolls back on its heel.

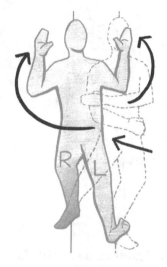

Push out as the weight rolls forward onto the left leg. Step through with the right foot and then shift your weight to the right leg as you push out to point with flat hands.

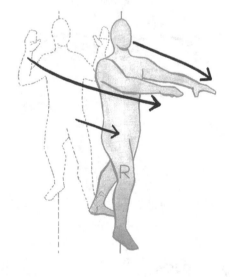

Push Turn and Carry Tiger to Mountain, #7

Carry Tiger to the Mountain, as with other movements, reminds us of our connection to nature as we mimic the grace of noble beasts.

With your weight on the right foot and your hands pushed out flat, your weight comes off the left foot until only the toe is touching as your pushing hands circle flatly (as if on a table top) to the left as the left foot pivots on the toe.

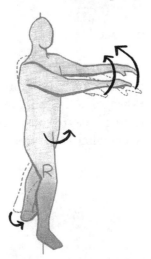

At ¾ of the hands circling to the left, your weight begins shifting to the left foot as the empty right foot pivots on the toe.

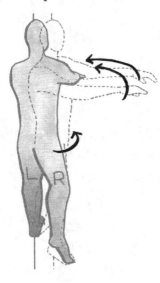

With the 180° turn complete, your weight settles back on the right foot. Only the left heel touches, as your left toes come up off the floor and your right fist rests over the thumb of your open left hand in front of your abdomen. Note the two figures in this sketch depict the same posture, only shown twice so you can now view it frontally.

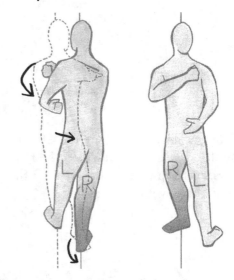

Spiraling Hands to Focus Mind Toward the Temple to Parry and Punch, #8

This movement encompasses the spiritual image of Focusing Our Mind Toward Our Temple, which is the heart, while providing a protective shield for the vital/vulnerable areas of the body.

With your hands open, the palms should be parallel to one another and pointing straight as the left heel lifts (your weight is still on the right leg) and the left heel lightly retouches the ground.

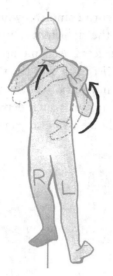

Your weight slowly shifts up to the left foot as your hands begin a clockwise corkscrew downward. (Keep your hands relaxed at the wrists so they pivot facing straight.)

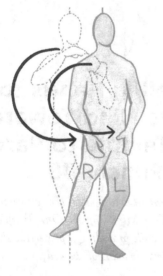

As your weight shifts completely to the left foot, your hands begin the upward part of a clockwise rotation, lifting the right foot up from behind, as if a string were attached from your hands to your feet, and reaching the top as the right heel touches the ground in front of you.

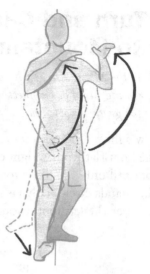

Repeat this stepping/shifting/spiraling hands with the right foot out this time, and repeat left foot out, and then right foot out (for a total of five times stepping forward on this Spiraling Hands Movement, alternating feet each time, of course).

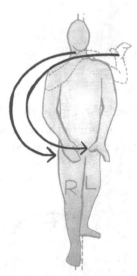

Remember not to "bob up" as you shift up into the front leg. In T'ai Chi, you always stay "down" in a slightly bent-knee stance.

However, on the fifth step, which is with the left foot out, don't shift your weight to the left foot. Leave it out and empty as the hands corkscrew one last time all the way around.

Then allow the right hand to fall to your side, forming a fist as the left circles in front to parry.

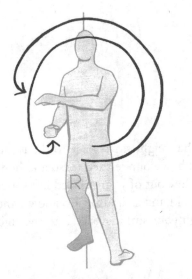

Now parry and punch, with your weight shifting about 65 percent onto the left foot.

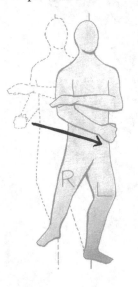

Fist Under Elbow, #9

With your weight still mostly on the left foot (in the Parry and Punch position), drop your right fist down under your left elbow.

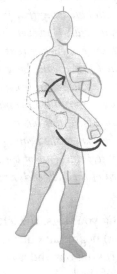

As your right fist is pulled up with the palm facing your chin, the left parry hand drops to the palm up position to rest at the left hip.

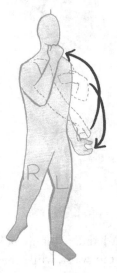

Repulse the Monkey, #10

Repulse the Monkey can be a powerful martial arts tactic of blocking an incoming blow, yielding to the opponent's force, and allowing that force to carry the opponent off to your side. However, it also fosters a very healing exchange of energy that Traditional Chinese Medicine (TCM) calls Long Qi when the open palms pass one another in front of the heart chakra, an energy center called the middle dan tien. According to TCM, this has a supercharging effect, opening the body to the healing force of Qi, and practitioners feel this sense of opening release through that area of the body each time they practice.

Without moving your legs, the left hand (palm up at your waist) begins an outside arc up to the left ear, as if stroking out and away over a large orb at the side of the body.

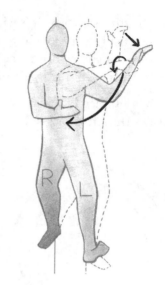

Now the weight shifts back to the right leg. Notice how your relaxed torso and body allow Qi to flow out of your relaxed left shoulder, arm, and hand as it also flows down and through your sinking back into the right leg.

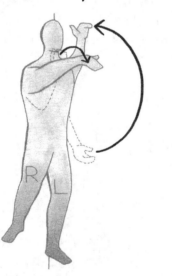

Now the right hand, palm up, pulls back to the right side of your waist, while the left hand, palm facing front, pushes outward from your chest; simultaneously, weight sinks back into your right leg, as shown in the following figure.

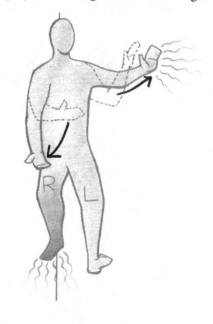

Prepare for the next three moves by moving the opposite leg back as your palm at your waist circles up near the ear, poised to push when the other hand pulls back as you shift back.

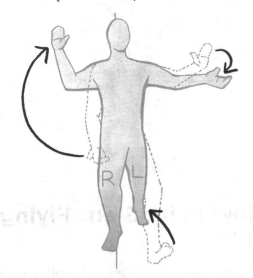

Repeat with the right hand pushing, the left hand pulling as you sink back.

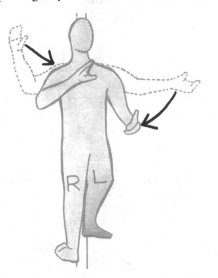

Shifting back to the left leg, Qi flows out of your relaxed torso, right shoulder, right arm, and right hand.

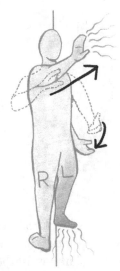

Repeat with the left hand pushing and the right hand pulling, shifting back to the right leg (see the third and fourth figures of the Repulse the Monkey movement).

Repeat with the right hand pushing and the left hand pulling, shifting back to the left leg (see the sixth and seventh figures of the Repulse the Monkey movement).

Stork Covers Its Wing/ Sword in Sheath, #11

After completing the last Repulse the Monkey with the right hand pushed out and the weight back on the left, back foot, the right foot now pivots on the heel to follow the extended right arm out to point diagonally 45° to left/front, as shown in the following figure.

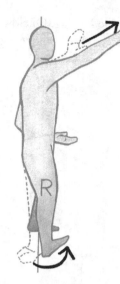

Upon completing the pivot, the weight shifts to the right foot while pivoting on the left ball and dropping the left heel in toward the right foot a bit.

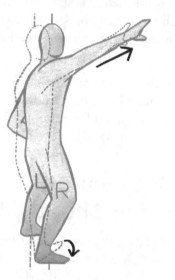

Now, as the left palm up turns into a sheath (palm turns in to face body), the weight shifts back to the left leg, and the right extended hand pulls back into the left hand's sheath between the left palm and the left hip. The right toe simultaneously pulls back to rest at the left instep, as shown in the following figure.

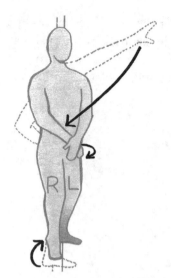

Slow Palm Slant Flying, #12

Slow Palm Slant Flying is one of the most beautiful and uplifting movements in the entire series.

The right heel goes out diagonally.

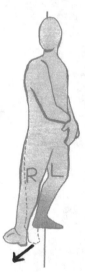

As your weight shifts to your right foot, the right palm extends slowly outward from your left hand's sheath as your left hand extends back to the opposite corner, as shown in the following figure.

Raise Right Hand and Left: Turn and Repeat (Part I), #13

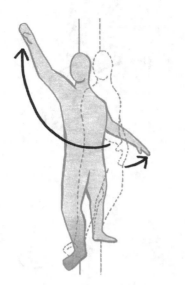

Although each movement has powerful martial applications, the goal of T'ai Chi is to "soong yi dien," to loosen the mind, heart, and body. This movement loosens the abdominal area, back, and shoulders by performing Long Qi. The palms passing one another healthfully stimulate the dan tien energy centers within the body, also relaxing the solar plexus.

Extend your arms fully with your weight totally on your right leg; the right arm begins a great arcing circle around a bit behind your body, while the open left palm arcs up from behind until both open palms meet in front of the chest. Lift the left foot to place the left toe lightly a couple inches in front of the body below your parallel palms.

Your left heel extends forward as your left arm curls around (as if hugging a tree), and your weight continues rolling up onto the left foot, as the heel of the right wrist begins to descend. (A soothing Long Qi experience can be felt in the abdomen as the right palm passes the left palm as the right hand drops.) Now the right hand forms a Duck's Beak and begins to lift upward.

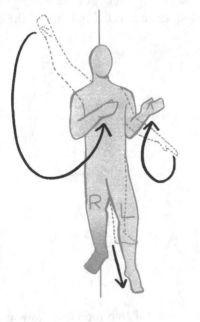

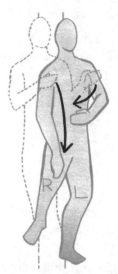

The right hand's Duck's Beak rises, as if pulling a string attached to the right foot, and pulls the back right foot up in front to touch the toe. When the Duck's Beak is above the head, the palm opens.

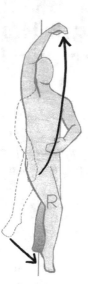

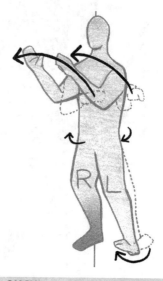

Now the right hand drops down as the right toe reaches back behind, until the right and left palms are once again parallel, facing one another in front, and the weight has shifted back to the right foot, with only the left heel touching.

OUCH!

While moving, remember to breathe deeply into the diaphragm, but also easily and naturally. This conditions you to breathe through life's changes just as through T'ai Chi's changing postures.

As the 180° turn/pivot completes, the weight sinks completely back into the left leg, and the hands fall again parallel in front of the chest.

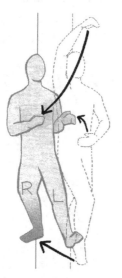

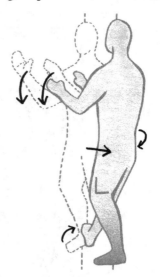

Turn to the right, pivoting on the (empty) left heel, palms arcing across in front of the chest, still parallel and facing one another.

(The following sketch merely gives you a frontal view for easier viewing.)

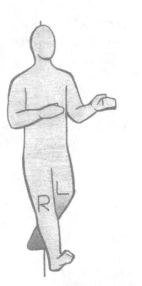

Now the left wrist begins its descent as the right arm parries as if hugging a tree and the weight begins shifting up onto the right leg.

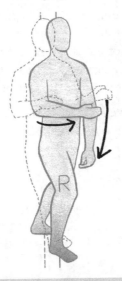

💡 **T'AI SCI**

T'ai Chi can accomplish the seemingly paradoxical goal of fostering deep relaxation *and* martial arts training simultaneously, teaching that effectiveness in all aspects of life can be effortless.

Your left hand forms the Duck's Beak, pulling the imaginary string up, bringing the left toe to touch in front as the left hand raises overhead and the weight completely shifts to the right leg.

Although this movement is very soothing to the upper body and therapeutic for the hand and arm, its martial application is powerful. As the right hand blocks a punch, the left hand lowers to block a kick. The left hand then rises to strike an opponent's face or nose as the left knee rises to kick the groin. Ouch!

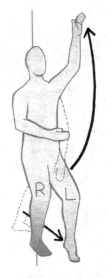

As the left hand opens and descends, the left toe reaches back, and the weight shifts back to the left foot as the palms face, parallel, in front of the chest (the right heel touching in front).

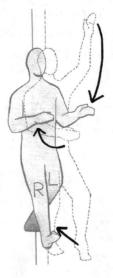

Wave Hand Over Light/ Fly Pulling Back, #14

With the palms parallel and facing each other, they rotate as if over a ball so the right palm is over the left palm.

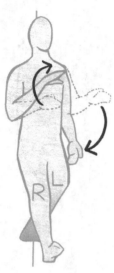

The right fingers extend straight out from chest level at your shadow opponent's throat level, as the weight shifts forward onto the right leg. The right palm curves around downward as if it has gone over and is now curving back under a sphere of light, to rest in front of the dan tien, cradled in the left palm, as the right toe pulls back to rest by the left instep.

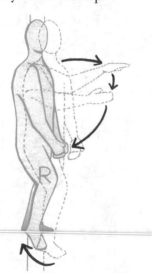

The right heel extends out front as the right palm circles, this time from "beneath the sphere of light" …

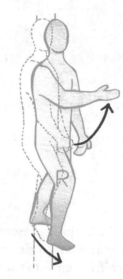

… and continuing up and over the back of the sphere of light until the back of the right hand rests in front of the chest. As the right hand is completing the circle, the left foot pulls up to rest with the toe at the right instep.

Fly Pulling Back extends your Qi forward and out in an expressive motion and then relaxes your Qi, sinking back into a retreat.

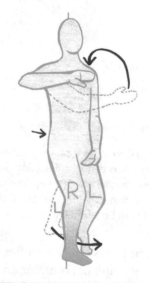

As you extend or strike, the upper-body torso muscles relax and loosen as you exhale. A cadence of breath timing can be further refined using video or live class instruction, but the figures help you see very precisely where your weight shifts occur.

Fan Through the Arms, #15

With the back of the right hand facing the chest and the open left palm in front of the dan tien, the left palm arcs outward to the left at shoulder height, and your weight shifts 60 percent to the left.

Your left fanning arm relaxes away from the body as the weight shifts toward the left leg. The dan tien carries the arm outward as it sinks over the left leg. Your arm moves out and up like a clock hand moving from 6 to 3 o'clock as you relax and exhale.

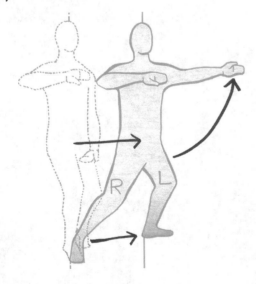

Green Dragon Rising from the Water, #16

Your weight shifts back to the right foot as the left foot pivots on the heel to point the left toe catty-corner toward the right. Your left arm follows so the entire body is turned catty-corner to the left now.

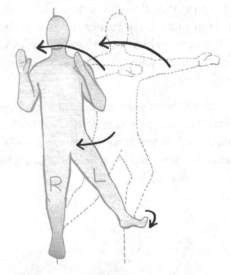

With the right and left palms falling parallel in front of the chest, weight settles back onto the left leg, and the right foot comes to the heel as your right toe comes up.

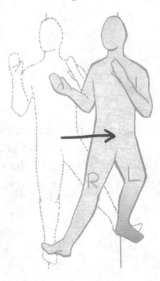

SAGE SIFU SAYS

Each time your weight settles or *sinks* into a leg, exhale and allow every muscle to let go of whatever tension it had unconsciously squeezed within it. This conditions your mind and body to stop straining through life, getting things done in a healthful, effortless way.

Lift your right heel slightly and replace it to extend out more catty-corner to right, then reaching open palms upward and outward while the weight shifts about 65 percent up toward the right foot.

This Green Dragon move teaches you to push and lift from your dan tien, keeping the back heel planted down, thereby reducing back pressure. This creates more power and less chance of injury while performing daily tasks.

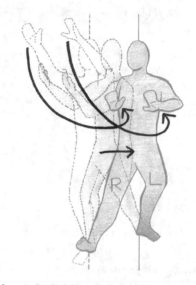

Then the right heel goes out and the hands push out from the torso.

The weight shifts on up to the right leg as you complete the push and then the hands turn to the right side, where the Duck's Beak begins for Single Whip.

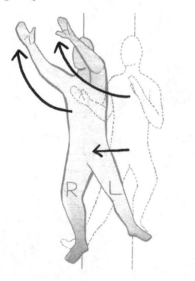

As if the hands are pulling a sphere of light back down into your heart, the weight settles back onto the left leg and the right toe pulls back to touch at the left instep.

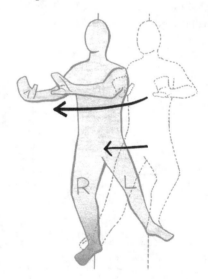

Single Whip (Part II), #17

The right hand is in a Duck's Beak (the fingers touching the right thumb), and as the left fingers stroke the inside of the right arm, the left palm pulls across the body. (Refer to the second, third, and fourth figures of the first Single Whip [Movement #3], and to the Web Video Support for this movement.)

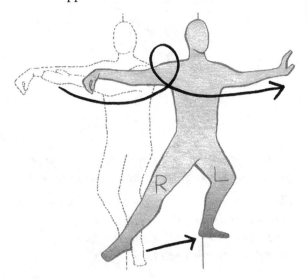

On the Duck's Beak, all the fingers on the right hand extend down to touch the right thumb. Modern carpal-tunnel-prevention exercises include movements like these. So among its many benefits, T'ai Chi appears to be an ergonomic carpal-tunnel-prevention exercise as well.

Wave Hands Like Clouds (3), #18 (Part I, Linear Style)

T'ai Chi connects us with nature as we rise up from the water to Wave Hands Like Clouds (parentheses indicate number of repetitions).

As your hands draw in from Single Whip extension, turn both palms to face down. Shift the weight to the right leg, bringing the left toe out to touch in front, as the right hand comes parallel to ground at shoulder height to the center chest and the left hand comes down to arrive at the center dan tien level.

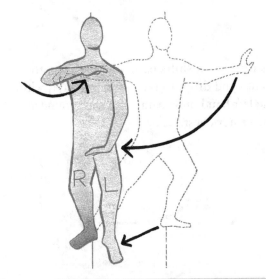

  OUCH!

You'll know you are doing movements correctly if it feels good. If you feel undue strain in a knee, leg, or anywhere in the body, you're probably forcing the position. All T'ai Chi positions are designed to enable you to relax into the position. If you feel lower-back pain in Wave Hands or other moves, it's usually because your lower back is overarched. Be sure as you exhale you allow the tailbone to *relax* down.

As the left toe goes straight out to the left, both hands reach straight out to the right at shoulder level.

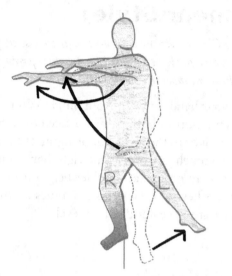

Your weight shifts to the left leg as the right leg is drawn toward the left leg and the hands reach out to the left at shoulder level.

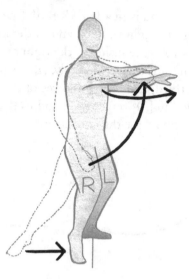

As the weight shifts back to the left leg, the right hand drops to the dan tien center, while the left hand pulls parallel to the ground across the center chest.

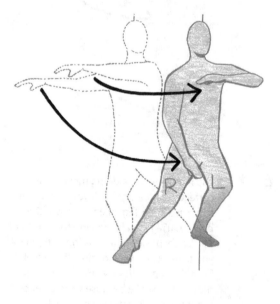

Your weight shifts to the right leg as the hands come to center (right at chest, left at dan tien).

Though obviously martial, there's also a soothing quality of imagining the hands waving like clouds. The thought unlocks an effortlessness flow throughout the mind and body.

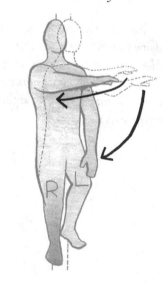

As the left toe goes straight out to the left, both hands reach straight out to the right at shoulder level.

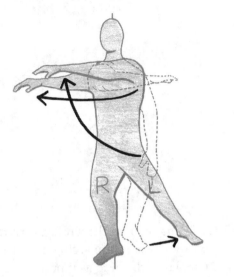

Repeat the second through sixth figures of this movement two more times (for a total of three repetitions for Wave Hands Like Clouds). However, on the last repetition, leave off the action from the sixth figure of this movement, because you will be going right into a Single Whip from there. All Wave Hands Like Clouds (and there are four of them in this style) begin and end with a Single Whip.

SAGE SIFU SAYS

T'ai Chi is taught in three stages. First, the movements are learned. Second, the breath is incorporated into the regimen by learning an inhalation or exhalation that is connected to each movement. Third, a relaxation element or awareness of the flow of energy through the body is learned. Although the first step offers many benefits from the first day, the benefits get richer and deeper with each level you learn.

Single Whip (Part III), #19

Refer to Movement #3's (the first Single Whip) second, third, and fourth figures, and to the Web Video Support for this movement, if needed, although if you are this far, you should know the Single Whip by heart by now. If not, go back and review. It's not a test, only a game. Enjoy!

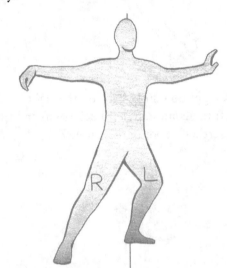

High Pat on Horse/ Guarding the Temples, #20

From the Single Whip pose, the torso rotates to the right and the arms begin to curve into a horseshoe shape in front of the body. While the torso turns, you pivot on the ball of the right foot, as shown in the following figure.

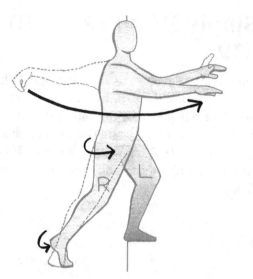

The weight now sinks back on the right leg as the left toe comes up (left heel down) and the arms settle in front of the chest.

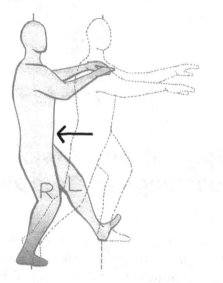

With the weight settled on the right leg, raise the left foot a bit and then touch the left toe in front, the palms patting downward a little as if patting a pony's hindquarters, as shown in the following figure.

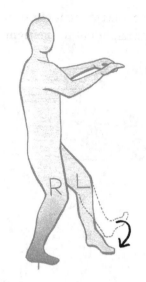

While shifting up onto the left leg, turn the palms outward, each palm arcing up to the side of the temples of the head as if protecting from a side blow, and then arcing down to form a low block by crossing the right wrist over the left in front of the dan tien. The right foot comes up to touch empty (without any weight on it) by the left instep (the left foot being filled with your weight on it).

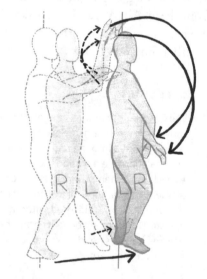

(The following sketch shows the front position of the preceding figure.)

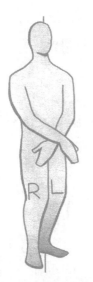

Lower Block/Upper Block, Separation of Right Foot; Lower Block/Upper Block, Separation of Left Foot, #21

With the wrists crossed at the dan tien in the preceding figure, now lift the wrists to cross them at mid-chest block (the palms still facing in toward the chest).

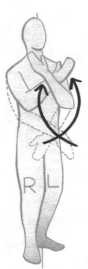

The arms continue rising as the palms turn out, causing the wrists to twist and forming an up block (with the palms facing out). It takes a 7-count to go from the low block to the up block and the kick that follows.

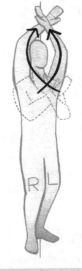

 OUCH!

Remember, there is no correct height to kick at. The kick may be only a few inches off the ground or, if you're a soccer player, the kick may be 2 feet higher than in the next figure. There is no wrong or right; the only rule is to relax and enjoy.

Kick the right foot up and out to the right side as the right hand chops down to meet the foot (at whatever height is comfortable—don't force it; the kicks will get higher over time). Catch the foot on its descent, and slowly settle the descending right foot down by the left foot, as shown in the following figure.

Your hand may not touch the kicking foot at first. That's okay; just kick as high as is comfortable.

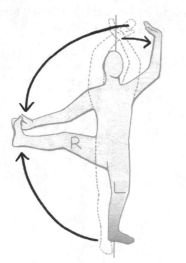

The weight shifts back into the right foot as the left wrist crosses over the right this time.

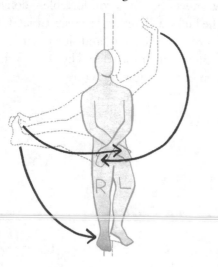

Begin the low/mid/upper block, the left leg preparing for the separation kick.

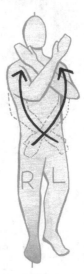

As the up block completes, the left hand begins to slip sideways to the left as the left foot prepares to kick out and up to the left.

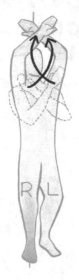

Kick the left foot out and up to the left side as the left hand chops down to meet the foot (again, kicking only as high as is comfortable) and catches the left foot as it drops to slowly settle "behind" the right heel, as the hands lower to your sides.

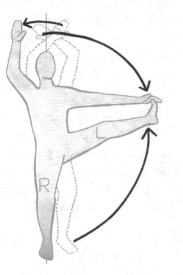

Turn and Kick with Sole, #22

The hands complete lowering to your sides, as the left foot settles behind the right heel, the body turns ¼ turn to the left. The left leg fills and the right leg empties as you complete the ¼ turn.

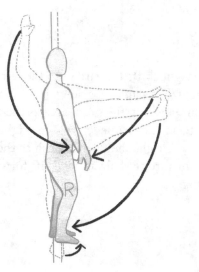

(The following sketch presents a frontal view of the pose in the preceding figure.)

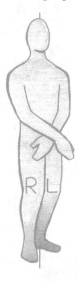

The weight shifts into the right leg as the low block rises to mid block.

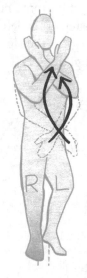

A T'AI CHI PUNCH LINE

T'ai Chi breath is fully exhaled from the chest to the abdomen, with the tip of the tongue lightly touching the roof of your mouth so that a *full inhalation* accompanies preparations, and full *exhalations* accompany shifts, kicks, or punches.

The weight sinks fully into the right leg as the mid block rises to high block as the palms twist out.

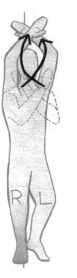

Kick the left leg up and out to the left as the left hand swings out in front and around to the side to slap the instep of the left foot (or the inside of the left leg), as the right hand chops out to the right slightly.

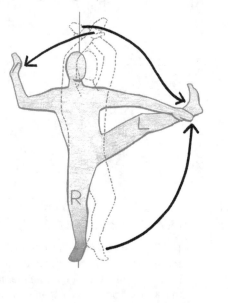

Wind Blowing Lotus Leaves (4), #23

This is an exquisite move. It is artistically beautiful and feels fantastic because it loosens the entire torso. It also helps the body learn to push the lawn mower or perform other tasks with much less pressure on the lower back. Correct T'ai Chi movement shifts strain from the lower back to the thighs, which are much stronger and less delicate than the back's vertebrae.

After the left hand smacks the instep or the inside of the left leg, it pulls back to the head just off the right ear, and the right hand pulls behind that, as if holding a beach ball off to the right side of the head. Place the left heel down at a 45° angle to the left/front.

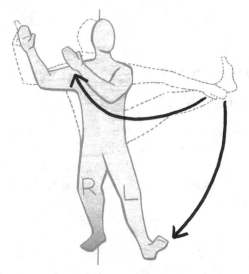

The weight shifts forward onto the left leg as the front/left arm drops down in a circular motion, blocking the groin area as the torso turns to shift over the left leg, the right hand still by the right shoulder to push as the body shifts forward. Exhale as you shift forward, relaxing.

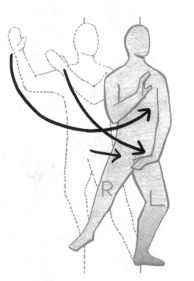

Now imagine holding the beach ball off to the left side of the head (the right hand forward of the left this time) as the right heel goes out 45° to the front/right.

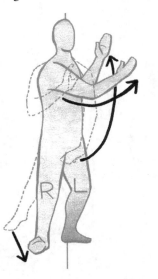

The weight shifts forward onto the right leg as the front/right arm drops down in a circular motion, blocking the groin area, with the torso turning slightly to shift over the right leg and the left hand still by the left shoulder. Exhale as you shift, relaxing.

Shift forward, as the breath seems to relax out of every cell. As your Qi sinks into the earth, its power also flows through you and out your hands. The dan tien pulls your relaxed body forward.

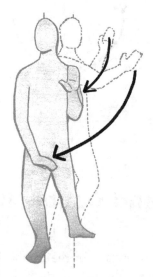

Now repeat the four figures of Wind Blowing Lotus Leaves for a total of four movements in this series, two from the right to left and two from the left to right.

Block Up/Fist Down, #24

Begin similar to the first two figures in the preceding Wind Blowing Lotus Leaves (Movement #23). However, this time, your right hand forms a fist and rises up and over to deliver a downward hammer-fist. Your left hand doesn't stop down at a groin block, but it continues circling up in front to a high block protecting your forehead, with the left palm down in a down block. As the block arcs out and up in front of the body, the palm continues to face away from the upper body even as the block is completed. (See the following figure.)

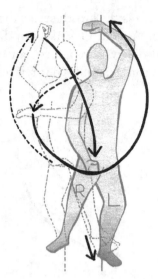

Turn and Double Kick, #25

Turn 180° to prepare for the Double Kick by shifting the weight back on the right leg and pivoting on the "empty" left heel as the body turns to the right.

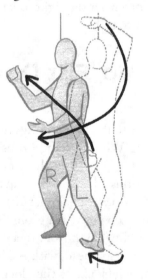

Sink back into the left leg as the pivot completes, allowing the right toe to come up, pivoting on the right heel. The left open palm rests at the left hip, facing up, as the right fist swings out in front of the right shoulder.

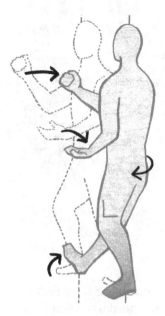

(The next sketch shows a frontal view of this last figure.)

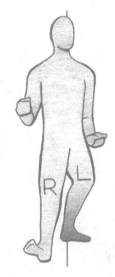

SAGE SIFU SAYS

The complexity and variety of movements may seem daunting at first, but just relax and learn the move you're learning today. You'll get it, one move at a time. *A lesson for life.*

From sunken down on the right leg, shift forward and kick the left leg up and out for a left front kick.

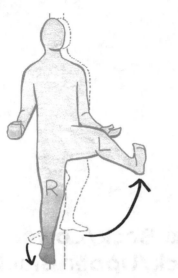

Remember that your kick does not have to be as high as illustrated. Then place the left leg out in front and shift up into the left leg …

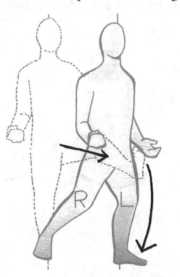

… kicking the right leg up and out front while opening the right fist and smacking the right palm down on top of the kicking right foot (or leg).

As the right leg kicks up, the right palm turns over and smacks down to slap the top of the right foot, or calf, or knee, or wherever your hand comfortably slaps without leaning forward.

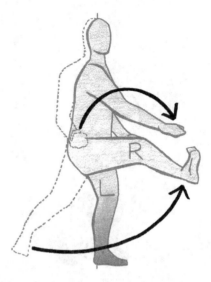

Place your right foot down in front after the kick, heel first.

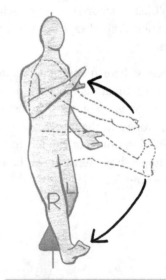

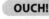

OUCH!

Never force or strain. Breathe easily. Let your mind and body learn to relax as you are absorbed in the silken flow of continuous movement.

Parry and Punch, #26

Step forward with the left foot while preparing the right fist near the right hip and dropping the left parry.

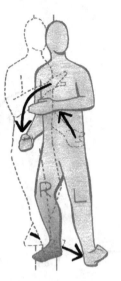

Then parry and punch as the weight shifts onto the left front foot about 60 percent forward. Again, don't lean forward as you punch. The body or Vertical Axis always stays stacked above the dan tien.

As the punch is thrown and Qi sinks into the forward left leg, breath is released in an easy sigh. This action is a wonderful stress release for both the hips and the upper body. Tension can be allowed to pour out the left foot into the earth, and upper-body tension can be released out the punching fist.

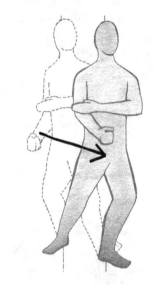

Step Back/Lower Block/Upper Block, Kick Front, #27

Shift the weight back to the right leg, rolling up off the left heel as the hands drop out to the sides.

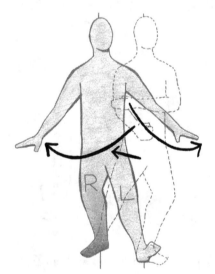

Bring the hands back down to center (the left wrist crossing on top) as the left foot comes back to touch at the right instep.

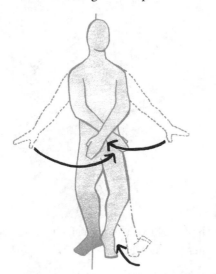

The low block rises to mid block as the left knee rises up.

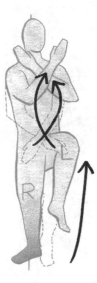

T'AI SCI

Timing on all low, mid, and upper blocks is a 7-count, but over time, the rate of your relaxed breathing will become your timer. Breath and motion become one, allowing effortless flow to fill and soothe your mind, as healing, soothing motion expands Qi and circulation through every relaxing capillary, cell, and atom of your being.

As the mid block becomes an upper block, your palms twist out and begin to strike up and out to the sides, as the left foot kicks out front.

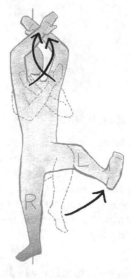

This kick is great for balance. You don't have to perform the kick as high as what's illustrated here. You may begin much lower. Go as high as is comfortable, without leaning backward out of your Vertical Axis. As with all movements, it is done very slowly, placing the foot out in front as you breathe. Observe your balance as you do this.

The hands slowly lower to the sides as the left foot slowly lowers to rest flat on the right side of the right foot.

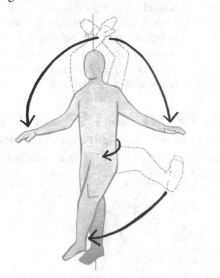

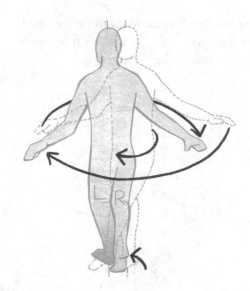

Shift the weight to the right foot as the ³/₄ turn continues to the right.

Pivot on the left ball as the ³/₄ pivot is completed.

> **SAGE SIFU SAYS**
>
> A relaxing exhale always accompanies the weight sinking into a leg to end a pivot. Let your motions become effortless as the breath relaxes out of you and the muscles beneath the muscles let go. Over time, it will feel almost as if the exhale were turning you effortlessly.

Pivoting clockwise, shift the weight slowly to the left foot, pivoting on the right ball (you are working to achieve a ³/₄-turn pivot).

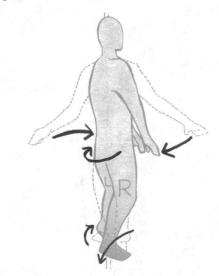

(The following figure is a frontal view of the previous figure, not more turning. See that the weight shifts back to the left foot as the right wrist crosses over the left.)

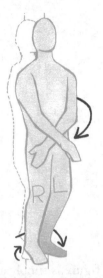

Lower Block/Upper Block Separation of Right Foot, #28

Perform a lower/mid/upper block with the right wrist crossed on top and the weight on the left foot so you can separate the right foot kick. (Refer to earlier lower/mid/upper block separation right foot kicks, and to the Web Video Support for this movement, if you need a refresher before proceeding on to this Parry and Punch.)

Don't psyche yourself into thinking this isn't for you. It's perfect for you. If you are in a wheelchair, this movement will involve your hand arcing down. If you are paralyzed to the waist, you'll give the right-side abdominal muscles instructions to extend upward toward the arcing right hand, and this intention of motion will exercise and coordinate mind and body, relieving tension.

Parry and Punch, #29

When Separation Right Foot completes, place the right heel out to the right side and shift into it, proceeding in to a Parry and Punch. (Refer to earlier Parry and Punch instructions, and to the Web Video Support for this movement, if you need a refresher.)

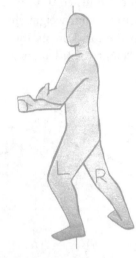

 SAGE SIFU SAYS

When punching or pushing in T'ai Chi, remember that these martial exercises can also be about how we move through our lives: cutting the grass, washing the dishes, or putting groceries in the pantry. If we adopt good postural habits by moving from the dan tien and Vertical Axis while punching, pushing, or pivoting, we will likely use these habits while mowing, lifting, etc.

Chop Opponent with Fist (Pivot and Rotate Fist)(3), #30

When turning, you must empty a leg before pivoting on it so you don't damage the knee. Once a foot is pivoted to the desired position, the weight can be returned to it. From Parry and Punch position, your weight shifts back to the right leg as the torso pivots 180° toward the right, and the "empty" left leg pivots on the heel to the right.

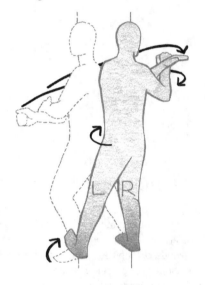

Sink back into the left leg, as the empty right leg pivots on the heel, the toes coming up, to result in a completed 180° turn.

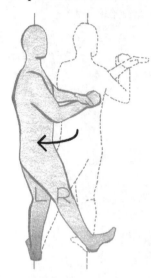

(The following figure is simply a frontal view of the preceding figure.)

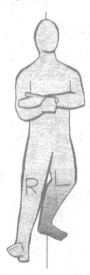

The dan tien sinks forward over the right leg, and the empty left leg comes up to place the empty left foot by the right instep.

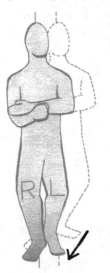

The weight now shifts onto the left leg, placing the empty right foot out, the heel first at a 45° angle front/right, simultaneously drawing the right elbow back to the left to prepare for the upcoming strike.

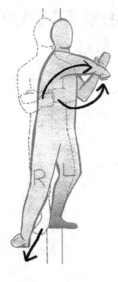

Now, shifting forward into the right leg, throw out the right elbow strike, exhaling and allowing the body to relax into the strike.

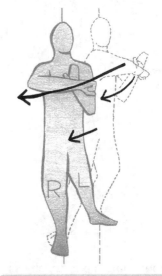

SAGE SIFU SAYS

Allow your mind to empty as you exhale and strike. This lets the pleasure of the relaxed muscle and tissue being gently massaged by the body's motion fill your empty awareness.

The weight continues shifting onto the right foot, with the left foot placed out at a 45° front/left angle.

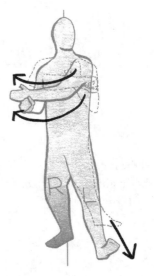

The weight shifts into the left foot as the right fist strikes a punch out to the left/front.

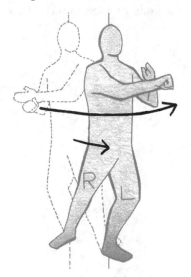

The right foot comes up to touch near the left instep and continues on out at a 45° angle to the front/right.

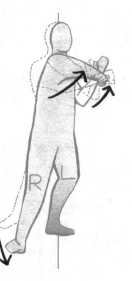

Sink the weight forward to the right foot, and throw another right elbow strike, as shown in the following figure.

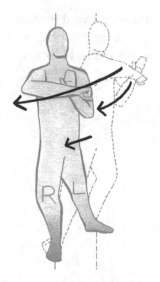

To recap, Chop Opponent involves an elbow strike stepping to the right, a punch stepping to the left, and an elbow strike stepping to the right. Over time, this movement, although martial in appearance, becomes soothing, healing, and almost dancelike in the way it lifts your mood to do it.

Sink to the Earth/ Backward Elbow Strike, #31

Now drop the weight back to the left foot and throw the elbow strike out left/behind. (Don't look back; it's supposed to be a surprise.)

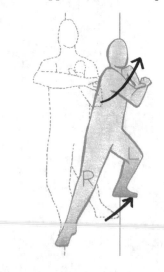

The depth of this strike is all in the bend of the left knee. If your knee feels comfortable with only a slight bend, then that is perfect for you. It will get deeper in time, and there's no rush.

Before coming up out of back stance, turn to the right and aim the right forearm to the front/right 45° angle.

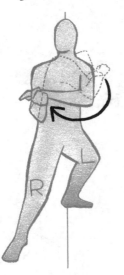

Now the right fist punches upward and the weight springs forward to settle over the right foot, the left wrist still crossed over the right fist, but then turning to follow the right hand to prepare for a Single Whip.

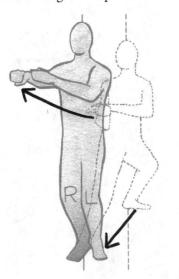

Single Whip, ³⁄₄ Single Whip (Part IV), #32

This begins like normal Single Whip.

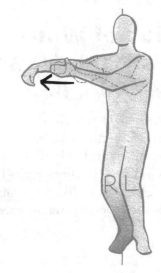

However, the left foot doesn't go all the way out to the left, but the heel touches out left/front at a 45° angle, and then the hand pushes out at that same left/front angle. (See the following figure.)

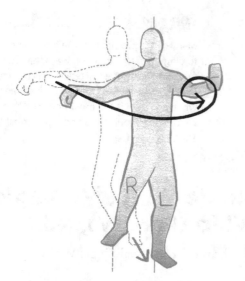

Now, as the left heel extends out front/left 45°, the fists begin to roll back behind/right. The left elbow rises as the right fist lowers. Again, this is much like the hand motion you learned for Wave Hands Like Clouds, except with fists, and Wave Hands Like Clouds steps sideways, while Partition of Horse's Mane steps out at 45° angles forward.

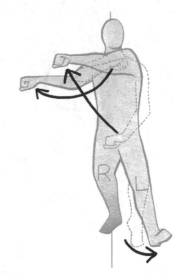

Partition of Wild Horse's Mane (4) and Single Whip, #33

Keep the eyes looking straight ahead (ideally). The right arm/fist settles back from the Single Whip at chest level, the left hand drops down to groin level, and the left toe touches in front of the body. This is much like preparing for the Wave Hands Like Clouds position, except with fists.

As the weight shifts up into the left leg, the left elbow strikes out.

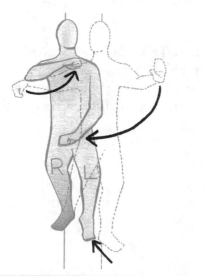

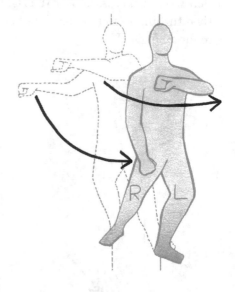

SAGE SIFU SAYS

Just as in Wave Hands, in Partition of Wild Horse's Mane (and all moves, really), the dan tien actually *pulls* the relaxed body and limbs into positions effortlessly as the dan tien sinks into/over the filling leg.

Now, with the left leg full, the right leg extends out to the front/right 45°, with the arms rolling back to the back/left this time.

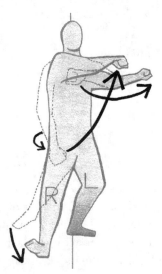

The right elbow strikes out as the weight shifts up to fill the right leg.

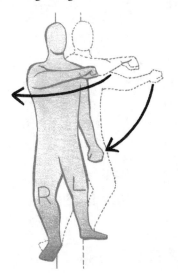

Repeat the second through fifth figures of this movement (for a total of four Elbow Strikes, left, right, left, right strikes in Part Wild Horse's Mane). End after the last right elbow strike by stepping up to form a Single Whip.

When striking forward, the "back" heel should stay down on the floor until the Vertical Axis is completely over the front filling foot. Also remember never to lean into a strike, but to maintain upright posture.

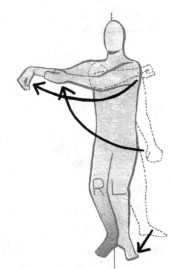

Fair Lady Works at Shuttles, #34

Fair Lady Works at Shuttles is actually a shadow-boxing routine involving blocks and punches used to spar with four opponents coming from four different directions.

From a completed Single Whip position, the right toe reaches back to behind the left heel. The left forearm points up to the sky, and the right arm comes across to rest the right open hand (palm down) just below the left elbow. (See the following figure.)

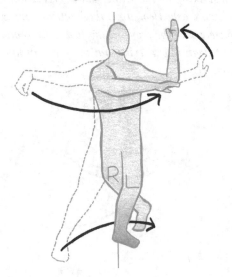

Now fill the right foot as the left pivots on the ball of the left foot. Both the body and the left foot are now pivoting toward the right for a ³/₄ pivot.

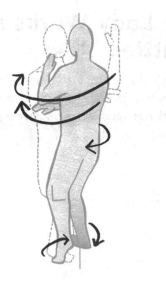

As the pivot completes, sink the weight back on the left foot pivot as the right toes come up, pivoting from the right heel. The left hand drops beside the waist to form a fist as the right hand arcs up to form an up block (palm out).

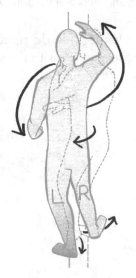

Shifting the weight forward about 60 percent into the right leg, the left hand punches out at about nose height, punching out front just beneath and beyond the blocking right forearm.

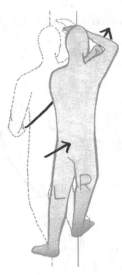

To prepare for the right-hand punch, first empty the left leg and bring it up to touch the left toe by the right instep, as the open left hand (palm down) touches under the right elbow and the right forearm points up to the sky.

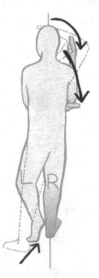

Now the left heel extends out front/left at 45°, the left arm rises in an arc to up block (palm out), and the right fist drops to the right hip, preparing for a punch.

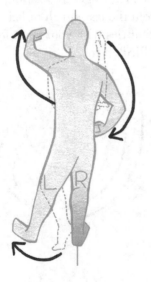

OUCH!

On all pushes, strikes, and punches, the back foot stays down until the front foot is completely full and the push or punch is complete. If you raise the back foot as you strike, the only thing behind that strike is a wobbly little ankle. However, if the back foot stays down, you have the whole planet behind it.

The weight shifts 60 percent forward into the left leg as the torso turns to the left slightly, to deliver the right-fist punch beneath the blocking left arm.

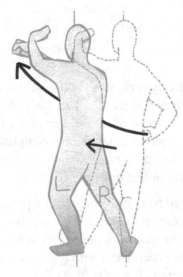

Again, note that the back foot remains down flat until the punch is complete. The body is in a state of "song" or relaxation, allowing the force of the earth to flow up through your body.

(The following figure presents a frontal view of the preceding figure.)

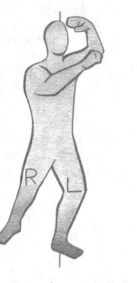

Repeat the movements shown in all these figures up to this point of Fair Lady Works the Shuttles—except, of course, beginning from this punch position, not from a completed Single Whip (as in the very first illustration/instruction of this movement).

To proceed from the punch in the preceding figure to Grasp the Bird's Tail, continue on through the punch, stepping forward out to left catty-corner with your right foot reaching hands up into Grasp the Bird's Tail.

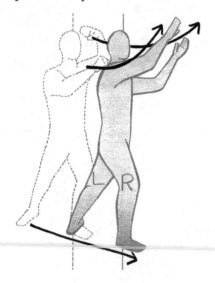

Grasp the Bird's Tail (Part II), #35

Notice this figure is simply a frontal view of the preceding figure. Refer to the earlier Grasp the Bird's Tail instructions, and to the Web Video Support for this movement, if you need a refresher.

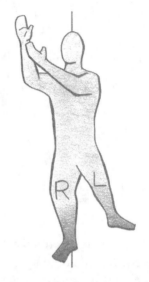

This is the same as the first Grasp the Bird's Tail, except that, to get in position, you step forward from the last punch of Fair Lady Works at Shuttles with your right foot out to Grasp the Bird's Tail.

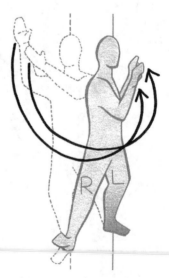

Caressing the Bird's Tail, Waving Hands Like Clouds, and so on, all can return upward cosmic experiences to the solid roots of Earth—and it feels great!

Single Whip (Part V), #36

From Grasp the Bird's Tail, push out to prepare for a Single Whip, with the left leg coming forward as the push completes.

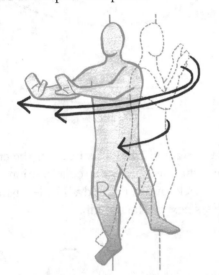

SAGE SIFU SAYS

As you push out on Single Whip, you can enjoy a nice cat-stretch feeling through the shoulders and back, while at other times you get more of a deep letting go feeling. Each time you do a movement, you can enjoy different sensations.

Refer to the first Single Whip instructions (Movement #3), and to the Web Video Support for this movement, if you need a refresher on Single Whip details.

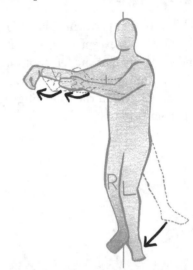

Wave Hands Like Clouds (Part II, Linear Style), #37

Refer to Wave Hands Like Clouds, Part I, if you need a refresher, but end with Single Whip "Down," as in the next figure.

Incorporate breath with each movement. This slows the movement and makes it a relaxing and centering exercise of and by itself. Be absorbed and loosened. Enjoy!

Single Whip Down, Return to the Earth (Part I), #38

Single Whip Down is performed just like regular Single Whip, except you step out left farther and on the ball of the left foot rather than the heel. Note that you do not have to go as low as what's shown in the following figure. Go to your comfort level.

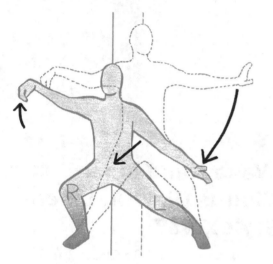

Golden Cock Stands on One Leg (×4), #39

From the Single Whip Down pose, shift the weight over to the right leg a bit more to the empty left leg completely so you can drop the left heel in slightly toward the body, as shown in the following figure.

Now shift the weight up into the left leg and bring the right leg/knee up while forming Duck's Beak with the right hand and sliding it down the top of the right thigh. The left hand falls palm up to the side of the left hip.

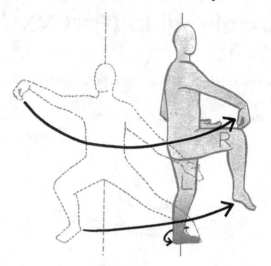

Slide the right hand Duck's Beak off the end of the right knee, up in a circular motion, and around back toward the body. The left palm up still rests next to the left hip.

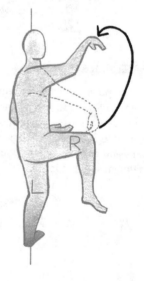

The hand completes a circle down to the chest, with the palm open and ready to push away from the body.

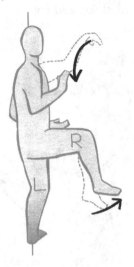

Then the right hand pushes out simultaneously as the right foot kicks straight out in front. Note that you don't have to kick as high as what's shown in the figure. Just go as high as is comfortable and balanced. You'll get higher in time, so just relax and enjoy.

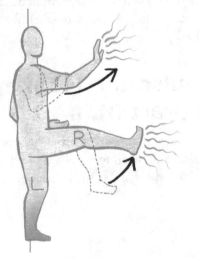

This movement may look tough if you are leafing through the book, but learning the previous movements changes your body and mind in ways that will make this movement feel easy. As always, each of us does it in our own way.

After the kick, place the right foot down slightly out in front of the body, and begin to shift the weight toward the right leg as the palm-up right hand begins dropping down to waist level and the left hand now forms a Duck's Beak.

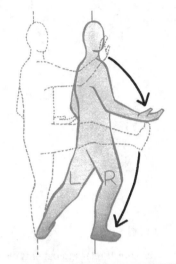

 T'AI SCI

A study by Emory University found T'ai Chi to be *twice* as effective in improving balance as other therapies. By the time you get to this move, your balance is much improved!

Now shift your weight completely into the right leg, and bring the left leg/knee up while forming a Duck's Beak with the left hand, which now slides down the top of the left thigh.

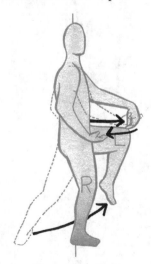

Slide the left-hand Duck's Beak off the end of the left knee, up in a circular motion, and around back toward the body.

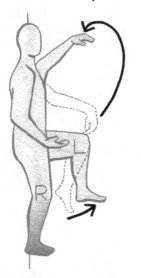

The left hand completes the circle down to the chest, with the palm open and ready to push away from the body.

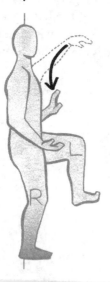

The left hand pushes out simultaneously as the left foot kicks straight out in front. Kick only as high as is comfortable and balanced; it'll get higher in time. Relax and enjoy!

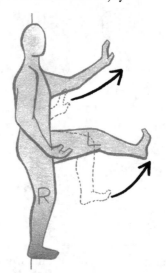

From here, repeat both right and left kicks again as in all the preceding figures for Golden Cock Stands on One Leg, but as you finish the last front kick with the left leg, put the left leg behind you and circle your right hand up from the right side to put you in position for Repulse the Monkey.

Repulse the Monkey (3) (Part II), #40

This Repulse the Monkey series begins with the right hand pushing out, so it's only three repetitions, not four, as in the first one.

Again, enjoy the soothing Long Qi as the palms pass one another, allowing a loosening of the back and shoulders.

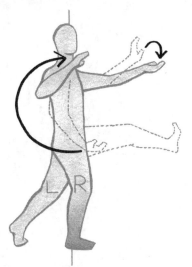

Movements #41 Through #44

You just did #40, Repulse the Monkey, so the next four movements are repeats of movement series 11 through 14. *You already know them!* But go back for a refresher, or just look at the Web Video Support for these movements, if needed. The movements are as follows:

- Stork Covers Its Wing/Sword in Sheath (Part II), #41

- Slow Palm Slant Flying (Part II), #42

- Raise Right Hand and Left: Turn and Repeat (Part II), #43

- Wave Hand Over Light/Fly Pulling Back, #44

Fan Through the Arms (Backhand Slap), #45

This Fan Through the Arms doesn't come up in a rising arc to the left (as the first Fan Through the Arms [Movement #15], did); instead, it swings out front and then to the left side like a back-handed slap. As always, dan tien turning left throws the slap/blow. Let the body loosen and relax the slap out from the dan tien up through the relaxed body and out through the hand.

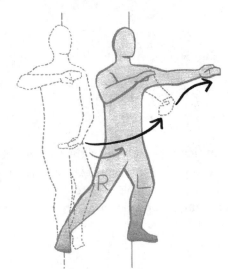

Step Push/Box Opponent's Ears/ Cannon Through Sky, #46

This series, a powerful advancing attack, involves three consecutive blows and three leg lunges forward, toward the opponent.

After the Back Hand Slap, the weight shifts totally to the left leg. This movement begins with the right foot stepping forward, as the hands begin to drop, preparing you to push away in front. (See the following figure.)

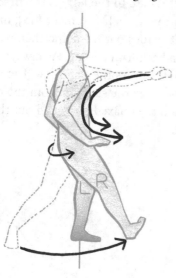

The dan tien now shifts over the front/right foot as you push out. The back heel stays down until the push is complete, before then touching the right instep as shown in the following figure.

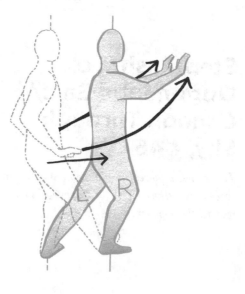

The weight completely fills the left leg so the empty right leg can come up. Now the right heel touches out front as the hands drop down and back, forming fists.

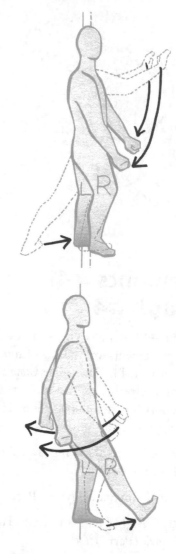

SAGE SIFU SAYS

Notice that on each of these advancing attacks, the hands drop back into a preparatory position as the heel touches out front. This is like cocking a crossbow before you pull the trigger.

The weight shifts toward the right leg while the fists begin to fly out and forward.

The fists arc around to drive into the shadow opponent's ears or temples, carried forward by the force of the dan tien shifting up completely into the right leg.

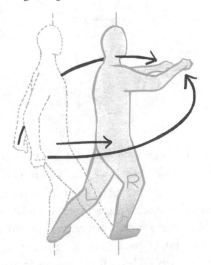

Just as Fanning Through the Arm allows deep tension releases through the hips, Box Opponent's Ears can foster releases through the spine, shoulders, and head.

(The following figure is simply a frontal view of the pose in the preceding figure.)

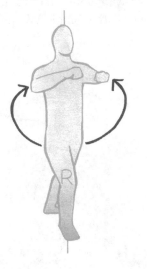

SAGE SIFU SAYS

Allow the blows or strikes to flow through your relaxed body, enabling the power of the earth, beneath your back heel, to pour through your hollow frame. T'ai Chi wisely recognizes that "you" are not powerful unless you let go of the illusion of your own power and control.

The left toe comes up to touch at the right instep as the fist drops down below the waist in front (slightly to the left of the body), and the weight shifts into the left leg.

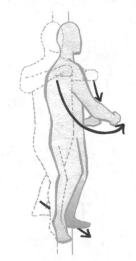

With the right heel touching out, the front (right) fist now circles up and out to drive forward as the weight settles up into the right foot.

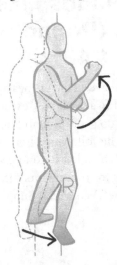

Be sure not to lean into the opponent as you box his ears, push, or strike. Remember, all punches come from shifting the dan tien forward rather than from a lunging upper body.

Single Whip (Part VI), #47

Finishing the right fist punch of Cannon Through Sky, step up with the back/left foot and turn the fist into a Duck's Beak for Single Whip, which begins the next Wave Hands Like Clouds sequence.

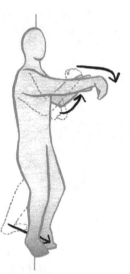

Wave Hands Like Clouds (Round Style; Part I), #48

Round Style Wave Hands is nearly identical to the original Wave Hands, except the hands are held palm up (bottom hand) and palm in (upper), as in the following figure. You already know Wave Hands, but if you need a refresher, see the figures for movements #18 and #19, and refer to the Web Video Support for these movements.

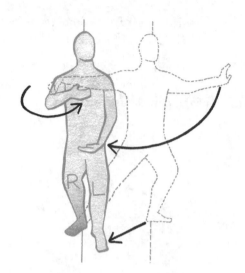

Beware of "creeping-butt syndrome" as you do this exercise. Any lower-back pain is likely caused by the sacral vertebrae (or butt) creeping out behind you, causing an over-arch in the lower back. As your breath relaxes out of you, allow your lower-back muscles to relax and your tailbone to drop. Don't force it—let it relax down.

Single Whip (Part VII), #49

As always, Wave Hands Like Clouds begins and ends here with a Single Whip.

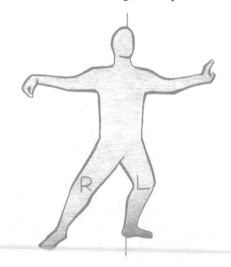

High Pat on Horse (Part II), #50

From Single Whip, the left hand stays in place as the right arm circles around. Once the right arm is around, bend both arms and relax like a horseshoe before patting the horse's behind in front. Shift your weight back to the right foot as the left toe touches out front. (If you need a detailed refresher, refer back to the first High Pat, and to the Web Video Support for this movement.)

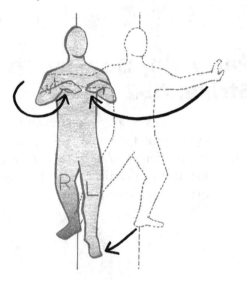

Cross Wave of Water Lily Kick (Part I), #51

From High Pat on Horse, the left heel steps out; then the weight begins to sink into it.

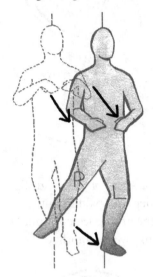

Then the right leg kicks up and out to the left side of front as the hands begin a clockwise circle up and out to the left of the body. The right leg is then pulled back across the body in an arc toward the left, where the now-descending hands circle to touch the foot or leg as it passes underneath, hearing a "pat-pat" sound as they lightly connect in passing, as shown in the following figure. Note that your "pat-pat" sound may come from tapping your shin or thigh rather than your foot. That's fine; don't force it. You'll gain flexibility over time.

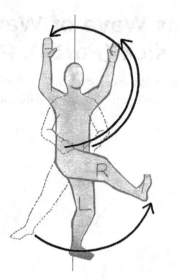

After the "pat-pat" of the hands lightly striking the foot or leg, the palms continue on out to the left as the arcing leg continues on to the right, passing by one another.

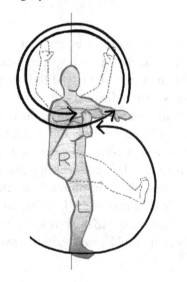

Place the right foot down in a normal Horse Stance, as the palms rise upward above the head to form a right fist and a left up block, preparing for the next movement.

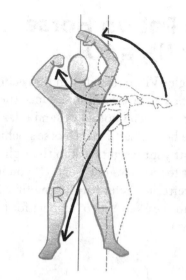

Parry Up; Downward Strike, #52

The right fist strikes down, and the left palm faces outward from the forehead. As you punch downward, try not to bend the back. Again, always maintain the Vertical Axis, aligning the three dan tien points vertically.

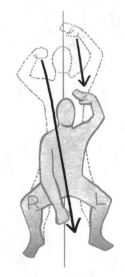

Now step forward with the right foot at a 45° left/frontal angle to Grasp the Bird's Tail.

Movements #53 Through #56

Movements #53, #54, #55, and #56 are a repetition of movements #35, #36, #37, and #38, with one exception: this time around, Movement #55, Wave Hands Like Clouds, is "circular/round" rather than linear (see Movement #48 for hand placement on Round Style Wave Hands if you need a refresher, and to the Web Video Support for these movements). *Wave Hands is a deep loosening of torso muscles and tissue when done well, and each time you do it, your body opens more deeply to be permeated by the expanding Qi energy.*

Step Up to Form Seven Stars, #57

Form Seven Stars and the remaining movement's complexity is at first a bit mind-boggling. However, as that complexity is absorbed into our beings, we grow from it, and that growth feels great! We learn to breathe and relax through seeming chaos, which stretches the mind's capacity to comprehend, absorb, and function. This ability carries over into all aspects of our lives.

OUCH!

Step Up to Form Seven Stars does not have to be done with your knees bent as much as what's shown in the figure. The height of stance or depth of knee bend, as always, is determined by your comfort. Many do this with only a slight bending of the knees, standing almost erect.

From Single Whip Down, shift up into the left foot, forming a fist from the Duck's Beak, and swinging it down and up into a groin punch.

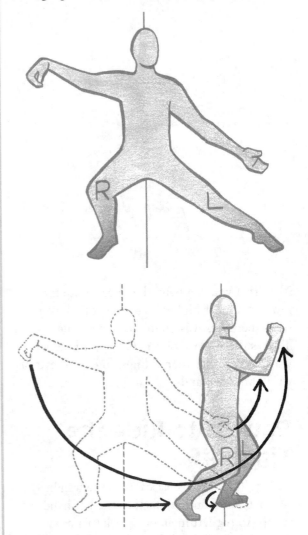

(The following figure is a frontal view of the preceding figure, to help you see the next move's details better.)

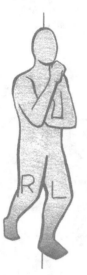

Note that you can bend the knees more for a lower strike, or higher if your knees ask you to bend them less. Listen to your knees and body. That is the essence of T'ai Chi—working with your body rather than riding roughshod over it with harsh demands.

Retreat to Ride the Tiger, #58

The right foot steps back flat so the weight is about 50-50 on both feet, as the left hand swings to the left in an out block (palm out, away from body) and the right hand drops back and down to form a Duck's Beak, as shown in the following figure.

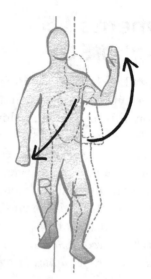

Slanting Body/Turn the Moon, #59

The weight sinks fully into the left leg so the empty right foot can pivot on the toe as the body turns to the right for a $1/4$ turn.

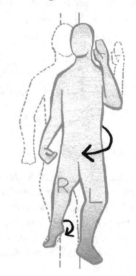

Complete the ¼ turn as the weight settles back on the right leg.

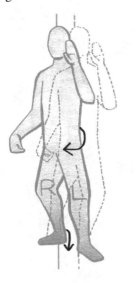

Although these blocks have very direct martial applications, they are soothing to the upper body. Breathe easily and enjoy the circular movement of the right arm blocking up and out while the left hand arcs easily down to form the Duck's Beak behind. As you memorize the movements, the silken flowing will be more and more soothing each time you perform them.

The arms exchange positions, with the right going up (palm in)/left going down (in Duck's Beak) as the left toe touches out in front.

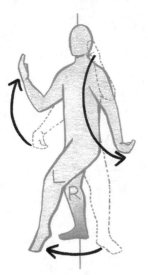

The left foot rises slightly, and as the body pivots, the left foot pivots on the empty left toe and the left heel drops in to the left (moving toward a 180° pivot).

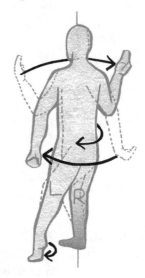

The pivot completes as the weight sinks back into the left foot and the right toe comes up, pivoting on the right heel.

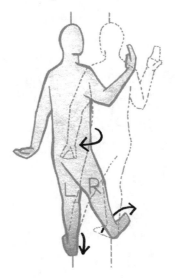

The weight shifts up into the right leg.

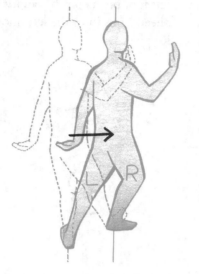

The weight sinks back up into the left leg.

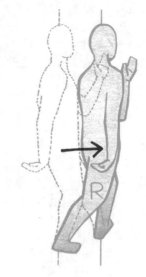

With the weight fully into the right leg, the arms again exchange places, with the left swinging up (out block, palm in facing body) and the right swinging down (side/down block) as the left foot touches the left toe out front.

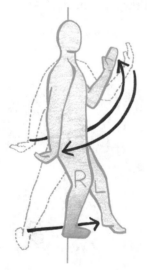

(The following figure is a frontal view of the preceding figure, to help you see the transition to the next movement.)

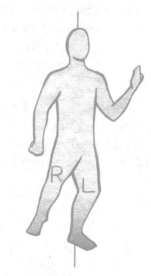

Cross Wave of Water Lily (Part II), #60

This movement is a repetition; see Movement #51 for details if you need a refresher, and to the Web Video Support for this movement.

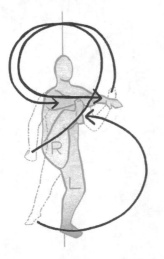

From Cross Wave Kick, keep the hands going out left for Stretch Bow to Shoot Tiger.

Stretch Bow to Shoot Tiger, #61

Imagine you're stretching a bowstring back with the right hand, while the left hand (palm out away from the body) aims the bow out to the left at a 45° angle.

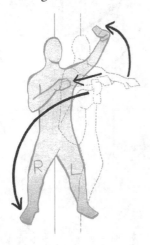

The right hand settles at the right hip.

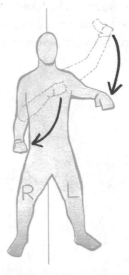

Now the right fist punches out and around to punch out directly in front of the chest.

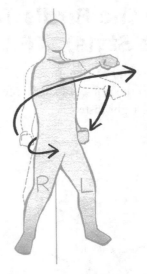

Then the left hand punches out and around while the right hand returns to the hip.

Punch three more times, right, left, right. Both hands punch and return for five punches total, beginning with the right fist and ending with the right fist. Note how the "hip" arrows indicate the punches' power ia in the turning dan tien.

As one hand punches, the other draws back to act as a pulley system. The hand pulling back adds power to the hand punching out. Stay loose; this is where your power is maximized.

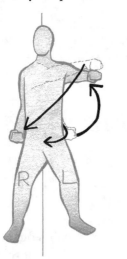

Grasp the Bird's Tail (Right Style), #62

From the last right-fisted punch, bring the fists down to the sides and the left foot over to touch by the right instep.

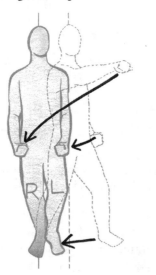

Then go into Grasp the Bird's Tail by dropping the left foot back and reaching up to the right. Complete Grasp the Bird's Tail, and if you need a refresher, go to figures for Movement #2 (the first Grasp the Bird's Tail), and to the Web Video Support for this movement.

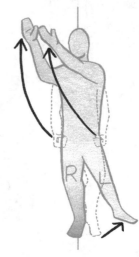

After drawing back the bird's tail, shift back to the left leg, and then shift forward to the right leg, performing a movement just like Green Dragon Rises from the Water. If you need a refresher, review the second, third, and fourth figures for Movement #16 (Green Dragon Rises), and see the Web Video Support for this movement.

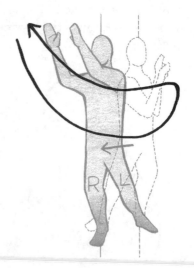

Complete the Green Dragon movement by drawing the arms back and bringing the left leg back, to now stand on both legs with fists at the sides.

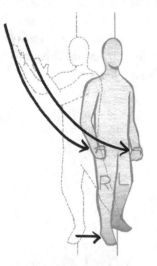

Grasp the Bird's Tail (Left Style), #63

This and the next figure mirror the Grasp the Bird's Tail and Green Dragon–like movement you did in the preceding figures, except, as you'll see, with opposite sides.

Reach up with the hands out to the left (with the left hand on top for this left-style movement and the right hand palm up underneath). The right foot goes out behind.

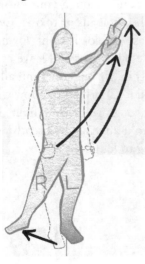

Draw the bird's tail back then push up into the Green Dragon–type movement, this time to the left/front.

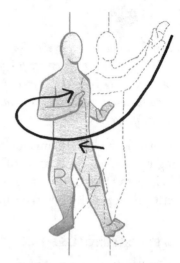

Complete the left-style motion before drawing back to the start point (as shown in the first figure for Movement #62), and now begin Grand Terminus, the very last movement.

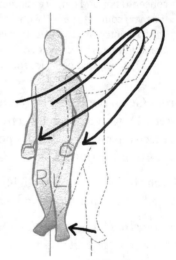

Grand Terminus; Gather Heaven to Earth, #64

Congratulations! You deserve a great, deep bow. Upon completion of learning the entire 64 posture series of the Kuang Ping Yang style form, you are now about to do the most wonderful movement of all, Grand Terminus.

This final move cleanses and reinvigorates the body, leaving you feeling about as terrific as a kid could feel, or as Dave Letterman might say, "Feeling better than people should be allowed."

A T'AI CHI PUNCH LINE

Grand Terminus is the last T'ai Chi movement and the name of that popular yin/yang symbol. The white wave interacting with the black wave symbolizes a balance of all things, hard and soft, force and yielding, concentration and empty awareness. Each time you complete your T'ai Chi forms, you will have integrated all aspects of yourself. Grand Terminus is a completion of renewal and a gateway to greater adventures.

1. From Grasp the Bird's Tail Left Style/ Green Dragon movement, return to the feet-together/fist-at-sides pose to start Grand Terminus.

2. Reach the hands out and slightly back, extending the arms back and outward.

3. As you stretch up, straighten the knees for the first time throughout the entire 64 posture series.

4. Gathering the Qi from all around, the light pours over your relaxing body as the palms turn down.

5. Slowly descend the palms, invoking the cleansing light to wash through every area as the palms pass through.

6. As the hands descend back to your sides, just bask in the soothing healing of this ocean of silken effortless energy washing over and through. Experience effortlessness.

"Experience the light!"

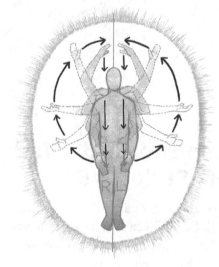

This movement is meant to gather all the light, or Qi, we have generated through the 64 movements. As the hands turn downward at the top of their arcs, allow the light to spill, washing over and through your entire being to cleanse any heavy loads or toxins. Let the feet open to release any loads right down into the earth's gentle pull. This will leave an expanding lightness within, throughout, and all around you in its wake. Continue to allow the light to expand through you throughout the day, touching into it anytime by breathing and being willing to let go.

The Least You Need to Know

- Practicing movements with full, easy abdominal breaths, relax each breath out of the entire body, allowing Qi to flow into and through your limbs as the weight shifts or sinks.

- Allow yourself to become T'ai Chi's natural elegance, as you feel at one with the world while each movement is transforming you.

- Push from your dan tien, not your shoulders or back. T'ai Chi's powerful self-defense moves can be soothing and can teach you to lift groceries or mow the grass correctly.

- T'ai Chi is effortless, showing that most battles are fought in our own minds and hearts, as we learn to let go of what's inevitable and to positively affect what is changeable.

- Adjust movements to fit your mobility. No matter how expansive or limited your mobility, T'ai Chi extends it. Don't force it.

- Pushing and punching with your back foot planted and your body relaxed guides the force of the earth through you, as you relax out of the way, as in Unbendable Arm.

T'ai Chi's Buffet of Short, Sword, and Fan Styles

In This Part

A mere 30 years ago, there was almost no T'ai Chi available to Westerners. T'ai Chi was a Chinese secret. However, today we are fortunate to live in interesting times, as the Chinese would say. In most cities today, you can find a variety of T'ai Chi styles, including not only basic forms, but the more artistic and challenging Sword and Fan Styles as well. In Part 5, feast your eyes on just a sampling of the wide variety of short forms, Sword Style, and Fan Style T'ai Chi now available to you, and then choose an adventure to embark upon. On the new Web Video Support, you'll find *exhibitions of the entire Mulan style basic short form* and an exhibition video of the *Fan* and *Sword Mulan styles* as well. Throughout the rest of Part 5, you are directed at various points to view the new Web Video Support, which enhances the text explanations.

Part 5 ends with a chapter on Push Hands, explaining how this ancient aspect of T'ai Chi is not only a sparring technique but, even more important, a way to observe our state of mind and the way we may *unconsciously* interact with the world around us.

Mulan Quan Basic Short Form

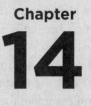

In This Chapter

- Discovering Mulan Quan-style T'ai Chi
- How Mulan Quan promotes grace, beauty, and health
- Understanding what Mulan Quan can do for your heart
- Web Video Support: *Exhibition of Entire Mulan-Basic Short Form,* and detailed video Mulan lesson excerpts

If Mulan Quan's main benefit could be put into one word, it would be *self-esteem*. The artistry of its forms and the mental healing of its practice expand and enhance our self-perception. Mulan's elegant promotion of grace and agility make it perfect for women, yet great for men, too.

See Web Video Support's *About Mulan Styles*, which shows brief samples of this chapter's Mulan Basic, and also the Fan and Sword styles that will follow in Chapters 15 and 16. The video speaks of expanding feminine power, but men should not feel excluded. In Chinese philosophy based on the Yin Yang symbol, both men and women share masculine and feminine aspects, and that we reach our maximum potential by finding balance between the two. This isn't a sexual issue, but a way of approaching the world, the Yin Yang represents the balance of nature: hard-soft, dark-light, force-yielding, etc.

Mulan Quan is a rather modern form of T'ai Chi, but it is derived from an ancient, nearly extinct form of Hua Chia Quan (*Hua* is "flower," *Chia* is "frame," *Quan or Chuan* is "fist"; together they mean "beautiful boxing style"). The Mulan Quan T'ai Chi short form comprises 24 powerful yet delicate movements that flow one into the other. This chapter introduces the first 10 movements of the Mulan style of T'ai Chi, which are also exhibited on the Web Video Support's *Exhibition of Entire Mulan Basic Short Form* where you can view the rest of the 24 Mulan movements as well.

Because T'ai Chi is constant movement, this edition of the book provides this highly useful Web Video Support to expand on the chapter's photos and general text descriptions of the Mulan basic short form. As you saw in Chapter 13, where we provided detailed step-by-step instruction of that

T'ai Chi long form, it took a lot of pages to flesh out all the details. Due to our limitation on page count, this Mulan Basic Style chapter won't break the form down with that intensive instructional detail. But I do want to expose you to various forms of T'ai Chi, so this chapter and the next two will give you overviews, and complete form exhibitions. However, this chapter's Web Video Support's *Mulan Step, Spread Wings, and Float* does provide a deeply detailed instructional on the first three basic Mulan-style movements, in addition to the video exhibition of the entire style, so you can have a rich understanding of Mulan and also a good idea of what class instruction might look like.

Mulan Quan Promotes Elegance and Health

The physical elegance of *Mulan Quan* gives the practitioner a regal appearance that is mesmerizing. The practice of its forms has a wonderful impact on its practitioners' self-esteem. However, the mental healing is just the beginning because this vehicle enhances our physical beauty as well as our physical health:

KNOW YOUR CHINESE

Mulan Quan translated literally is "wooden orchid fist," which means "strong, beautiful fist." (*Mu* is "wood," *lan* is "orchid," and *quan* or *ch'uan* is "fist.") This style is named after the brave young woman Mulan Fa, who selflessly took her aging father's place in the war to save his life. Her story was made famous by Disney's epic animated feature *Mulan*.

Mulan Quan is a highly effective beauty regimen for women. Its ability to simultaneously instill a sense of deep personal power and elegance in motion literally changes the practitioner's personality and outlook on life.

This living embodiment of power, grace, and artistry actually transforms the practitioner. No external cosmetic can come close to the beauty treatment Mulan Quan offers. However, with a more beautiful being within, anything you adorn yourself with externally will be very effective.

Mulan Quan is recommended for many ailments and chronic diseases, including obesity, heart diseases, insomnia, and lower-back problems. (Chinese T'ai Chi masters often say, "You are as young as your spine is flexible.") Reports from Chinese hospitals indicate Mulan Quan has been very useful in stroke rehabilitation treatment and as an adjunct therapy for cancer patients. The Beijing Cancer Center used Mulan as a physical therapy for patients, who then saw improved appetites, weight gain, and better overall health.

If you haven't already, begin this section by viewing the Web Video Support's *Exhibition of the Entire Mulan Style Basic Short Form* section to get a moving visual of the power and grace of Mulan T'ai Chi before continuing.

SAGE SIFU SAYS

Refer to the Web Video Support section for a moving visual video example of the following *Step East to Lotus, Spread Wings on Lotus,* and *Floating Rainbow* movements.

Step East to Lotus

This series of movements rotates both your upper and lower body joints while promoting a deep sense of tranquility. These movements improve your balance and promote an expressive attitude of elegance. The insights in this chapter go deeper than a video or live class could, due to the time limitation of classes and video. However, live-class moving instruction offers a right-brain quality that adds a sooth-ing and hands-free learning dimension. This chapter's Web Video Support gives you a video example of what live Mulan instruction might look like, with detailed instruction on the *Step in the Eastern Direction* and *Spread Wings to Lotus* movements in this section, as well as on the *Floating Rainbow* movement that begins the next section. Again, you'll have a good feel for what class instruction might look like after viewing this on the Web Video Support's *Mulan Step, Spread Wings, and Float* video.

Step in the Eastern Direction

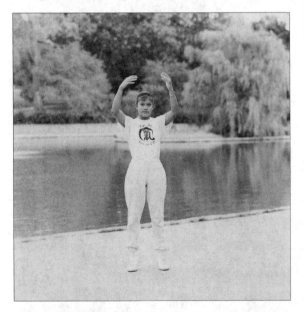

Step in the Eastern Direction helps you relax into your forms. This initial motion's liquid quality places the mind in a pool of tranquility as it prepares the body for what's to come.

Spread Wings on Lotus

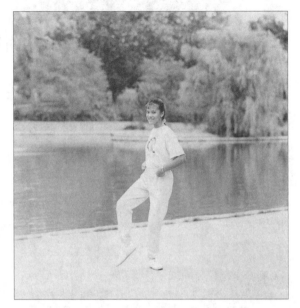

This motion fully rotates the shoulder joints, which can begin to loosen some of the daily stress that tends to accumulate there. This movement challenges and improves your ability to balance, as it carries you through a transitional move toward the next movement.

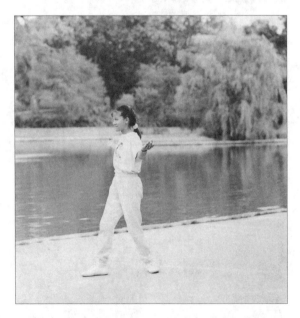

This is the preparatory movement leading to lifting the left leg.

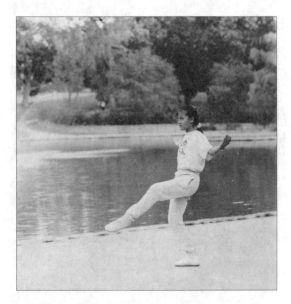

Elegance and balance are the hallmarks of this form. This movement rotates and begins to release deep tensions in the hip sockets and surrounding tissue.

Float Rainbow to Golden Lotus

This series begins with deep loosening throughout the upper body and out to the fingers. Yet it continues to open Qi's flow throughout the entire lower body as well.

Floating Rainbow

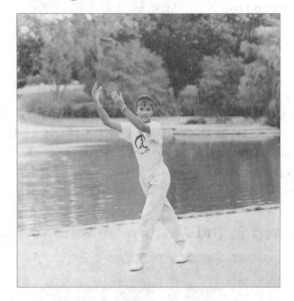

This beautiful extension lives up to its lovely name. Floating Rainbow tones the body and exercises the shoulder, elbow, wrist, and finger joints.

Sit on Golden Lotus

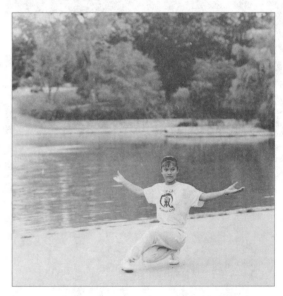

While promoting grace and balance, Sit on Golden Lotus works the thighs and legs. Some feel that the demands T'ai Chi puts on the thighs very effectively promotes circulation to the lower extremities, which allows the heart to work less hard to oxygenate the body.

OUCH!

A *Mulan-style "Ouch!"* cautionary tutorial is included in the Web Video Support. It explains how Mulan Style T'ai Chi can be modified for those who can't see themselves, or their knees, getting into the Sit on Golden Lotus position. T'ai Chi teaches us to be flexible, so the least T'ai Chi can do is be flexible to our needs, right?

Ride Wind to Dragon Flying

These motions promote a very subtle internal awareness of balance and movement. Every part of the body is worked and loosened in this series.

Ride With Wind and Waves

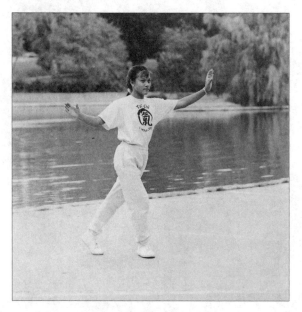

A very subtle shifting of the weight between the front and back legs exercises all the muscle groups in the lower body. The arm movements likewise loosen joints and tonify muscles throughout the upper body.

Dragon Flying Toward Wind

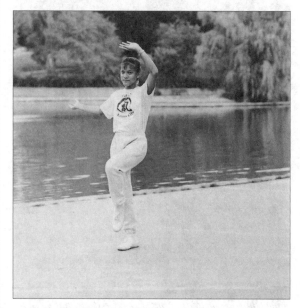

This movement is a very subtle internal motion that focuses awareness within.

Purple Swan Tilts Its Wings

See Web Video Support's *Purple Swan Tilts Its Wings* for a look at how movements might be broken down in a live class (www.idiotsguides.com/taichi).

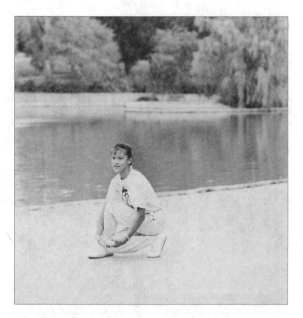

Nearly every muscle is loosened and strengthened by this move, but the abdominal muscles benefit especially. This series promotes spinal flexibility.

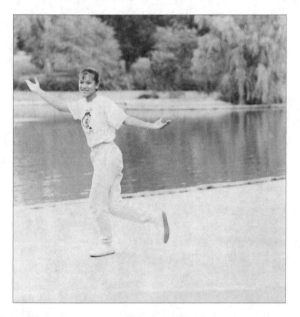

This exquisite movement is not only beautiful to the eye, but it also promotes health, balance, and flexibility through the torso and spine.

The Least You Need to Know

- Mulan Quan movements promote elegance and balance.
- Mulan Quan promotes flexibility through the spine and extremities, which may keep you feeling young.
- Mulan Quan can tone muscles and especially strengthen the thighs, which may be very good news for your heart.

Mulan Quan Fan Style

In This Chapter

- Discovering the benefits of Mulan Quan
- Using Mulan Quan as emotional therapy
- Finding the pearl within you through Mulan Quan
- Web Video Support: *Exhibition of Entire Mulan Quan Single Fan Style*

Mulan Quan is based in traditional T'ai Chi movement and *wushu* (Chinese for "martial arts"). However, it adds aspects of Chinese folk dance and gymnastics to provide a vessel of motion for the beauty of the practitioner to be poured into. Mulan Quan, therefore, reaches to the outward limits that the practitioner can express, both with the wushu aspects and even as a spectacular sword form (which I give examples of in Chapter 16). Yet it also explores the softest, most delicate aspects of the user, which is most beautifully expressed in the Mulan Quan fan style. (Note that several other T'ai Chi styles offer fan versions, in addition to the Mulan style; by exploring via www.worldtaichiday.org, other books, and Appendix C, you'll find much more on this.)

There are two fan styles: the single fan and the double fan. This chapter introduces you to the basic single-fan style, by exposing you to how the forms look and elaborating on how they're performed and what benefits each provides.

This chapter gives you an overview of some of the Mulan Fan Style forms; however, its Web Video Support provides the *Exhibition of Entire Mulan Quan Single Fan Style* video, showing all the movements in this form, meant to enhance your general knowledge of T'ai Chi fan styles.

Mulan Quan styles are rapidly gaining popularity and have been involved in exhibitions and competitions from Beijing to Kansas City. Work is being done to eventually introduce Mulan Quan as Olympic competition.

Flying Bees Through Leaves

This section's movement works and stretches the entire body. Refer to the Web Video Support's *Exhibition of Entire Mulan Quan Single Fan Style* as you look through the following descriptions.

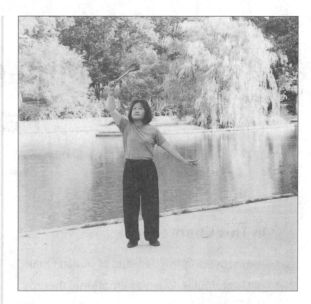

Flying Bees Through Leaves is quite graceful, but the movement is only a vessel through which to express yourself. Enjoy as you experience your own grace being poured into the vessel of your T'ai Chi. Furthermore, it tonifies the entire body from head to toe.

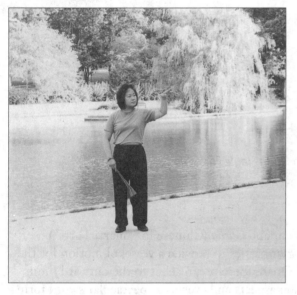

Notice here how this motion exercises the arm muscles and loosens the joints as you relax into the pose.

Stretching Cloud to Floating

Promoting equilibrium and refinement, this series is internal and subtle, yet externally strengthening to all muscles.

Stretching Left Foot

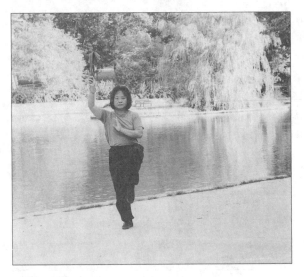

While strengthening the leg muscles, this movement fosters an internal awareness that improves your balance.

Cloud Lotus Floating

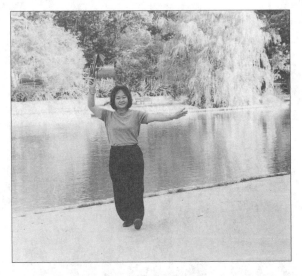

The external motion is refined by encouraging the practitioner to "feel elegant." Of course, besides that mental and spiritual benefit, it has a very practical purpose of working and loosening the arm's joints.

Miracle Touching Ocean

The beautiful names of this section are inspiring, but the movements hold even more. While creating very solid strengthening, these movements also affect the way we feel about ourselves. Mulan Quan can literally transform our self-esteem.

Miracle Dragon Lifting Head

Miracle Dragon Lifting Head is actually well named because moving in a posture of head-lifted self-esteem (which T'ai Chi requires) actually transforms the practitioner over time in ways that may seem miraculous. Mulan Quan may be a powerful adjunct therapy for the many emotionally affected conditions, such as eating disorders, facing some young people today.

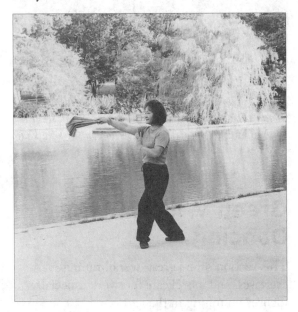

The Miracle Dragon Lifting Head encourages the practitioner to lengthen, thereby enhancing and promoting good posture.

In Chinese folklore, the dragon represents the *yang* (expressive) aspect of power and majesty, which may be why it's commonly used in T'ai Chi imagery to help practitioners access and evoke the limitless power of their dynamic nature.

Swallow Touching Ocean

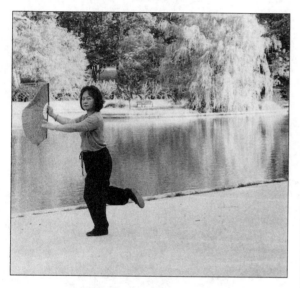

This movement powerfully strengthens the leg and back muscles while promoting release of tension through the back. (For a visual example of this movement, see it in the Mulan Fan Style T'ai Chi *section on the Web Video Support.)*

Green Willow Twigs Dancing

This section offers great overall toning exercises, and its delicate footwork especially focuses on toning in the leg.

Green Willow Twigs Swaying

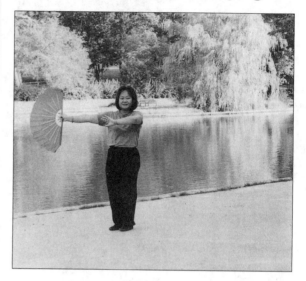

The deep rotation of the hip of Green Willow Twigs Swaying allows a subtle internal awareness of how the body shifts from its power point, or dan tien. (For a visual example of this movement, see it in the Web Video Support's Mulan Style T'ai Chi *section.)*

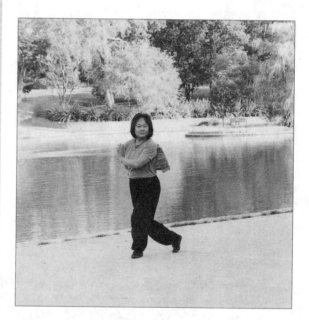

This posture works all the joints and muscles, offering great strengthening and toning throughout the entire frame.

Dancing in Wind

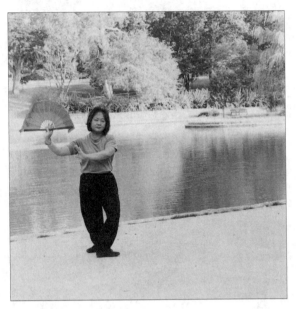

The delicate footwork of Dancing in Wind is a great toning exercise for the legs, and its subtlety offers a meditative quality as it's performed.

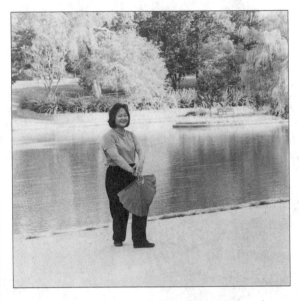

The shoulder and wrist rotations of this motion release stress and soothe your mind as you flow through its graceful ways.

Dun Huang Flying Dance

While challenging the lower body to maintain balance, the upper body is rotated and flexed in a soothing, relaxed way.

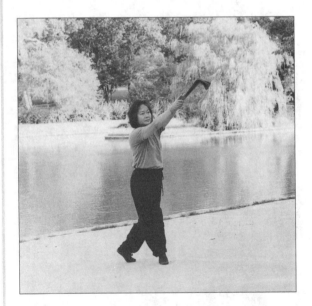

The spine and waist are flexed gently, promoting a litheness that is not only lovely but enhances all aspects of health, according to Traditional Chinese Medicine.

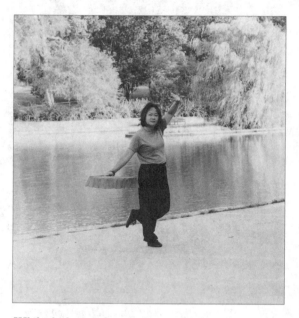

While the legs work and adjust to subtle posture changes, the upper body is gently stretched and loosened.

The Least You Need to Know

- Mulan Quan can change your self-image, which can positively change your physical appearance over time.

- Mulan Quan's self-esteem promotion may be a wonderful adjunct therapy to women facing emotional problems, as well as men.

- The elegance Mulan Quan offers is really within you right now! Mulan Quan only helps you to loosen up and express that part of yourself.

Mulan Quan Sword Style

In This Chapter

- Developing internal power using the sword form
- Promoting balance and strength through elegance
- Balancing raw power and subtle beauty within your mind, heart, and body
- Web Video Support: *Exhibition of Entire Mulan Quan Sword Style*

Mulan Quan is great for everyone, but women especially greatly benefit from the elegance and tender beauty it promotes. However, another profound benefit is its tremendous yet subtle power. The power of Mulan Quan is perhaps most dramatically observed in the performance of Mulan Quan sword style.

This chapter exposes you to some of the Mulan sword form postures, their benefits, and points to enrich your experience with the postures. Several styles of T'ai Chi offer sword styles as well as the Mulan. You can learn much more about various T'ai Chi sword forms from www.worldtaichiday.org, other books, and Appendix C.

This book's Web Video Support provides an exhibition of the entire Mulan Quan sword style, meant to enhance your *general* knowledge of T'ai Chi sword styles.

Preparation to Eye on Sword

This section quietly prepares the mind and body before launching into the expansive motion of the Mulan Quan sword style. Refer to the Web Video Support's *Exhibition of Entire Mulan Quan Sword Style*, www.idiotsguides.com/taichi, as you proceed through these descriptions.

Preparation Stance

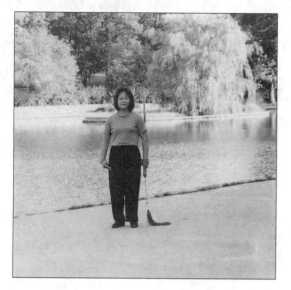

The Preparation Stance is meant to focus and relax the mind, body, and heart.

Left Foot Half-Step with Eyes on Sword

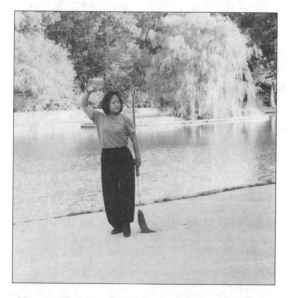

Here is a full rotation of the shoulder and arm as the sword arm goes into a clockwise rotation. (Again, for a visual example of this Mulan sword style movement, see the Mulan Sword T'ai Chi section on the Web Video Support.)

Forward Step to Low Jab

This series works the entire body, loosening and lengthening it from head to toe.

Forward Step, Holding Sword Under Elbow

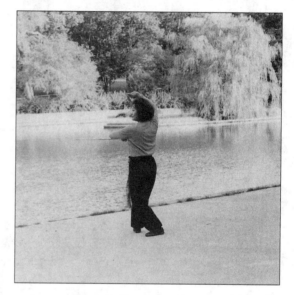

Your right foot steps right, with the weight shifting forward. Bring your sword-wielding arm straight out to the side and then around to the front, bent elbow. This movement helps to loosen the entire body as you breathe and allow your Qi to flow through all your limbs, as well as through the sword hand.

Sword Exchange, Turn Body, and Low Jab

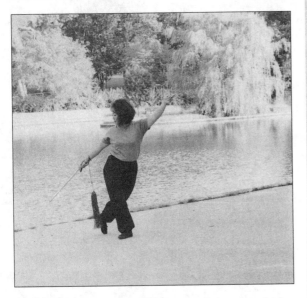

This movement fosters an elongation of the entire frame as the hips are rotated and the body loosens. (See Web Video Support.)

Sword Upright to Balance Body

In these motions, your entire body is strengthened with very desirable and select muscle toning.

Body Return, Step with Sword Upright

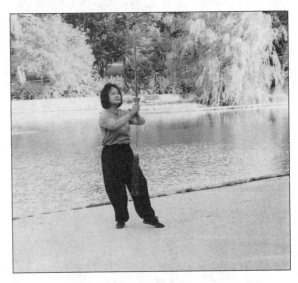

The abdominal muscles are toned in this movement as the back and legs are worked as well.

Vertical Sword and Balance Body

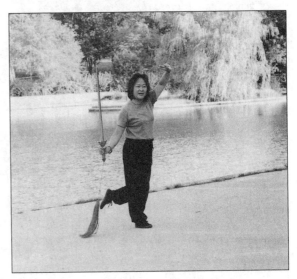

The shoulder and wrist joints are exercised here, which helps the practitioner avoid calcium deposit buildup in joints that might negatively affect flexibility. Mulan Quan enables you to age while maintaining fluid, elegant flexibility.

Turn Around to Up-Jab

Balance, posture, and leg strength are found in this set of movements.

Turn Around, Lower to Sitting Position, Sword Upright

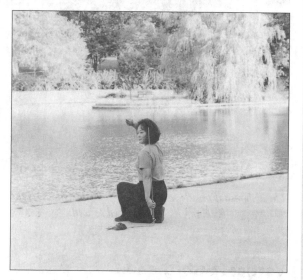

Leg muscles are both stretched and strengthened as you breathe and lengthen through this movement.

Step Up, Lower to Sitting Position, Sword Up-Jab

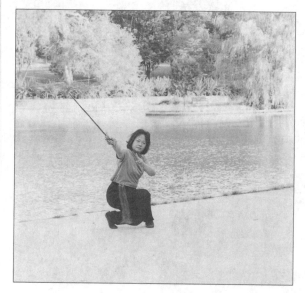

Practicing this movement with an attitude of elegance and style will have a wonderful impact on both your balance and your posture.

Level Sword to Lift Leg

The following set of postures tonifies and beautifies your body in many ways.

Level Sword, Turn Body, and Lift Knee

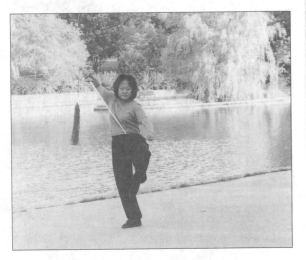

While improving your balance, Level Sword, Turn Body, and Lift Knee also tones and strengthens.

Lift Leg, Side Step, Side Chop with Sword

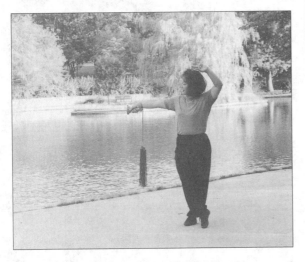

This may be the most beautiful of all Mulan Quan sword style movements, yet it also works to loosen the body's muscles and joints.

The Least You Need to Know

- The sword form promotes a sense of gentle power.
- Remember to make the forms fit your body.
- Let the thought of elegant power elongate your form through the practice of these movements.

The Art & Science of Push Hands

In This Chapter

- Learning the art of Push Hands
- Using Push Hands to learn about yourself
- Discovering how masters resist many opponents effortlessly
- Web Video Support: *Push Hands Shifting*

Push Hands is a paradox. It is a sparring technique in a way, but it's also a quiet tool of self-awareness. The way you see Push Hands says as much about you as it does about Push Hands. To one person it may look like a delicate dance, while another may see a physical contest not unlike a sumo-wrestling match. Actually, it can be a tiny bit of both.

By moving your dan tien in toward your opponent, your weight shifts toward your front foot and your Qi flows through the body, exerting a very relaxed force (like the unbendable arm). So as your hand pushes toward your opponent, if your opponent is stiff, this will likely uproot his stance, causing him to lose his balance. If he is supple and yielding, he will absorb your attack and respond in kind.

The goal, however, is not necessarily to forcefully uproot your opponent. Rather, the purpose of Push Hands is to become accustomed to the ebb and flow of physical energy expressed in motion and how *you* respond to it. If your opponent is pushy and abrupt, he will likely overextend himself as he attacks. This attack isn't violent; it's just his arm extending into your chest or heart area. When he overextends, he will come in off-balance *if you yield*. When he retreats to try to catch his balance, he is vulnerable. A slight push can send a larger, more powerful opponent reeling when he is out of center. The Web Video Support's *Push Hands Shifting* illustrates how the practitioner does not overextend when pushing or receding, but maintains postural alignment while flowing through the changing positions. It also will recap how QiGong breathing coordinates with motion, and how energy flow is part of each T'ai Chi or QiGong physical movement.

When pushing hands, you seek to maintain a delicate contact with your opponent while remaining flexible and calmly aware of yourself. Push Hands is mainly about observing and responding with the most power and least effort. The expanded awareness and practice of experiencing different aspects of self that Push Hands promotes makes us more fluid and better able to become whatever is required and most useful at any given moment. Push Hands is training in being all things.

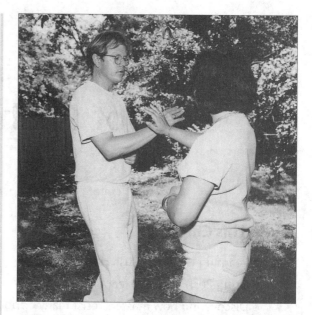

The photos are of right-handed Push Hands, and both the advance and the retreat take the form of body and arm counter-clockwise ovals, as you push with your right hand into their heart. They yield by letting their body shift back and toward their right, and then the oval goes back toward you from their right side, as you yield back and to your right. The goal of Push Hands is not to resist, but to yield and deflect incoming power. As you sink back into your back leg to retreat from the incoming push, the goal is to let your upper body loosen, so that the pushing opponent has nothing to push against. Remember to breathe (tip of tongue lightly touching roof of mouth, just behind top/front teeth) and let the body relax and loosen as you exhale and push, or inhale and yield, alternating pushes and your sinking retreats.

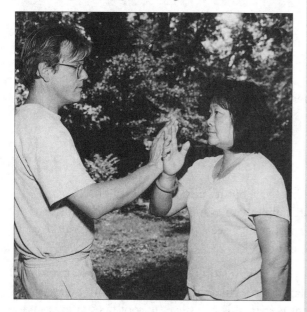

Notice that the pusher is focusing his energy toward the other by facing his palm toward the opponent as he pushes. The energy center, Lao Gong, on the pericardium energy meridian is in the center of the palm of the hand. This is a highly sensitive point and also projects energy outward. Also, notice how the push comes from the dan tien, or lower body, as it shifts forward toward your opponent. You don't lean out of vertical alignment, but rather let your body ride stacked up above the dan tien. The power of your push comes up from the earth, through your relaxed body carried effortlessly forward by your advancing dan tien, and out through your open hand.

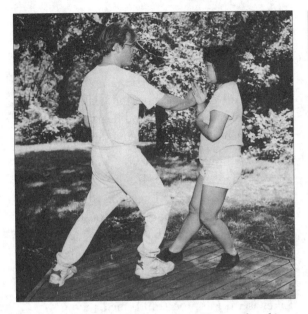

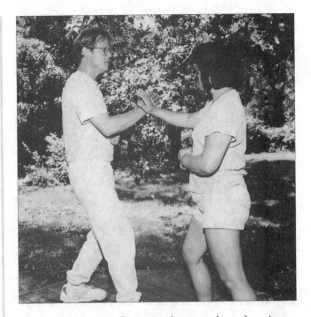

Remember the story of the snake yielding to the white crane's attacks? Your surrendering retreats, each time your opponent pushes toward you, yielding you out of the way as your pelvis/dan tien rotates to the side, removes any power of the pushing opponent. Again, this isn't done by resisting, or by pushing back with force, but by relaxing the body to let it turn more easily from the dan tien or pelvis, out of the way of the push. Then when the opponent has extended herself forward, her tendency will be to pull back to regain her vertical posture or balance point, as your now-pushing hand and body surges toward her as she now yields to your push. This practice will develop a subtlety of awareness of force and balance dynamics that will make your efforts in T'ai Chi and life ever more powerful and yet more effortless.

Think of a butterfly resting between the exchanging hands or wrists as you push or retreat from your opponent. Try to be sensitive enough to anticipate motions so your advancing opponent does not crush the butterfly as you lithely retreat. And in turn, as you advance on your opponent by pushing with your right hand, you will apply pressure to his wrist, but he will deflect you and avoid crushing the butterfly by yielding as his body rotates in a relaxed surrender off to his right (your left). This pushing and retreating motion will take on a counter-clockwise oval-shaped motion when you and your opponent use your right hands/wrists to push and yield. When using the left hand, it will be a clockwise oval, as you push toward your partner's heart, and he deflects you off to his left (your right), and he then pushes into your heart and you deflect him to your left (his right).

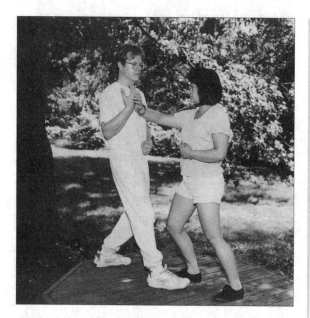

Realize that, just as with all T'ai Chi, Push Hands is not physical force as we usually think of it.

SAGE SIFU SAYS

When pushing hands, envision a butterfly poised between your wrist and the wrist of your opponent. Try to have just enough pressure between them so the butterfly doesn't fly away, yet not so much that you crush it. Your goal is to maintain subtle contact, yielding when attacked and advancing when your opponent yields.

Push Hands is done with the same effortless power as the Unbendable Arm presented in Chapter 3. Also notice that, in this exercise, the unused hand is a fist held at the ready near the chest. In T'ai Chi, as in all martial arts, nothing is done without reason. The resting hand is ever ready to spring into action. Don't think in fear, but in relaxed alertness.

The Psychology of Push Hands

Push Hands is about observing. As with all T'ai Chi, it is all-encompassing and has as much to teach us about our mind and heart as it does about our physical balance and dexterity.

You know how people say you can tell a lot about someone by his or her handshake? That's not an old wives' tale. The same is true of Push Hands. If I am aggressive, pushy, and overpowering in life, this will show up in my Push Hands technique. I will often find myself overextending or over-emphasizing the attack, with little thought of staying centered. Likewise, if I am too timid, the dancing exchange of Push Hands will seem limp and lifeless—not much fun. The goal, as always, is to strike a balance between the raging bull and the shrinking violet, the Yin and the Yang, that resides within all of us. Both aspects of self are perfect and absolutely necessary to making us a whole being, just as nature is perfect because it contains these extremes and everything between.

Practicing Push Hands can raise the raging bull from the shrinking violet and bloom delicate petals from the raging bull. As T'ai Chi expands your beingness, Push Hands can help by illustrating in an external social element the internal tendencies you may not have noticed about yourself or others.

Eventually, Push Hands may become a powerful business or marriage-counseling tool because it helps illuminate how people interact. It's not about labeling one person's technique as good or bad, but rather about becoming aware of people's tendencies so we can interact more effectively, no matter where they're coming from.

Different Forms of Push Hands

There are several different forms of Push Hands. Some incorporate very directly applicable martial techniques that involve deflecting blows and tripping your opponent as he loses his balance. These are fun but not necessary for most T'ai Chi training. If you're curious about these techniques, shop around for an instructor well versed in Push Hands. If your instructor doesn't do Push Hands, you may find weekend workshops that teach the techniques, or video instructionals, or perhaps there may be someone who knows at T'ai Chi club gatherings. Contacting the T'ai Chi organizations listed in Appendix A or at www.worldtaichiday.org may help lead you to teachers or events that specialize in Push Hands.

OUCH!

For people in a more frail physical condition using T'ai Chi as therapy, more martial Push Hands techniques are not advised and really not necessary. You can play a basic Push Hands routine with a partner you can trust to be gentle enough. Or you can skip Push Hands altogether. These tools are toys to play with. We play only with toys we enjoy and that make us feel good, which is the point of toys in the first place.

Legends of the Masters

There are stories about T'ai Chi masters who exhibit almost superhuman strength when being pushed or when pushing others. Bill Moyers' documentary on the healing mind showed an old Chinese master who could withstand the onslaught of a half-dozen pushing students without being budged and seemingly without really exerting himself. This same master also sent those students flying off across the lawn with hardly any indication of movement on his part. I met such a master, a Russian T'ai Chi teacher named Vladimir Pankov, who had mastered this skill, and he stunned my large athletic son when he visited us in America and demonstrated some techniques on him.

There is an area of T'ai Chi that focuses on energy projection, called *fa-jing*, and it is claimed that some masters (like the one Bill Moyers met) can use the force of their Qi to withstand attacks and send opponents flying. However, there may be a physically explainable element to this ability as well.

Master Henry Look, one of the great T'ai Chi masters, was an engineer by trade, and he saw T'ai Chi from that angle. If the human body is a structure like a building, engineering principles may explain some of this. If just the right structuring of materials in just the right way can build buildings that resist massive pressure in weight-bearing demands, can't the body likewise do so? If a T'ai Chi master were very attuned to how his body aligned bones and muscles with the support of the earth beneath, he would be more able to resist great external force by using internal engineering principles by relaxing his body out of the way between opponent and earth (see Unbendable Arm). Also, as in Push Hands, if one was so self-aware of these principles, one could be subtly attuned to when this opponent offered the slightest break in solidity. Then the master would be able to uproot the opponent with the least bit of force. This would seem magical to the untrained eye, just as a remote control would seem magical to a caveman. However, it may really be just a matter of developing a subtle physical awareness.

The Least You Need to Know

- Push Hands helps you become self-aware.
- Push Hands improves your balance and power.
- For those rehabilitating from injuries or with balance problems, Push Hands may best be avoided.
- Masters' feats may seem magical, but at their root is a high human science evolved in China.

Life Applications

In This Part

Part 6 demonstrates how T'ai Chi can change your life and our world. T'ai Chi becomes a gateway to looking at life and health in a completely different way. By seeing our world and ourselves in a proactively empowered way, we can literally change the course of our lives and make our world a much better place.

Part 6 details illnesses T'ai Chi can help treat. It also explains how corporations can support their employees' development of healthy lifestyles while maximizing profits by increasing productivity. You'll also learn how, in addition to business savings, society may save big on avoided social problems by incorporating T'ai Chi at all levels of society, beginning with elementary public education.

Last but not least, you'll discover how T'ai Chi and QiGong can help literally change our world by enabling all of us to maximize our ability to be healing forces.

T'ai Chi as Therapy for Young and Old

In This Chapter

- Kids, seniors, women, and men—everyone can benefit from T'ai Chi
- T'ai Chi and sports: a winning combination
- T'ai Chi as a health therapy

T'ai Chi is for everyone, and this chapter provides details on how T'ai Chi benefits specific people, their health conditions, and their athletic activities—with even more information in this fourth edition. In fact, anyone, but especially health professionals and T'ai Chi/QiGong teachers, will find the last part of this chapter a powerful reference, with maladies listed in alphabetical order and details on how T'ai Chi or QiGong might help.

If you are treating a specific condition, you will find here an introduction to how T'ai Chi might assist your ongoing therapy. Seniors will find out why T'ai Chi is the very best thing they can do for themselves. Specific reasons why children, men, and women should practice T'ai Chi are provided as well.

This chapter will also assist parents and T'ai Chi teachers who want to start a T'ai Chi class for kids. Kids are taught differently from adults, and this chapter gives teachers or parents some great insights into helping their kids make the most of T'ai Chi—and have fun doing it. It also provides specific information on new research regarding T'ai Chi's benefit to young people with attention-deficit and hyperactivity disorder (ADHD).

T'ai Chi for Kids

Kids are the embodiment of change, and change can be very stressful. Their minds and bodies grow at phenomenal rates, so they are constantly having to work with new and different bodies, making coordination and balance a big issue. T'ai Chi, with its emphasis on balance, is well suited to address these challenges.

Preparing for Athletics and Life

T'ai Chi works to integrate the mind and body, skeletal and muscular systems, and left brain and right brain. In physical terms, this centering is built around an awareness of moving with good posture and from a low center of gravity, or the Vertical Axis and the dan tien.

Some people, such as gifted athletes, are naturals at this kind of self-awareness and movement. Because most of our kids are not naturals, T'ai Chi can be a most effective way to help them prepare for athletics and simply be comfortable in their rapidly changing bodies.

Treating Attention Deficit Disorder

Attention deficit disorder (ADD) is a growing problem, not only with children but with adults as well. T'ai Chi is a wonderful adjunct therapy for treating ADD because it augments many of the mood-management techniques recommended for ADD sufferers. A University of Miami School of Medicine study shows T'ai Chi is a powerful therapy for ADHD. The children participating in the study saw a drop in ADD symptoms and an enhanced ability to focus, concentrate, and perform tasks.

Edward M. Hallowell, MD, and John J. Ratey, MD, experts on the management of ADD, wrote, "Exercise is positively one of the best treatments for ADD. It helps work off excess energy and aggression in a positive way, it allows for noise-reduction within the mind, it stimulates the hormonal and neurochemical systems in a most therapeutic way, and it soothes and calms the body."

T'ai Chi's slow, mindful movements have much to offer people who suffer from ADD. The following table explains why T'ai Chi may be a perfect ADD therapy.

T'ai Chi and ADD

What Experts Suggest	What T'ai Chi Offers
Set aside time for recharging batteries, something calm and restful, like meditation.	T'ai Chi is a mini-vacation.
Daily exercise that is readily available and needs little preparation can help with the blahs that occur and with overall outlook.	T'ai Chi is easy, requires no preparation, and is a daily mood-elevator.
Observe mood swings; learn to accept them by realizing they will pass. Learn strategies that might help bad moods pass sooner.	T'ai Chi is a tool for self-observation of feelings and for letting those feelings go.
Use "time-outs" when you are upset or over-stimulated. Take a time-out; go away, and calm stress.	T'ai Chi can be performed in the bathroom at school or work, giving you a break from the down.
Let go of the urgency to always finish things quickly by learning to enjoy the process.	T'ai Chi's slow, flowing routine is about letting go of the outcome and learning to love the process.
ADD usually includes a tendency to over-focus or hyperfocus at times, to obsess or ruminate over some imagined problem without being able to let it go.	T'ai Chi teaches the practice of letting go on a mental, emotional, and physical level with each exhale.

Teaching T'ai Chi to Kids

All kids—not just kids with ADD—usually have difficulty with the slowness of T'ai Chi. Therefore, you simply speed it up when teaching children. But do teach each child at his or her own pace; some can go slower than others.

SAGE SIFU SAYS

T'ai Chi for kids with ADD will not look like T'ai Chi for adults. It will be faster.

Give kids constant recognition for their T'ai Chi accomplishments. Ask each kid to demonstrate her new movements for the class at the end, and have everyone applaud. If a kid forgets a move, jump in and do it with her. Over the weeks, she will look forward to the recognition and will practice more.

T'ai Chi is a loose thing, not a rigid thing. It can work for everybody and can be taught in many fun ways. Keep a kid's T'ai Chi class moving, and include stretching exercises from yoga or aggressive calisthenics to use up excess energy. Then, as the kids get more tired, ease them into slower movement.

Kids can do QiGong meditations, too. It isn't anything like adult meditations; more and different images work. Try the children's meditation CD (see Appendix C) for examples.

T'ai Chi for Seniors

Seniors can find no better exercise in the world than T'ai Chi. *Prevention* magazine has reported that "T'ai Chi may be the best exercise for people over the age of 60 … providing cardio fitness, muscle strength, and flexibility all in one simple workout that is easy on the joints." According to some studies, T'ai Chi may help build bone mass and connective tissue, with zero joint damage. Other studies show T'ai Chi is twice as good as any other balance exercise in the world. Because complications from falling injuries are the sixth-largest cause of death among seniors, this is a very big deal. For seniors with chronic conditions, T'ai Chi can help treat many maladies. (For details, see the section "The Therapeutic Powers of T'ai Chi and QiGong" at the end of this chapter.)

If your mobility is limited in some way, even if you're in a wheelchair, that's no problem. There is a T'ai Chi class for you, and if you are persistent, you'll find a teacher and a class perfect for you.

OUCH!

Each condition is different, so discuss with your physician T'ai Chi's potential benefits to your case. T'ai Chi is extremely gentle and should not be confused with the harder martial arts, but consult your doctor before beginning the class.

T'ai Chi for Women

T'ai Chi is the ultimate exercise for women, in part because of its ability to cultivate both elegance and power. In today's working environment, where women are competing with men and trying to break through the glass ceiling, T'ai Chi's ability to cultivate an inner sense of confident power can be very helpful. However, T'ai Chi can be helpful to women for many biological reasons as well.

Halting Bone Loss

Bone loss is a big problem with many women. Studies indicate that stress may be a major factor contributing to the loss of bone mass in even relatively young women. The daily stress relief T'ai Chi promotes provides a powerful preventive therapy to help ensure a long, active life for women.

Studies have shown that QiGong practice raises estrogen levels in women, including those over 45. This is highly desirable because reduced estrogen levels after menopause cause a loss of calcium from the bones and increase the risk of osteoporosis and heart disease.

Treating Eating Disorders

Women suffer from eating disorders 10 times more often than men. Although often thought of as an adult problem, anorexia and bulimia most often start in the teenage years, while the sufferer is still living at home. Although I am unaware of any studies on the effectiveness of T'ai Chi as therapy for anorexia or bulimia, the underlying issues and symptomology seem to suggest that T'ai Chi practice embodies much of the treatment criteria for eating disorders.

For example, it is recommended that anorexia and bulimia sufferers strengthen their inner core of self and self-worth. The self-esteem T'ai Chi practice builds and encourages can be a highly effective way to discover the power within one's self. The need for a restoration of biochemical and hormonal balance may be facilitated with T'ai Chi's ability to create a homeostatic effect throughout the body, not

only physically, but also mentally and emotionally. T'ai Chi addresses the need to balance internal rhythms and needs with life's demands by those who practice it so they can become quietly mindful of subtle feelings and needs before they suffer a crisis born of acute stress or panic.

> **OUCH!**
>
> Do not attempt to self-treat any disorder, including an eating disorder. Suggest T'ai Chi and QiGong to your physician or therapist as an adjunct therapy. It may be a powerful addition to your ongoing treatment, but discuss it with your doctor.

Mood swings and depression are a part of bulimic bingeing, and feelings of lack of personal control are a part of many teenagers' anorexia or bulimia. Food, or denying ourselves food, provides us with a feeling of self-control over an out-of-control world. T'ai Chi's regular practice is designed to help us realize that we have a great deal of control over how we are impacted by the world. This centering enables us to feel more accepting of the fact that much of the world is beyond our control.

Preparing for Childbirth

T'ai Chi has much to offer a pregnant woman, if practiced very gently and with care. Most pregnant women can practice its slow and gentle movements. Its gentleness and relaxed motion promote the circulation of energy and blood throughout the body, while its smooth abdominal breathing fully oxygenates the bodies of both mother and child. However, *only practice when it feels good*, and *never strain yourself.* Rest whenever you need to, and modify or forgo any movement or exercise that doesn't feel right.

T'ai Chi breathing is a wonderful way to prepare for delivery. The famous Lamaze breathing technique is based on QiGong breathing techniques and pain-management tools. This aspect of T'ai Chi makes it perhaps the most effective exercise to prepare you for a safe, natural childbirth. Remember to breathe.

> **SAGE SIFU SAYS**
>
> Although T'ai Chi is very gentle, some postures may be too low or somewhat strenuous for pregnant women. Do not practice these postures, or else adjust them so they are less strenuous for you. As your pregnancy progresses, change your T'ai Chi to make it less strenuous with each passing month. Always go slow and listen to your body. Don't do anything that doesn't feel good. Be sure your physician approves of T'ai Chi before beginning classes.

T'ai Chi for Men

Just as T'ai Chi can help women develop their powerful dynamic side, T'ai Chi helps men develop their passive or receptive side as well, thereby helping men become better homemakers and parents.

T'ai Chi's goal is to strike a balance between our dynamic (male/yang) side and our receptive (female/yin) side. Men and women have both qualities, and T'ai Chi helps balance them.

T'ai Chi helps us let go of old self-concepts and prejudices, just as it teaches us to let go of tensions and fears. As our physical bodies relax and become more fluid, we become more flexible mentally and emotionally.

However, T'ai Chi can help you be that big, strapping stud of an athlete as well. In fact, maybe it can help you keep up with the women who are advancing in every sport today.

T'ai Chi and Sports

T'ai Chi is the ultimate sports training tool because its goal is to cultivate balance, calm, and power—the basis for excelling in any physical activity. T'ai Chi can enhance any athletic performance. T'ai Chi's cultivation of awareness of the dan tien, or center of gravity, can be especially helpful for surfing, skateboarding, snowboarding, and skiing. In fact, T'ai Chi instructor Chris Luth conducts "T'ai Chi Skiing Workshops."

However, the self-awareness, or biofeedback, element of T'ai Chi and QiGong can bring out the giant in any athlete. Several blind golfers are very accomplished. Yes, you read right—*blind* golfers. When asked, they explain that golf is more of a game of "feeling" than sight (as are most sports at their core). They explain that the sighted golfer is handicapped in a way because of their obsession with *outcome* rather than *process*, or *feeling*. T'ai Chi takes the awareness of the athlete internal to the nth degree, maximizing the power of any athlete in any sport, blind or sighted.

Weight Training

Gil Messenger, a student of Master Kuo Lien-ying, was a sports trainer as well as a T'ai Chi instructor. He often taught a form of QiGong meditation to weight trainers, who were surprised to discover that they could then lift more weight. We think when we are pumped and straining we are more powerful, but these weight lifters discovered that by allowing the body to let go, to fill with light, and to move from a calm center, they increased their physical power.

Golf

At an American QiGong Association conference in San Francisco, I had the pleasure to meet a golf coach who had worked with Tiger Woods and had written a book about Tiger's incredible, almost superhuman golf swing. His book theorized that the reason for Tiger's immense power was that as a young child he had practiced QiGong exercises with his dad. This introduced him to "feeling" his swing in a heightened way and also taught him to swing from the dan tien at a very young age. You see the results, as Tiger has dominated professional golf for many years of his career. That's yet another reason all children should be learning T'ai Chi and QiGong from kindergarten through university!

In golf, instructors encourage you to "swing with the belly button." This is another way of saying to swing with the dan tien. Many golfers discover that they can drive the ball much farther after practicing T'ai Chi for only a few months.

OUCH!

The concept of swinging from the dan tien may also help reduce "golfer's back" problems. By thinking of swinging from below the navel (or dan tien) rather than from the navel, your lower back twists less.

Also, T'ai Chi's relaxed motion allows the limbs to be swung by the dan tien's motion with no muscle resistance. This, in turn, allows the entire force of the dan tien's turning to be projected outward through the hands and club into the ball.

Tennis and Racquetball

The same force used in golf is brought to bear in tennis and racquetball. If you play either of these racquet sports, you will also find an increased sense of control. Sometimes tennis players describe a sense of slowing down, as if T'ai Chi practice made the game seem a bit slower than before.

Tennis players also often discover less pressure in the knees after practicing T'ai Chi. Consciously moving from the dan tien can bring less pressure to bear on the knees when coming to an abrupt halt because when the head or upper body leads the movement, the knees must work harder to stop your momentum. T'ai Chi can also give you an off-day exercise that is soothing to the joints but still keeps the mind and body working together at a fine edge. You may be able to have fewer days on the court while still improving your game, which may save your knees as well.

Baseball

The concept of swinging with the dan tien is exemplified in baseball's batting motion. Many batting coaches speak of "squashing the bug," which is another way of saying swing with the dan tien or body: as the body pulls the bat around and the back foot pivots, an imaginary bug beneath the back foot is squashed. When performed correctly, the most powerful swings appear almost effortless. The mental calming and focus T'ai Chi promotes can also improve the hit-to-strike ratio, as well as improving defensive reactions when fielding.

T'ai Chi's ability to improve balance is excellent for infielders, who must move on a dime and reach outward to make plays. However, pitchers are probably the greatest beneficiaries of T'ai Chi training. Just before going into a pitch, pitchers must hold their balance on one leg for a moment. This moment of balance is the most crucial point in a pitcher's windup and can determine both force and accuracy. Therefore, the amazing balance improvement T'ai Chi provides can be the most powerful weapon in a pitcher's arsenal.

The "Hard" Martial Arts

In the 1970s, the world was surprised to see a 19-year-old Canadian win the World Karate Championship. His secret? T'ai Chi. The centering, balance, looseness, and focus T'ai Chi promotes greatly enhance the power and speed of any boxer or martial artist. More than any other exercise, T'ai Chi promotes increased reaction speed because it's therapy, not just for external muscular performance but for the mental and neural processes as well.

T'ai Chi as Therapy

The following sections provide an introduction to how and why T'ai Chi and/or QiGong may be an effective therapy for your condition. If you or your doctor is interested in more in-depth explanations, refer to the end of this chapter for an alphabetical listing of maladies found to benefit from T'ai Chi or QiGong therapy. Master Ken Cohen's book *The Way of Qigong: The Art and Science of Chinese Energy Healing* may be very helpful as well (see Appendix B). The QiGong Institute's QiGong Computerized Database, at www. qigonginstitute.org, is also a great resource, as is www.worldtaichiday.org's medical research library. Find a link to this library in the Web Video Support's Appendix section.

Cancer Treatment

In Chinese hospitals, T'ai Chi and QiGong are often used in conjunction with chemo or radiation therapies. QiGong and T'ai Chi therapies can lessen the side-effects of radiation treatments, but T'ai Chi has many other benefits to offer. For example, a sense of hopelessness or helplessness can diminish the effectiveness of standard treatments. T'ai Chi, however, engages the patients in the healing process, giving them a sense of empowerment. I teach a class for people with cancer, who often come up to me after class expressing how profoundly these tools have shifted the way they feel. T'ai Chi and QiGong don't always make symptoms disappear, but by lifting our laser-like focus away from our challenges and toward the larger, lighter energetic nature of our being, we feed that rather than feeding our symptoms.

In China, QiGong is used as a primary therapy for advanced, inoperable, and medically untreatable cancer. It can slow the progression of the disease while maintaining appetite and helping with pain management. Beyond that, the emotional and mental clarifying aspects of T'ai Chi and QiGong can help patients prepare for life transition in a more meaningful and spiritual way. By helping them become more at peace in their lives, they may find the transition to death a less fearful event, thereby enabling them to make the most of their remaining days.

Cardiac Rehab and Prevention

Many cardiologists prescribe T'ai Chi as an adjunct therapy for treatment of heart problems or as preventive therapy, and the British Heart Foundation said, based on emerging research, T'ai Chi could be adopted into treatment programs for cardiac rehabilitation. T'ai Chi provides a gentle exercise that promotes circulation, but its meditative quality may offer even more benefits. T'ai Chi's stress-reduction qualities foster a feeling of self-acceptance and safety in the world, enabling practitioners to let go of the control issues that can make life seem like an endless state of panic, thereby untightening their hearts. Notice that when you feel panic, your heart feels constricted. T'ai Chi's breath and ungripping techniques do the opposite.

> **SAGE SIFU SAYS**
>
> When you release a deep breath, think of the muscles letting go of the bones. On the next exhale, think of the brain, the mind, and the cranial muscles letting go of thoughts and worries. On the next release of breath, think of letting the heart and the muscles around it relax. Each release of breath becomes a deep cleansing and letting go on many different levels: physical, emotional, mental, and other levels you're not conscious of.

T'ai Chi gives us a daily dosage of homeostatic feelings of well-being. As we become familiar with this feeling of optimum health, we get more attuned with what foods, drinks, or activities promote or detract from that wonderful feeling. This biofeedback feature can be instrumental in helping people make lifestyle changes that may extend their lives by many years.

Stroke Recovery

Doctors often recommend T'ai Chi for stroke recovery because T'ai Chi's soothing demands of left brain/right brain interaction and mind/body interaction can epitomize a physical therapy for stroke victims. T'ai Chi challenges patients to coordinate movement, but at the same time helps them feel at ease in the face of the frustration this challenge might cause. If balance is a severe problem, a spouse or friend can spot you to help maintain balance.

For years I have been advocating a new approach to T'ai Chi for stroke victims with balance problems. By securing a mountain-climbing harness to the ceiling by a hook, a patient may perform T'ai Chi without fear of falling. One of the main balance benefits all T'ai Chi practitioners get comes from constantly testing the limits of their balance. As one drifts in and out of balance, the mind and body exchange data that effortlessly improves the balance, which often continues to improve for life. The following figure shows the harness approach. Note that the harness pictured is only illustrative and is not sufficient to prevent falls; *a full-body harness, including a shoulder harness that secures in front of the upper chest, is required to prevent falling.*

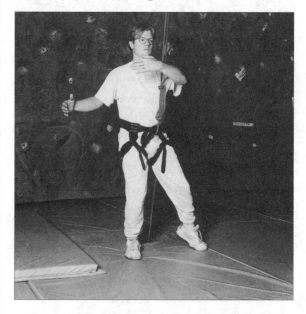

Do not use this harness to prevent falls. Use a caving-harness with upper-body support straps for fall-prevention training.

Hospitals all over the world eventually will provide rooms filled with hooks for climbing harnesses so that stroke rehab or other balance-challenged patients can come and practice T'ai Chi without fear of falling. These same patients may want to have a qualified contractor install harnesses in their homes. Contact your hospital and show them this section of the book. Physical therapists can consult with mountain-climbing supply stores to find the optimum full-body harnesses.

OUCH!

If you have a balance disorder and want to use a climbing harness to prevent falls, discuss the exact purpose of the harness with a climbing expert so he or she can ensure that the harness you use is appropriate to keep you from falling. This security will help you relax more, enabling you to get more benefit from T'ai Chi. Ask the expert about a full-body harness, often used in caving as well as climbing.

Addictions

T'ai Chi, as well as acupuncture, is being successfully used to help people break addictive patterns. A research program working with heroin addicts revealed that withdrawal symptoms decreased much more rapidly than in non-QiGong control groups.

Furthermore, breaking an addiction, whether it's to cigarettes or heroin, is a very stressful endeavor. The body and mind crave and yearn constantly. This study also showed that the QiGong group had much lower anxiety and was able to find restful sleep five times faster than non-QiGong-practicing addicts in recovery. The reason QiGong is so powerful lies in the essence of what an addict, or any of us stuck in unhealthful behaviors, craves.

What is it that they crave? Ultimately, it is life energy. When a smoker gets a cigarette or an addict gets a fix, the first thing this person does is sit back, enjoy the moment, and relax into the pleasure of the cigarette or fix. This moment of relaxed, focused awareness opens the mind and body to an increased flow of Qi or energy. This is why a raging drunk can have so much energy, even when filled with alcohol. The problem is, the cigarettes or drugs are destroying the body to open up to Qi; when the drug wears off, the body clamps down, squeezing off the flow even more. So learning to open to Qi in a healthful, expansive way is one means of healing an addiction.

Note the steps common with a pattern of addiction:

1. A prospective user is looking for access to Qi, or life energy, whether he or she realizes it or not. When Qi is flowing through us, we feel good, at peace, and capable.

2. When cigarettes, drugs, or alcohol are first used, the ritual of using them and/or the chemical they put in the body causes the user to relax and open to Qi flow. But this is a false and unhealthful way to open to it.

3. Because this is an artificial way to open up to the flow of Qi, the mind and body don't learn how to keep the flow open.

4. In fact, when the drug, whether it's nicotine or heroin, is gone, the body and mind tighten up even more than before. The chemicals and their reactions in the body are unhealthful and cause the mind and body to get tighter, squeezing off more Qi than ever before.

5. The user is then required to use more of the drug or to use it more and more often, because now it takes a more forceful dose to open the mind and body's gates to allow the Qi to flow through.

6. Eventually, the user's dosages, no matter how large, do not open the user to increased Qi flow or a feeling of "highness." Eventually, even the largest dosages give the user only a lower-than-normal flow of Qi.

7. People who are heavily hooked on cigarettes or alcohol (even more so with harder drugs) have a look of lacking life. They are becoming void of Qi. Their mind and body have become tight.

> **SAGE SIFU SAYS**
>
> The more we can tap into ways to fill our bodies with life energy using tools such as T'ai Chi, the less we will have to look outside ourselves for satisfaction. Our consumption level drops as our needs diminish. Therefore, T'ai Chi can also help the environment because less consumption means less trash.

T'ai Chi and QiGong provide us with a healthful pattern of access to life energy, or Qi. This is what we all want. When we hug a loved one, we feel their Qi mingling with ours. When we pet our dog or cat, they revel in feeling our loving intention in our Qi flowing from our hand to their body. T'ai Chi and QiGong are tools to fill us with life, and they can be very effective tools for helping addicts find their way out of the maze they have stumbled into, finding a way back to being truly alive.

The best drug program is preventive. T'ai Chi and QiGong will eventually be taught in schools worldwide. By teaching the mind/body awareness and powerful stress-management tools these health sciences offer, many future drug, alcohol, or other addicts will avoid the desire for mood-altering drugs or addictive behaviors or substances. Educating every student from kindergarten through university in mind/body internal awareness and health development techniques like T'ai Chi and QiGong as a matter of standard education makes perfect sense.

The Therapeutic Powers of T'ai Chi and QiGong

Although T'ai Chi and QiGong can play a positive role in many existing conditions, each condition is different, and you must discuss T'ai Chi or QiGong as an adjunct therapy with your physician.

The following list contains some conditions T'ai Chi and/or QiGong may help. Realize that some of the research mentioned is sourced from research being done worldwide, with varying qualities of scientific method, sometimes involving QiGong medical treatment by professional QiGong doctors or therapists using "emitted Qi." (Refer to the "Allow Healing Qi to Flow Through You" section in Chapter 8 to give you some idea of what emitted Qi is, but given there are so many forms of QiGong therapy, the one explained in Chapter 8 may or may not necessarily be the treatment type used in the studies referred to below.) The following section is meant to encourage a more expansive dialogue of treatment options between you and your physician, and is not meant to replace your standard care.

Many of the following listings are based on information provided by the QiGong Institute's Computerized QiGong Database, which contains over 3,500 research abstracts. You, your teacher, your doctor, or anyone else can obtain this excellent research tool at www. qigonginstitute.org. This QiGong Database is a must for every health professional/health reporter in the world today. You should recommend this database to your doctor or health center. Other research came from the resource library at www.worldtaichiday.org. There you can visit the library to obtain article references for some of the T'ai Chi research referred to in the following list and to keep abreast of new research on T'ai Chi and QiGong as it emerges from research centers worldwide. Also, visit the Headline News section of www.worldtaichiday. org for the latest breaking health news on T'ai Chi and QiGong.

ADD and ADHD. Research at the University of Miami School of Medicine has shown that adolescents with ADHD displayed less anxiety, daydreaming behaviors, inappropriate emotions, and hyperactivity and showed greater improved conduct after a T'ai Chi class two days per week over five weeks. T'ai Chi meets many of the criteria for mood-management techniques recommended for ADD (see the "Treating Attention Deficit Disorder" section earlier in this chapter).

Aging, slowing the aging process. Research at Baylor Medical School has found that some cells from the bodies of long-term QiGong practitioners live *five times longer* than the same cells from non-QiGong-practicing test subjects.

Other research from The Shanghai Institute of Hypertension looked at several aspects of aging. They determined that QiGong is an effective measure in preventing and treating geriatric diseases and delaying the aging process.

AIDS. Studies indicate that regular T'ai Chi practice may boost one's T-cell count while improving outlook and providing a soothing, gentle exercise. The relaxed forms effectively oxygenate the body while moving blood and lymph throughout.

Allergies and asthma. The stress-reduction benefits of T'ai Chi and QiGong help the body maintain elevated DHEA levels. Low DHEA levels have been directly linked to allergies. High stress levels are linked to the frequency and intensity of asthmatic reactions as well. One of my students used allergy remedies every year for many years before beginning my classes. She recently informed a magazine reporter doing a T'ai Chi story that she no longer needs medication.

Angina. Biofeedback aspects of T'ai Chi and QiGong can help students learn to regulate blood flow by awareness of warmth in the hands and feet. Evidence suggests that this skill may alleviate some forms of angina.

Anorexia/bulimia. See the "Treating Eating Disorders" section earlier in this chapter.

Anxiety, chronic. The relaxed abdominal breathing T'ai Chi and QiGong promote can be a beneficial adjunct to therapy, especially when used in combination with the loosening physical motions and soothing visualization practices of Sitting QiGong.

Arthritis. T'ai Chi's low impact causes no joint damage (unlike other higher-impact exercises), while its weight-bearing aspect may encourage development of bone mass and connective tissue. *Note:* Those with arthritic knees may want to do modified T'ai Chi forms, sharing weight on both legs rather than fully centering the weight over one knee.

Back pain. *Prevention* magazine reported a study in which, after one year of T'ai Chi classes, a group of men and women ages 58 to 70 found increased strength and flexibility in their back, helping to reduce the odds of back pain.

Balance disorders. T'ai Chi practitioners fall only half as much as those practicing other balance training, as reported by an Emory University study, among others.

Baldness, premature. QiGong and T'ai Chi promote stress management and blood circulation. Some QiGong exercises, such as Carry the Moon, specifically promote circulation in the scalp.

Behcet's Disease. Behcet's Disease is a chronic, recurring disease. Neijing Central Hospital of Management (China) claims to have cured five patients of Behcet's Disease. It believes this was due to QiGong's ability to build up immunological function and increase blood-flow volume, and by promoting saliva flow and increased oxygen intake.

Brittle bones/bone loss in women. Research from the National Institute of Mental Health reports that the stress hormones found in depressed women caused bone loss that gave them bones of women nearly twice their age. T'ai Chi and QiGong are known to reduce depression and anxiety, and provide weight-bearing exercises to encourage building bone mass and connective tissue.

Bronchitis/emphysema, chronic. Over time, Sitting QiGong and/or T'ai Chi may show positive results in appetite, sleep, and energy levels, but also rather dramatically and healthfully in decreasing breaths per minute.

Burns, healing of. Researchers at the Navy General Hospital of Beijing, China, studied emitted Qi on burned rats. They noted that the QiGong treatment in some ways expedited the healing ability of burned rats.

Cancer. Several clinical studies reported that a combination therapy of drugs with personal practice of QiGong provided a better outcome than drug therapy alone.

Carcinoma. The Guangzhou College of Traditional Chinese Medicine, Guangzhou, China, researched the effects of emitted Qi on carcinoma. It reported, "The emitted Qi may promote normal function of human immune cells while killing the tumor cells, suggesting that QiGong is a feasible means to the treatment of carcinoma."

Cardiovascular benefit. Research has shown that the extremely gentle and low-impact T'ai Chi exercise can provide the same cardiovascular benefit as moderate-impact aerobic exercise. The *Harvard Women's Health Watch* reported, "Studies support T'ai Chi [use] for heart-attack and cardiac-bypass patients, to improve cardio-respiratory function and reduce blood pressure."

Chronic Fatigue and Immune Dysfunction Syndrome (CFIDS). In 2008 the National Fibromyalgia Association reported that tai chi has been found to help some Chronic Fatigue Syndrome (CFS) patients and is prescribed for symptom management. (For more information, contact the CFIDS Association of America.)

Chronic Fatigue Syndrome (CFS). Research in the *British Medical Journal* showed 84 percent of CFS patients adding exercise to their CFS standard care got "very much" or "much" better, as opposed to only 12 percent of patients receiving only standard care. CFS's chronic pain limitation may make T'ai Chi and QiGong's gentle motions and deep breathing (with its pain-management benefits) an optimum exercise for CFS sufferers.

Chronic pain. Students often find anything between mild pain relief and complete alleviation of chronic pain by using T'ai Chi and/or QiGong. In some cases, patients find complete relief from long-term chronic pain conditions. The *Wall Street Journal* reported that neuroscientists are finding mind-body approaches, such as T'ai Chi, are effective in diminishing chronic pain.

Circulation and nervous system disorders. T'ai Chi promotes circulation and can have a very integrating effect on the mind and body.

Compulsive, obsessive disorders. T'ai Chi and QiGong's mindful awareness of self and constant reassurance that we can breathe through and relax into any situation may be a helpful adjunct to therapy for OCD, which gently exposes patients to their fears. Again, introduce T'ai Chi and QiGong only with your therapist's approval.

Concentration/QiGong uses in education. Although researchers in a study in Xinjiang, China, admit limitations in their research, they find encouraging signs that QiGong exercises could greatly enhance the educational experience for primary school children and beyond.

Coronary disease. Ganshu College of TCM in China claimed to have found strong evidence that QiGong exercises may help with coronary disease.

Depression and mood disturbance. Regular (daily) T'ai Chi practitioners usually find lower incidence of depression and overall mood disturbance.

Diabetes. T'ai Chi's stress-management and increased circulation qualities make it ideal for diabetes. A Beijing University of Chinese Medicine and Pharmacology study found that blood sugar could be lowered successfully by doing QiGong exercises. In the study,

42.9 percent of patients were able to take less medicine while having more staple foods. Nanjing University's study found that T'ai Chi exercise helped regulate metabolic disorder of type-2 diabetes mellitus with geriatric obesity by regulating the nervous-endocrine system in the body.

Digestion, improving. T'ai Chi's gentle massage of internal organs and stimulation of blood circulation and Qi promote healthy digestion.

Dementia. *The Washington Post* reported that research has shown that regular physical activity can help prevent dementia, heart attacks, strokes, type-2 diabetes, and certain cancers … The American College of Sports Medicine (ACSM) recommends "functional fitness" activities such as T'ai Chi.

Drug uptake. The QiGong Institute reviewed voluminous studies done worldwide and concluded that QiGong and drug therapies are superior to drug therapy alone. The reason for this is believed to be found in QiGong's ability to enhance Qi and blood circulation to that area so nutrients may more efficiently be delivered to the affected cells. Also, waste products in the stressed tissue can be removed more readily.

Fibromyalgia. Fibromyalgia is a modern epidemic, a chronic pain condition affecting 3 to 6 percent of the U.S. population, according to Arthritis Today. According to *The New York Times*, a clinical trial at Tufts Medical Center released their results in 2010, showing that after 12 weeks of T'ai Chi, patients with Fibromyalgia did significantly better than a comparable group given stretching exercises and wellness education, in measurements of pain, fatigue, physical functioning, sleeplessness, and depression.

Flexibility enhancement. *Harvard Women's Health Watch* reported an Emory University study showing that T'ai Chi may possibly improve elasticity in ligaments and tendons, create stronger knee flexors and extensors, and create better posture.

Gallstones. The Navy General Hospital, Beijing, China, did a study using emitted Qi to determine whether a particular emitted Qi therapy could help people pass gallstones. It found a positive treatment rate of 93.33 percent.

Gastritis. Chronic atrophic gastritis (CAG) is a common yet difficult illness, according to researchers at the Institute for Industry Health in Xian, China. Studying the effect of a combination of QiGong exercise with Tuina (Chinese therapeutic massage), researchers found that 97.1 percent of patients gained some benefit.

Gastrointestinal malignant tumors. The Department of Chinese Medicine, Second Affiliate Hospital with Jiangxi Medical College, found that a group of patients using QiGong exercises with their standard chemotherapy, radiotherapy, and Chinese medicine had a significantly higher survival rate than those getting only standard medical therapy with no QiGong exercises.

Geriatric fitness. *Prevention* magazine reported, "T'ai Chi may be the best exercise for people over the age of 60 … providing cardio fitness, muscle strength, and flexibility all in one simple workout that is easy on the joints." Other studies show that T'ai Chi is by far the best balance conditioner. Research finding that T'ai Chi may also lessen tissue brittleness further adds to the case that T'ai Chi is the best possible exercise for seniors.

Heart disease. At the Institute of Psychology, Academia Sinica, a research study found that T'ai Chi and QiGong practice can positively affect the states of mind of subjects to lessen the incidence of type-A behavior patterns, believed to increase the risk of heart disease.

Hemorrhoids. Some QiGong breathing involves the sphincter muscles, which may directly alleviate hemorrhoid symptoms. T'ai Chi's ability to reduce constipation lessens the aggravation of hemorrhoid symptoms.

High blood pressure. T'ai Chi can significantly lower high blood pressure in many cases.

Infections. Regular T'ai Chi practice is believed to increase the T-cell count. T-cells are thought to consume viruses, bacteria, and even tumor cells.

Insomnia. Insomnia is a growing problem in our rushed and digitized world. T'ai Chi and QiGong students often remark of improved sleep and reduced insomnia after a few weeks of regular T'ai Chi and QiGong practice. Researchers at the QiGong Department of Ningbo Hospital of TCM in China gave 78 patients suffering from insomnia treatments involving QiGong Meditation (Sitting QiGong), coupled with QiGong self-massage of several acupressure points, including in the wrists. After 1 course of treatment, 35 cases were cured (good sleep for more than 6 hours a day, no concomitant symptoms anymore), 22 cases showed obvious effect (sleeping for 4 to 6 hours per day, with other concomitant symptoms ameliorated obviously), 9 cases showed some effect (better sleep than before, with other concomitant symptoms ameliorated a little), and only 2 cases showed no effect (just like before). So *76 out of 78 found relief from insomnia using QiGong without the need for drugs.*

Knee strengthening. Knee problems are common as we age. The University of Illinois at Urbana-Champaign conducted a study on older adults using 20 weeks of T'ai Chi training. The overall findings suggest that T'ai Chi training improves knee extensor strength and force control in older adults.

Leukemia. The Immunology Research Center, Beijing, China, studied the effects of externally emitted Qi to see how it affects leukemia cells in mice. It found the mice treated with Qi emission had reduced numbers of L1210 cells (malignant tumor cells). However, researchers cautioned that the mechanism and the way emitted Qi does this need to be further investigated.

Liver disease, hepatitis B, and the like. Researchers at Lixin County Hospital of TCM in Anhui province, China, found that 10 kinds of liver diseases, especially hepatitis B, could be cured with the combination of drugs and QiGong.

Lou Gehrig's disease. Many support groups of neuromuscular diseases recommend T'ai Chi. Check with your doctor to discuss introducing T'ai Chi as an adjunct to your therapy.

Low blood pressure. At Lixin County Hospital of TCM, researchers believe QiGong combined with standard drug therapy to be good for low blood pressure.

Menopausal therapy. The QiGong Institute reviewed voluminous studies done worldwide and concluded that QiGong combined with drug therapy is superior to drug therapy alone, including in the case of menopausal treatments. This mechanism of enhanced drug delivery suggests that QiGong could make possible smaller doses of drugs, which would cause fewer adverse side-effects. For example, QiGong is reported to restore estradiol levels in hypertensive menopausal women, leading to the possibility that estrogen-replacement therapy might not be necessary or might be used at reduced levels.

Menstrual disorders. Researchers at PLA General Hospital in Beijing, China, used acupressure, massage, and emitted Qi to treat 76 cases of various gynopathic diseases. The results were that 52 cases (68.42 percent) were nearly cured, 14 (18.42 percent) were markedly effective, and 10 (13.16 percent) found the treatment to be effective.

Mental health. The Institute of Psychology, Chinese Academy of Sciences, Beijing, China, conducted studies to see how QiGong practice would affect mental health. The result was a group that had practiced QiGong for more than two years had a curative rate on symptoms of psychosomatic disorders about *twice* as high as that of a QiGong group practicing less than two years.

Migraine. Biofeedback aspects of T'ai Chi and QiGong can help students learn to regulate blood flow by increasing awareness of warmth in hands and feet. Evidence suggests this skill may alleviate some forms of migraines.

Multiple sclerosis. MS support groups recommend T'ai Chi.

Muscle wasting (and other tissue deterioration). Studies indicate that T'ai Chi may be an ideal exercise to help older people suffering muscle wasting.

Neurotransmitters, QiGong's effect on them, and how that impacts health. Researchers at Anhui College of TCM assert that their research indicates that QiGong practice affects neurotransmitters in such a way to help regulate the function of the neuralgic system to prevent and help cure diseases.

Ovarian cysts. Researchers at PLA General Hospital, Beijing, China, found a high success rate using a combination of acupressure, massage, and emitted Qi in curing or positively affecting the majority of cases of various gynopathic diseases, including ovarian cysts.

Paralysis. Researchers at the PLA General Hospital of Beijing, China, studied the effect of emitted Qi combined with QiGong exercises in treating paralysis. The effect of the treatment judged by the indexes of rehabilitation commonly used was "excellent" in 23.25 percent of cases, "good" in 46.5 percent, "fine" in 23.25 percent, and "bad" in 6.99 percent of cases, with an overall effective rate of 93.01 percent.

Parkinson's disease/improving motor-skill control. Parkinson's support groups recommend T'ai Chi, and many students claim significant reduction in tremors with T'ai Chi practice. *The New England Journal of Medicine* recently reported on a new study showing that Parkinson's patients using T'ai Chi found dramatic balance improvement over those in the control groups.

Posture problems. T'ai Chi's gentle, mindful awareness of postural adjustment makes it a wonderful therapy for posture problems and for alleviating the pain or chronic tension associated with them.

Psychotherapy. A German researcher points out that QiGong is gradually gaining prominence as a therapeutic tool in Germany and pointed to positive effects of QiGong exercises for those dealing with neurosis, depression, anxiety, psychosomatic disorder, and psychosis. The researcher cautions that a wrong practice of the exercises, as pertains to especially sick people, can have bad effects, and these subjects require competent guidance and assistance.

Psychiatric Treatment. Roger Walsh, a psychiatrist at the University of California College of Medicine in Irvine who authored "Lifestyle and Mental Health," which was published in *American Psychologist*, is wary of the [psychiatry] profession's tendency to reduce diagnosis, prevention, and treatment to biochemistry … Walsh found convincing evidence that "self-management skills" (mainly stress-reducing practices such as yoga, tai chi, and meditation) confer psychological advantages.

PTSD (Post Traumatic Stress Disorder). 89 percent of VA medical centers offered alternative forms of therapy in 2011, including T'ai Chi and meditation. Some veterans/patients reported that these therapies have allowed them to rely less on pain medication and sleeping pills, but the VA indicated that more research needs to be done to fully determine PTSD benefits.

Rehabilitation and immunity strengthening. The Institute of Medical Science at Wonkwang University, Korea, found that of those patients who used QiGong, 84 percent of respondents reported improvement in recovery time, 66.6 percent reported reduced inflammation after QiGong, and 50.3 percent reported no scarring as compared to before. In addition, 59.9 percent of respondents reported an increase in resistance to the common cold after four months of QiGong.

Respiratory diseases, chronic. A collaborative study with the Research Institute of TCM, Tainjin College of TCM, and Tianjin Thorax Surgery Hospital was done on patients suffering from chronic bronchitis, asthma, pulmonary emphysema, and cor pulmonale. A group treated with QiGong exercise and drugs fared better than the one treated only with drugs.

Rheumatism. *OT Week* magazine reported, "Areas where T'ai Chi has proven effective include rheumatism, weight management, treatment of back problems, management of high blood pressure, and stress reduction … and may speed recovery in postoperative patients …."

Sexual performance. T'ai Chi's stress reduction and promotion of circulation can make it a very healthful way to improve sexual performance.

Stomach carcinoma. The General Navy Hospital in Beijing studied the effects of emitted Qi on NK cells, which they believe play a role in cancer. They found a statistically remarkable effect of emitted Qi killing both adenocarcinoma cells of the stomach and the NK cells.

Strength enhancement. After one year of T'ai Chi classes, a group of men and women ages 58 to 70 found increased strength.

Tears, cleansing mechanisms, and QiGong. *Psychology Today* reported that the Tear Research Center has discovered crying may cleanse chemicals from the body that build up during emotional stress, including ACTH, a hormone that is considered the body's most reliable indicator of stress. Sitting QiGong's progressive relaxation therapy often leaves practitioners wiping away tears, perhaps explaining why we feel clearer and lighter after practice.

Thrombosis. At the Department of Pathology, Weifang Medical College in Shandong, China, researchers claimed their research indicates that "QiGong exercise could reduce thrombosis, RBC aggregability, and blood viscosity, and could prevent and treat cardiovascular and cerebrovascular diseases."

Ulcers. QiGong relaxation therapy coupled with reductions in external stress factors has shown substantial success, even with long-term ulcer problems.

Weight loss. *OT Week* magazine reports that T'ai Chi has been proven effective with weight loss. T'ai Chi promotes healthful weight loss in many ways: it burns calories but also helps reduce stress levels. This stress reduction helps reduce nervous snacking. Furthermore, T'ai Chi's slow, quiet mindfulness helps us get in touch with our *homeostatic* or healthful potential and what that feels like. That steers us away from foods or activities that don't promote health and toward those that do.

KNOW YOUR CHINESE

Modern psychologists refer to a state of mental and emotional well-being as homeostasis, or a homeostatic state. T'ai Chi promotes this by smoothing our Qi, the life blood of our mental, emotional, and physical being. T'ai Chi is the epitome of a homeostatic exercise.

Hopefully, this book will be shared with physicians throughout the world to encourage more worldwide research on these health tools. In my first edition of this book, I wrote that the Department of Physical Medicine and Rehabilitation at the Medical College of Ohio had aptly stated that "research into the efficacy of T'ai Chi, QiGong, and Yoga clearly is in the beginning stages. What little has been conducted thus far is promising. These methods may serve to add valuable contributions to the continuity of care of ambulatory and nonambulatory patients." Since then, T'ai Chi and QiGong have begun to be taught in many major medical schools throughout the United States. A QiGong workshop I did at a local hospital was covered by the Blue Cross and Blue Shield premium plan, enabling those who had such coverage to attend for free. T'ai Chi and QiGong are at the center of a health revolution that will save our nation trillions in future health costs as these tools become integrated into society at all levels. This could happen quickly by teaching T'ai Chi, QiGong, and other proven mind-body techniques in schools, teaching them in age-appropriate ways from kindergarten through higher education.

The National Center for Complementary and Alternative Medicine (NCCAM) in Bethesda, Maryland, funds T'ai Chi, QiGong, and other natural remedies research. However, at this time, complementary medicine research (which includes T'ai Chi, QiGong, Yoga, massage, reiki, etc.) only receives a tiny percentage of NIH research funding (far less than 1 percent). Given the stunning findings that have emerged over the years since this book's first edition was printed, it would behoove our nation's institutes of health to apply serious funding to discover just how extensive T'ai Chi and QiGong's potential is in reducing health costs given the skyrocketing cost of healthcare in America and around the world. T'ai Chi and QiGong are extremely inexpensive, and yet highly effective, therapies.

The Least You Need to Know

- T'ai Chi helps kids with physical development and focus.
- Teach kids faster T'ai Chi, and spice it up with harder exercises.
- T'ai Chi is perfect for all ages—and athletes, too.
- If your physician or therapist is unfamiliar with T'ai Chi and QiGong, show him or her this book!
- No matter what ailment you have, T'ai Chi and/or QiGong can probably help.

T'ai Chi's Philosophy of Balance and Flow

In This Chapter

- Following a T'ai Chi diet plan
- Discovering herbs and teas as medicine
- Increasing health and prosperity by using Feng Shui
- Learning about yourself with the *I Ching*
- Using T'ai Chi to really enjoy life

T'ai Chi is not an end in itself. T'ai Chi is a passageway to a more healthful lifestyle. Dietary changes, the inclusion of regular massage therapy, acupuncture tune-ups, and the power of positive thinking can all catapult you forward into even greater rewards T'ai Chi offers. This chapter exposes you to many interesting and wonderful tools to further your life adventure in self-awareness and limitless growth.

The Yin Yang of Diet

T'ai Chi's movements are a blend of hard and soft, exertion and relaxation, force and yielding. In fact, the T'ai Chi symbol is the yin/yang symbol—the symbol of balance. Just as T'ai Chi and QiGong are built upon the concepts of balance, so is every other aspect of healthful living.

Chinese cooking adheres to these same principles. In Chinese cooking, a good cook balances the use of yin foods and yang foods to create a meal that is not only delicious, but also provides optimal health benefits. In a way, a good Chinese chef is almost like a pharmacist, blending nutrients, herbs, and Qi into a prescription that treats the eyes, palate, and health.

Green vegetables are yin food. They are cool and easily digested, and helpful for certain parts and functions of the body. Meat and some other protein sources are yang foods. Yang is power and provides great energy to the body, but it is less easily digested. Chinese herbs are divided into cool and hot, dry and wet, each of which is good for certain conditions. Your food becomes not only a culinary treat, but also a prescription for optimum health.

A principle benefit of T'ai Chi and QiGong are that they take stress off the body. As mentioned previously, in my classes I recommend a documentary called *Forks Over Knives*, which explains how a whole-foods vegan diet is much less stressful for the body to digest, thereby freeing up energy to focus on immune system function, etc. Don't think you have to be a vegan to enjoy the benefits of T'ai Chi and QiGong. However, as T'ai Chi and QiGong help your mind, body, and heart loosen up and change more easily, you might be drawn to explore even more ways to support your body's needs, including playing with new dietary adventures. If you do change your diet, let it happen in a way you can live with. It doesn't have to be an all-or-nothing game. You can simply start to "play" with vegan, whole-foods dishes, dipping your toe in at first. Over time your habits and patterns can change as you discover tasty whole-foods recipes. More and more supermarkets are now carrying organic foods as well, and local farmers markets are popping up everywhere with locally grown organic foods.

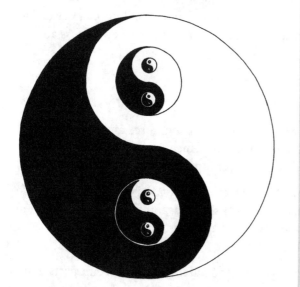

This ancient yin/yang symbol is actually called "T'ai Chi." It represents two things: that everything in the universe exists within each individual thing (including you), and that we should seek balance in all things.

> **SAGE SIFU SAYS**
>
> Many nutritionists see the traditional Chinese diet as optimal, encompassing approximately 40 percent grain (rice), 40 percent vegetables, 10 percent meat, and 10 percent fruits and nuts. Be aware there are healthful and unhealthful Chinese foods as well. Use your own good judgment and remember that each person is unique. Ask your physician or a qualified dietician to discover your optimal diet.

Chinese Herbs and Teas for Health Conditions

Ginseng tea is made from ginseng root, which resembles a person's head and body. Ginseng has yang qualities. If a person's condition is overly yin, or cool and damp, an herbalist may suggest herbs promoting the yang qualities of dry and hot. For example, fresh ginger tea may be good to treat some early cold symptoms. Bitter melon soup, a yin food, may be used to treat an overactive yang condition such as nosebleeds. Consult a qualified herbalist for more detailed information. Be sure your physician is aware of any herbal therapy you may engage in.

> **OUCH!**
>
> The Chinese health philosophy frowns on iced drinks because they introduce too much yin into the body too quickly. This shocks the body and upsets the balance. Hot or tepid drinks are preferred because the body is naturally warm.

Feng Shui: Architectural T'ai Chi

The Chinese believe that Qi, or life energy, flows not only through living things, but through *all* things. According to this belief, we move in a great ocean of invisible energy that affects and interacts with energy from other beings, nature, and even buildings. In fact, the Chinese have developed an architectural style to affect the way energy flows through your home or business to maximize health, happiness, and prosperity. *Feng Shui* (pronounced *fung shway*) is like architectural T'ai Chi, or T'ai Chi for your house.

KNOW YOUR CHINESE

Feng Shui means "wind" and "water." Wind represents universal forces, while water represents Earth forces. Balancing the two creates optimum health and prosperity.

Have you ever noticed how almost all Chinese restaurants have aquariums, many near the front door? This arrangement is based on Feng Shui because running water is very good for the room's Qi.

Western architecture often uses running water for decorative purposes. However, science is now suggesting that the use of water in architecture is also functional. Many homes and geographical areas are bombarded by positive ions in the air. This can aggravate allergies or cause other physiological or mental discomforts. Some of this positive-ion overload is because of modern electricity, but some is a natural phenomenon. Running water produces negative ions, which can balance the ions in a room, home, or business, making it more pleasant and more healthful. If a restaurant makes you feel more at ease, you will likely come back there more often, making the restaurant more prosperous. So Feng Shui works on principles based on a subatomic understanding of the energy dynamics in a room, which, in the end, can lead to a happier, more prosperous existence.

The *I Ching*

There are many ways to use the *I Ching*, and there is some debate about what it really does. Some think it is a fortune-telling device, while others see it as a tool for self-analysis or self-contemplation. There are 64 possible hexagram combinations, which represent all the possible ways life can transform.

Some modern analysts compare the *I Ching*'s hexagram system to the Rorschach test, where the person reading the hexagrams is really defined by how she sees them. To read your *I Ching*, you throw out the hexagrams or shake yarrow sticks from a cup, and the way they fall tells you what to look up in books that list the hexagrams' meanings. The meanings are often just vague enough so you must interpret for yourself the detailed meaning for your life. Therefore, when you use this method of divination, you are compelled to introspection, to understand who you are, what you want, and where you want to go in life. Seen in this light, the *I Ching* can be a very healthful and potentially invaluable tool. Some bookstores will have books, or even kits, so you can practice using the *I Ching* system yourself.

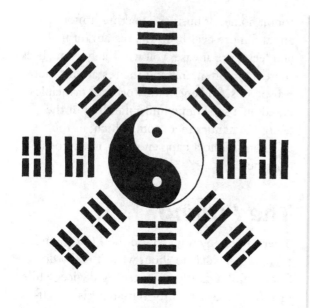

The 64 possible hexagram combinations represent all the possible forms of life's changes, just as styles of T'ai Chi, like the one with 64 movements, represent all possible physical changes we go through. (See Chapter 13 and the T'ai Chi Long Form Exhibition *on the Web Video Support to view the flowing changes.)*

A T'AI CHI PUNCH LINE

One day my wife and I went to a temple in Hong Kong, and while there, we had our fortunes forecast by a priest using the *I Ching.* After divining our fortune, the priest told my wife, "You are pregnant." We laughed because we knew we had been careful. Two days later, my wife got dizzy, so we rushed her to a clinic, where the doctor did blood tests. The doctor came back and announced, "You are pregnant."

Rest and Rejuvenation

T'ai Chi's yin and yang symbol reminds us that we must balance our natures in our bodies and in the world around us. In our modern, fast-paced lives, we are too reliant on busyness and constant noise. We consider television a form of relaxation. While a small amount can be, the number of hours most Americans watch television is actually unhealthful. In fact, the American Medical Association has stated that more than two hours per day is unhealthful, and can increase chances of type 2 diabetes and cardiovascular disease, perhaps caused by the exercise time lost to tv viewing, as well as our in-front-of-the-tv eating habits.

However, emerging research is also showing that the quick scene cuts and rapid disorienting segues which comprise much modern television in their attempt to "capture" our attention, affects the alpha and gamma brainwaves by disrupting them. This is particularly significant because meditative experiences bring the mind into relaxed alpha brainwave states while also cultivating the gamma wave states of consciousness, which involves higher consciousness function, as well. So, hours and hours of stimulation and disruption of these states of consciousness may add up to more stress, rather than the *relaxation* we often associate with tv watching.

Just as activity is important to our health, so is absolute rest. Most of us probably find it difficult just to sit, to simply be and serenely enjoy the absence of stimulation. At first, the slowness and quiet quality of T'ai Chi and QiGong drive many people a little nuts.

SAGE SIFU SAYS

A famous Vietnamese monk once said that we are like glasses of dirty water. Each day the dirt gets shaken up, and we become cloudy and unclear. If we take time to sit still, our stress settles down, and we again can see clearly.

This is a cleansing process. The more anxiety we feel, breathe through, and let go of, the more we settle into a clarity and calmness that we eventually learn to enjoy. By sitting still, we become aware of anxieties and tensions we may have buried in our subconscious mind, and thereby squeezed unconsciously in our cells. These repressed feelings can manifest as muscle tension, asthma attacks, volatile emotions, and so on, unless we become aware of them, feel them, and begin to breathe through them by physically letting the muscles let go and the mind relax. The cleansing pleasure of that "empty awareness" is perhaps the most healthful thing we can do for ourselves. It gives our mind a chance to rest, heal, and recharge. This also gives our spiritual nature an opportunity to come forth. We can get a new perspective on life just by sitting. Just as a drug addict must go through a period of anxiety to let go of the craving for drugs, those of us who are addicted to "busyness" and constant stimulation (TV or whatever) must go through that same anxiety period. But eventually we tap into the bliss of stillness of mind. As always, remembering to *breathe* makes the transition more tolerable.

T'ai Chi Teaches Mindful Living

T'ai Chi's slow process and seemingly endless progression from one movement to the next teaches us to let go of the outcome and be in the moment. In the West, this is called "stopping to smell the roses." With T'ai Chi, we don't just think about stopping to smell the roses; we simply must do it. You cannot stand to perform a 20-minute slow-motion exercise like T'ai Chi and stay in a rush-rush-hurry-hurry mentality. It is impossible. Therefore, T'ai Chi is like a magic formula that actually changes who you are. Its methodology forces us to love the act of living, just as we must love the feel, the sensation, *the breath*, and the motion of each T'ai Chi movement so we don't anxiously wait for it to be over. Life becomes a sacrament, and every moment and every person we touch becomes sacred and a miracle. As T'ai Chi's slow mindfulness causes us to subtly attune to the miracle of our own existence, we see the world as miraculous. On a physical level, as we daily immerse ourselves in Qi, or life's energy, we connect with that quality in all living things.

The mindful living T'ai Chi teaches spills out into every aspect of our lives. To help bring forth T'ai Chi mindfulness, practice the following exercises:

Savor the smell and taste of liquids. When you take a sip of water with a lime twist or hot tea, really smell the rich aroma as you drink. Let the fragrance fill your awareness. As you swallow it, feel the heat or cold go down your throat. Experience its descent all the way into your stomach.

When you hold a hot cup of tea, watch the steam rise. Get your face right up next to it. The steam is agitated atoms that burst free of the surface and scream outward into space, just like the huge bursts that erupt from the surface of the sun. Enjoy this fabulous display of erupting atoms.

Simplify your diet. Drink more water with a lime twist and less soda or beer. Take the time to really taste and smell the lime. Lime is an exquisite gift we've been given. Usually we drink very sweet, over-flavored things because we don't slow down enough to really taste them. When we're not really tasting our liquids, that's when we need the shock value of 13 sugar cubes and the other sticky stuff that comes in most cans of soda.

Eat more fruits and vegetables. Really stop and chew them. Feel their texture, sense their temperature, and savor their subtle flavor and smell.

When you cook, feel the food as you cut it up. Listen to the sizzling as it cooks, and really smell the richness of its aroma. Pretend for a moment that this was your last day on Earth and you would never be able to smell these smells, hear these sounds, or taste these tastes again.

Sit and watch nature. Nature cannot be analyzed or fixed. Nature simply washes over you. Watch the clouds move, the trees sway, and the weather unfold. This world is a miracle placed here for your enjoyment. Don't take its beauty for granted.

Just listen when your spouse (or children or friends) talks to you. Observe their faces and the excitement in their voices. Let the images of their day wash over your mind. Don't worry about how you are "supposed" to respond. Enjoy their presence.

> **SAGE SIFU SAYS**
>
> The T'ai Chi symbol, or yin yang symbol, literally means the supreme ultimate point in the universe. When you follow the suggestions to allow T'ai Chi to weave its mindfulness into your life, you begin to feel more and more as though you are in the center of the universe.

Observe people; experience them. Imagine for a moment that you were the only person on Earth and there was never ever going to be anyone else but you. You probably would be filled with desire to speak to others, to enjoy their existence. Here they are, now. Enjoy.

Let life wash over you. Do what needs to be done, whether it's washing dishes or paying bills, with a sense of unhurried pleasure, like the way T'ai Chi movements are done. If we don't run from what we must do, it can be pleasant, and all things simply work out, as if we did nothing at all. It doesn't mean we don't do anything; it means we allow our endeavors to become more effortless and less angst-driven.

The Least You Need to Know

- Balance your diet; balance your life.
- Traditional Chinese diets are based on a *food as medicine* approach to eating.
- According to Feng Shui, an open, flowing interior design does much more than just look good.
- The *I Ching* may help you understand yourself better.
- T'ai Chi teaches you to savor life and smell the roses.

T'ai Chi as Corporate Wellness

In This Chapter

- Understanding the benefits of starting a T'ai Chi program at work
- Learning why T'ai Chi is a natural for the office
- Web Video Support: exhibitions to show how T'ai Chi fits in at the office

Corporations all over America are integrating the powerful health and personal growth tools of T'ai Chi into the fabric of the workplace. Why? Because T'ai Chi can save companies big money, is very applicable to the office, and can lessen workplace injury, reduce stress, and boost performance. I have done T'ai Chi ergonomics classes for some of the world's largest corporations, as are many other T'ai Chi teachers I've talked to.

This chapter details how T'ai Chi accomplishes these goals so you can speak with authority to your company's wellness director about incorporating T'ai Chi into your workplace. Many companies will pay for a T'ai Chi program, making it well worth your time to suggest it to your wellness director.

The Bottom Line on Stress Costs to Business

You can help your company understand how sponsoring T'ai Chi classes is in its best interest as well as yours. One of corporate America's highest unnecessary production costs is in lost productivity due to *employee stress*. U.S. businesses are losing $300 billion per year due to stress (that's more than $7,500 per employee, per year), which may be why the Occupational Safety and Hazard Administration (OSHA) has declared stress a workplace hazard.

Using T'ai Chi as Stress and Pain Relief

Companies and corporations are increasingly turning to T'ai Chi as a solution to stress. Companies that have offered T'ai Chi to either their employees, clients, or executive staffs include Sprint, Hallmark, Inc., Black and Veatch Corp., Associated Wholesale Grocers, BMA (Financial), and Columbia Hospitals, to name a few.

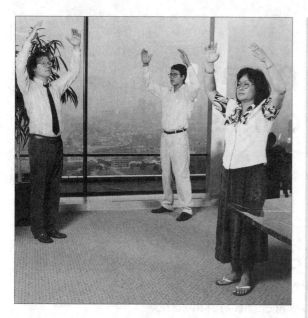

Penthouse T'ai Chi at BMA's headquarters became a popular wellness program. Approximately 100 employees attended the introductory stress-management-with-T'ai Chi workshop, setting a new record for employee attendance for a wellness workshop.

A community college near Kansas City provides T'ai Chi classes as a wellness program to its staff, and many participants are finding alleviation of chronic pain conditions, less stress, and fewer sick days. T'ai Chi is rapidly becoming the most popular wellness program for many companies. Isn't it great that some companies are realizing that what is good for the employee is good for the company's profits as well?

Investing in Creative Potential

If T'ai Chi can help employees recover from illnesses and thereby reduce absenteeism, that can also mean major savings. But what about creativity? T'ai Chi's meditative quality enables practitioners to become more creative as they let go of being locked into old patterns.

Although now largely considered cliché, a popular corporate expression is to "think outside the box," or look beyond the established way of doing things. It's a useful concept, but how do you really think outside the box? You have to release the old ways of doing things. Again, T'ai Chi is about letting go of everything—mentally, emotionally, and physically. That requires releasing prejudices and preconceptions, making you clearer and more open to new possibilities and potential. If T'ai Chi can help employees think outside the box, this will open them to fresh, innovative approaches and may boost profits more than anything you could begin to measure.

> **SAGE SIFU SAYS**
>
> Albert Einstein said, "Imagination is more important than knowledge." When T'ai Chi and QiGong help us let go of physical, emotional, and mental tension, our "imagination muscle" literally expands. As we let go of old patterns, we open to new and exciting concepts that our old, tense bodies and minds couldn't comprehend. We also learn more easily and are more creative in using what we learn.

Helping with Lower-Back Problems and Carpal Tunnel

A large part of costly, unscheduled absenteeism is due to employees' lower-back problems. T'ai Chi is very effective at helping with chronic lower-back pain, as well as other chronic pain problems.

Because T'ai Chi is the very best balance training in the world, causing participants to be half as likely to suffer falling injuries as other exercises, T'ai Chi can reduce workplace injuries dramatically. Tell your company's safety director to look into Emory University's T'ai Chi study on balance. It will get his or her attention.

Some T'ai Chi exercises are very similar to exercises designed to prevent repetitive stress injury, such as carpal tunnel syndrome. You may be hitting several birds with your well-thrown T'ai Chi stone.

T'ai Chi Is a Natural for the Office

One thing that makes T'ai Chi uniquely ideal for the workplace is that it requires no special clothing or equipment. If you have 15 minutes and a quiet room, you are all set to experience some amazing stress reduction and energy boosting.

Because T'ai Chi is so slow and gentle, you often need not work up a sweat when taking a T'ai Chi break. By simply loosening your tie or kicking off your heels, you are ready to play. (See the *Exhibition of T'ai Chi Long Form* and *Exhibition of Entire Mulan Basic Short Form* on the Web Video Support to see how T'ai Chi can be done anywhere, in little space, and with no special wardrobe needs.) In fact, Sitting QiGong or simple Moving QiGong can be done right at your desk. As employees become more adept at these tools of breath and relaxation, they'll use them throughout the day to reduce stress and boost performance.

 A T'AI CHI PUNCH LINE

British dominance of the seas in the 1700s can, in part, be linked to the simple discovery that citrus fruits cure scurvy. Feeding British sailors limes, therefore, made it possible for British ships to stay at sea for much longer missions than enemy ships. Today's captains of industry who realize that stress is the greatest threat to their crews and who give their people tools such as T'ai Chi to avoid illness and burnout will dominate in business.

The Least You Need to Know

- T'ai Chi at work can save companies big money in avoided stress induced office politics; missed sick days; and increased creativity and flexibility.

- T'ai Chi can be done in work clothes in an office. Just loosen your tie or kick off your heels, and you're ready to go.

- T'ai Chi can help employees get along better by helping them relieve stress internally, rather than externalizing it to fellow workers.

- Companies can increase productivity by offering T'ai Chi classes to their employees.

Do T'ai Chi and Change the World

In This Chapter

- Lowering unemployment and healthcare costs
- Helping schools
- Reducing crime and violence
- Cleaning up the environment and healing our world

T'ai Chi is widely misunderstood. Is it an exercise, a martial art, or a meditation *technique?* Actually, T'ai Chi is all those things, but it also offers so much more. T'ai Chi can be a key to discovering our personal empowerment. As we find that we can take control over our body's circulation, our blood pressure, and our stress responses, we are empowered. This empowerment begins to resonate out to every aspect of our lives—work, relationships, and society.

As we feel empowered and T'ai Chi works its clarifying magic, we find learning easier and more exciting. We become drawn to learning as the world becomes fresher and more magical because of our new attitude of well-being. T'ai Chi cultivates and supports our childlikeness, curiosity, and zest for life. When we treasure each moment of our lives, we are much less likely to engage in acts that endanger our health or our freedom. When we feel at peace within ourselves, we are much less likely to hurt others. Much violence is the act of someone in personal pain who externalizes that pain on others. T'ai Chi can help heal that pain, thereby reducing much violence.

Since the first edition of this book came out over a decade ago, T'ai Chi and QiGong, as well as other meditative mind-body practices, have spread rapidly around the entire planet, which I learned from organizing World T'ai Chi and QiGong Day (see Chapter 22). Psychologist Steven Pinker's book *The Better Angels of Our Nature* offers research showing that our planet is now less violent than at any time in human history. Yeah, I know, hard to believe that, given the steady stream of violence we get from the shiny box in the living room, but true, nonetheless. As mentioned in the previous chapter, emerging research has shown that human consciousness is actually physically connected on an energetic level, and that we actually impact the state of the planet by clarifying and calming our own consciousness.

The reason this is mentioned in a *Complete Idiot's Guide to T'ai Chi and QiGong* is because Chinese Taoist philosophy, which T'ai Chi and QiGong philosophy are based upon, has been saying this for centuries. Each of us is the microcosm of the macrocosm of humanity, and by changing ourselves, we change the world. For example, by using tools like this to create a calmer household for ourselves and our family, we may actually be helping to lower future unemployment rates.

T'ai Chi and Unemployment

Because, according to research, people who grew up in high-stress households have higher unemployment rates, T'ai Chi may help both parents and children change that pattern. Furthermore, because the modern economy forces many people to change careers several times, T'ai Chi's promotion of letting go of the past and relaxing into change can be helpful to adults in today's job market.

England's Royal Academy of Pediatrics College released a study that concluded that "stressful" households caused problems for children that could last a lifetime. One thing it discovered was that children from such households endured higher unemployment levels than kids from more peaceful households. We know stress limits our creativity and can affect our self-esteem. T'ai Chi's ability to provide children with a tool that can help them find a calm place within, even when home is less than calm, can be of powerful help to them.

It is estimated that most of us will change, not jobs, but careers more than five times in our lifetime. For people who find change difficult,

this can be excruciatingly stressful and even life-threatening over time. In a world of constant and relentless change, T'ai Chi's ability to help us mentally, emotionally, and physically let go can be a great help.

> **SAGE SIFU SAYS**
>
> Change in and of itself is an essential and wonderful part of life. Our unhealthful responses to change are the problem. T'ai Chi is a tool to lubricate our way into the challenging and exciting future that awaits those who rise to the occasion.

The economy is in constant changing flux today. We've seen massive economic shifts in our lifetimes that would have taken centuries to evolve in the past. Changes in environment, energy, and society are being demanded of our generation like no other generation in history has seen. Change is the order of the day. If you're one of the unemployed, you might be thinking: What good does it do to be adaptable if there aren't any jobs out there to get, at a time of high unemployment?

Again, back to the microcosm of the macrocosm of T'ai Chi philosophy. By society using and expanding mind-body tools like T'ai Chi and QiGong into our lives and our culture, it can have an impact on our entire nation becoming more fluid, so we can flow into a new economy that will nurture us all.

By being able to let go of the past and being open to new information and self-definitions, we can be ready to flow into our next occupation. This flowing can happen not only less stressfully, but with an adventurous anticipation, just like when we were kids. This is what T'ai Chi can help us do as individuals and as a society. View the *Exhibition of the Entire Long Form* and *Exhibition of the Entire Mulan Basic Short Form* (Chapters 13 and 14 respectively) sections on the Web Video Support to see how the physical model of flow and release can provide a daily example of how we can begin to flow with less resistance through all aspects of life.

Research indicates that even just watching T'ai Chi can trigger relaxation responses in your body. Why this happens may be explained by genetic studies showing that humans, other higher-thinking species like dolphins and primates, and even mice according to research at the Pain Genetics Lab at McGill University, have an *empathy gene* that causes one to actually feel what the person or creature they are watching is experiencing. As you watch the T'ai Chi exhibition videos, feel yourself breathe and loosen as the T'ai Chi practitioner is doing so in the video.

When you catch yourself considering worst-case scenarios while engaged in a task or project, take a deep breath and let your entire body release thoughts, tensions, and fears. Then make a list or flow chart of what is required for your success. This will let you realistically decide whether to proceed rather than resist change because of irrational fears. T'ai Chi promotes a sense of being in the moment, of dealing with the tasks at hand, and of letting go of fear-based projections of the future.

T'ai Chi and the Healthcare Crisis

According to Dr. David Sobel, commenting on a long-term study by Kaiser Permenete, approximately 80 percent of the illnesses that send us to the doctor are due to stress. The six leading causes of death are stress-related. Today's healthcare crisis is literally due to stress. Stress can be managed, and perhaps no more effective stress-management tool exists than daily T'ai Chi and QiGong meditations. If these tools were taught on a massive scale in education, our healthcare crisis could end in one generation. This isn't some airy mystical T'ai Chi vision, it is scientific fact.

Thankfully, hospitals and insurance carriers are incorporating T'ai Chi and QiGong into what they offer clients. Physicians, neurologists, cardiac and hypertension specialists, and mental health providers are prescribing T'ai Chi for a host of physical, emotional, and mental conditions. Medical universities are now introducing T'ai Chi to their students as part of their training.

SAGE SIFU SAYS

To get the maximum benefits from T'ai Chi and QiGong, make time to practice every day. After a while, it won't be a chore at all. You will relish and savor your T'ai Chi moments, looking forward to them like a schoolkid looks forward to the weekend.

T'ai Chi begins to show us that we have a healthcare crisis simply because we choose to have a healthcare crisis. Each of us has it within our own power to dramatically lower our dependence on general healthcare, pharmacology, and surgery. The fastest-growing investment industry in the United States today is pharmaceuticals. The three top-selling medications are ulcer, high blood pressure, and mood-altering medications. T'ai Chi and/or QiGong can have significantly positive effects on all three of these conditions, in some cases.

T'ai Chi and QiGong are not at odds with modern Western healthcare. They are partners with it. You don't decide between medication or surgery and T'ai Chi. If you need medication or surgery, then use it. However, medication and surgery should not be the first line of defense. If we practice T'ai Chi, we might never develop the need for certain medications or for heart surgery. If we daily water our "T'ai tree" roots with the soothing balm of life energy, we will be less likely to ever need that medication or surgery, saving ourselves pain and money, while saving society a great financial burden.

We cannot afford to ignore our body's signals and our health until we are in a crisis situation and then expect society to lavish money upon us for expensive surgery or medication. This isn't just about Medicare alone; *all* our health insurance premiums are skyrocketing due to a national need to become mindful of our health. T'ai Chi can save us all big money and help us feel good while doing it. And by this evolution occurring, it will bring down the cost of surgery and drugs, so that when we do need them, we'll all be able to afford them.

T'ai Chi in Education

I mentioned that by training all students in schools in these techniques it could end our nation's health crisis, but it should also happen because it would improve their education.

Studies show that change, even change for the better, is stressful. A good example is when you upgrade your computer. The newer program gives you new tools to make your work faster and more efficient, but letting go of the old ways and learning the new is often stressful.

In many ways, each day our children are learning new ways to do everything, both at home and at school. Kids today are under tremendous stress because the world is changing very fast, and they will see changes we never dreamed of in our lives. Therefore, the best tool we can give them to launch out upon the world with confidence and health is, you guessed it, T'ai Chi.

Helping Students Stay Current in a World of Change!

T'ai Chi brings you back to the calm center, no matter how fast life's carousel is spinning. In today's rapidly changing world, this is a very important tool to give our children. No matter how much math, science, and economic facts we give them, they will be lost if they don't know how to thrive healthfully in a world of change. Why? Because our understanding of math, science, and economics is changing on an almost daily basis. The world is only getting faster with the explosion of the information age. Therefore, children with mind/body training that can help them adapt to new ways more easily and more healthfully will have a distinct advantage over kids *who learn only* the current ways things are done or the current textbook facts.

Chronic stress can even inhibit our thinking processes, literally shrinking parts of the brain. So by teaching children T'ai Chi, we help them be calm and provide them a physical model to relax through changes, which thereby can improve their mental function and their educational experience.

A T'AI CHI PUNCH LINE

If you look at many long-term T'ai Chi practitioners, Chinese or Western, you will find very vibrant people, often at the pinnacles of their professions. T'ai Chi practitioners don't fear and run from change, but find it essential to a full life.

Studying Health from the Inside Out

Hopefully, every school will begin providing T'ai Chi instruction through all levels of education and to teachers as well. T'ai Chi is a cross between physical education and health science, and should eventually become a staple of health science. What better way for kids to learn about their bodies and health than by paying attention to the laboratory they walk around in every day, their own miraculous minds and bodies, through practicing T'ai Chi's mindful exercises?

Although most of the high school T'ai Chi classes I've taught have been in health science, instructors in physical education, art, and drama are considering T'ai Chi as an adjunct to their classes.

Helping Students Avoid Drugs

Some schools are already providing T'ai Chi to students. I have taught T'ai Chi and QiGong relaxation therapy to students in elementary, junior high, high school, and university levels through health science, college-preparatory programs, and drug-abuse-prevention programs, as well as for developmentally disabled

students. Health science teachers have told me that students claim the main reason they begin smoking or using drugs and alcohol is to alleviate stress. Of course, those of us with more life experience know that, in the end, drug abuse creates more stress, but it's not enough to simply tell kids to "just say no." We must take the next step and provide them with tools to manage the enormous stress they face in an increasingly complex world.

T'ai Chi and Crime and Law Enforcement

T'ai Chi is now being taught in prisons, as well as in court-sponsored rehabilitation programs. T'ai Chi's ability to build self-esteem, heal childhood trauma, and manage potentially violent stress makes it an incredible coping tool for anyone trying to change. If we want to reduce crime, finding ways people can become productive parts of society is a cost-effective and just plain effective way to do it. It costs twice as much to send a child to prison as it does to send that child to Harvard. Per capita, the United States has incarcerated more of its children than any nation in the world. It's time to find creative solutions such as T'ai Chi and mind/body fitness training to heal the very roots of crime—*the potential criminals.* Doing this before the crime occurs will save us all much pain and vast amounts of money.

A T'AI CHI PUNCH LINE

Many people using T'ai Chi to rehabilitate from drug-abuse problems like the fact that T'ai Chi gives them something to replace the old habits with. Rather than just denying themselves the high they loved, they are growing toward a new life as T'ai Chi helps them improve each and every day.

Law enforcement officers work in constant danger and often see only the worst sides of people. This can be very stressful. Historically, law enforcement officials have suffered from stress-related maladies such as alcoholism, drug abuse, coronary heart disease, diabetes, and suicide, according to *Police Chief Magazine* and the U.S. Public Health Service. T'ai Chi may be an effective, multipurpose way to help law enforcement officers deal with job-related stress. T'ai Chi's martial applications are an added bonus to officers learning T'ai Chi's soothing stress-management tools.

T'ai Chi can help in several ways. First, it can help officers dump job stress after work. Then if they do go out for a drink after T'ai Chi class, they will be doing it for pleasure rather than for stress reduction. This can mean the difference between a couple of social drinks and a mind-numbing binge.

Second, if officers are less stressed on duty, they will likely see more options in any given situation. Problems can be defused more easily when in a calmer, clearer state. Even in difficult situations, T'ai Chi's calming effects can resonate, especially if it helps the officers sleep better, which T'ai Chi is known to do. T'ai Chi's calming aspects can help defuse potentially dangerous situations, which leaves the officer with less stress to take with them off duty. Less stress begets less stress, and so on and so on.

Hopefully, departments will eventually provide officers with seven-hour shifts and use the last hour for T'ai Chi decompression time. This will make business sense for all the reasons listed in Chapter 19 on corporate T'ai Chi, but these benefits are magnified because law enforcement officials' stress can be even higher.

T'ai Chi and Violence

Most domestic violence is a very ineffective form of stress management. Domestic violence is a way a very unhappy person takes out personal stress on his or her loved ones. It's ineffective because as we tear down those around us, that eventually tears us down. We create a sanctuary of pain rather than a loving home.

T'ai Chi can change that from many angles. If children begin to use T'ai Chi's mind/body fitness stress-management tools to self-heal in school, the cycle of pain at home will be changed and diminished in some ways. Then if parents are encouraged to learn these tools through community services, they can change the cycle even more effectively. There is a great spider web of connection in a community that will be affected as well. If one parent breaks a cycle of abuse and pain, his or her children will not spread that pain by being mean to the children around them at school or by growing up and passing it down to their kids by being violent to them.

A T'AI CHI PUNCH LINE

Many T'ai Chi practitioners hear others tell them they have "changed," "are calmer," or "are easier to be around" before they even notice the changes in themselves. Even when you are feeling stress, others may see you as "mellow" in comparison to the rest of the world.

Alcohol and other substance abuses aggravate much domestic violence. (The benefits of T'ai Chi for drug rehabilitation are discussed in Chapter 18.) Substance abuse and domestic violence all set a destructive dynamic in motion that reaches far beyond the home. A famous "kick the cat" story shows how a community is affected by one person's calm or rage:

An executive gets a traffic ticket on the way to work and then fumes at his administrative assistant. She, in turn, snaps at the other executives and employees she deals with. They get ticked off and snap at their co-workers, who are testy with people in the other companies they deal with on the phone, and so on. Eventually, thousands of people who have had a lousy day hit the freeway and begin to give the one-fingered salute to other motorists. And so it goes.

Finally, all these seething people get home and yell at their spouses, who yell at the kids, who walk upstairs and kick the cat.

T'ai Chi can invert this process, and thousands of family cats can get a loving caress by kids growing up in a more loving world, nurtured by parents who work at companies that provide health tools to them like T'ai Chi. Sound far-fetched? Not really. Stress is the source of much of our communal pain, and stress management such as T'ai Chi can act as a balm and dramatically heal it.

> **A T'AI CHI PUNCH LINE**
>
> Once you learn T'ai Chi, you'll begin to notice people practicing everywhere you go, in any country in the world. T'ai Chi is an international language. My students have done T'ai Chi with people in England, France, Japan, Vietnam, Mexico, China, El Salvador, and Cuba, to name a few. As you travel, T'ai Chi will give you a pleasant vehicle to interact with and meet other people, even if you don't speak their language.

A study done by the Transcendental Meditation Foundation (which teaches an excellent form of stress management called Transcendental Meditation, or TM) found that when a small percentage of the population of a community, school, or organization practiced TM, it had a positive impact on that entire social body. Therefore, even though many people will never practice T'ai Chi, those who do may change the entire community in positive ways.

T'ai Chi and the Environment

At first, it may not seem like T'ai Chi has anything to do with our world's environment, but it does. The words *T'ai Chi* mean "the Supreme Ultimate Point in the Universe." Every single part of the entire world exists within each and every thing, even you and me. Modern physics demonstrates this by explaining that all things are made of energy—*the same energy.* You, I, the sun and moon, and Earth's oceans and mountains are all made of the same energy. We are connected. This is brought home even more as science explains that you and I and everyone on this planet have breathed an oxygen atom breathed by Jesus, Buddha, and Mohammed. The world gets smaller.

> **SAGE SIFU SAYS**
>
> Each time you walk outside, look up at the sky and at the trees or grass. Let the full breadth of nature's beauty wash over you. Think of opening your body to the universal energy as if you were an open, airy sponge that could fill with the life around you, and likewise you can expand out to merge with it. If you make this a habit and take 30 or 60 seconds to do this each time you walk in or out of your home, it will change your life.

When you practice T'ai Chi and especially Sitting QiGong, you often feel at peace, somehow connected to the world around you, as if you were the center of the universe. This experience leaves you feeling as though you matter, yet it also leaves you feeling as though every other person and every other thing in this world are of vast and profound importance as well.

T'ai Chi and QiGong remind us that we are energy by immersing our mind and body in the experience of it each day. This constant immersion reminds us how closely we are linked to all things. This isn't an illusion. The illusion is that we think we are separate from the world. The rainforest and ocean are the earth's lungs and thermostats. Without them, we perish. To feel connected to the world is to become real. T'ai Chi and QiGong help us become more and more real.

Our decisions about how to live in our world will be healthfully influenced by the realness that T'ai Chi cultivates. This will be a powerful asset to building a cleaner, healthier world. As with all things, the world's environmental health begins with our own state of health. Your heart beats to supply oxygen to your entire body. However, the first thing the heart feeds is itself because if it is healthier, stronger, and clearer, it is more useful to its world (your body). By feeding yourself the healing force of life energy every day, you enable yourself to be a healing force as you flow through the world *around you*.

The Least You Need to Know

- T'ai Chi helps heal our society, our world, and us.
- T'ai Chi saves money in healthcare and may lower crime and unemployment rates.
- T'ai Chi helps us all "just get along."
- T'ai Chi influences our environment in a positive way.

Celebrating World T'ai Chi and QiGong Day

In This Chapter

- Unleashing your power to change the world
- Connecting to T'ai Chi and QiGong world events, teachers, and resources with one source: www. worldtaichiday.org

Legendary poet Rainer Maria Rilke wrote: "If we want to make something truly spectacular of our world, there is nothing whatsoever that can stop us." Most people who practice T'ai Chi and QiGong for decades look back and realize that their lives would have been so much more constricted and less spectacular had they not discovered these mind-body tools. As the techniques help us un-grip on old perceptions of ourselves, they enable us to open to the fact that our lives offer much more potential.

Not only are *you* truly profound and unique, but you are holding a truly profound and unique book: the first edition of this book actually launched a world event, changing the world in a healing way. World T'ai Chi and QiGong Day, through coverage by *CNN, The New York Times, The South China Morning Post, and media worldwide,* has educated millions about T'ai Chi and QiGong. Therefore, this book doesn't just "talk the talk"—it *walks the walk* of T'ai Chi's expansive personal power.

Since this global phenomenon was launched, T'ai Chi has rapidly expanded throughout the world, with many leading T'ai Chi and QiGong professionals crediting World T'ai Chi and QiGong Day's annual global health-education event as a catalyst to this rapid global expanse of awareness of these ancient mind-body tools. In 2012 media announcements of T'ai Chi's ongoing permeation of popular culture included famed actor Keanu Reeves' landing a contract to create a major motion picture titled "Man of T'ai Chi," and film star Jet Li's announced collaboration with the Chinese Wush Association to promote T'ai Chi's benefits worldwide. See the full breadth of this massive, unprecedented worldwide event, which this book's first edition helped create, as a video montage at Web Video Support's *World T'ai Chi and QiGong Day—A Global Healing Phenomenon,* www.idiotsguides. com/taichi.

Too often in our lives we underestimate and undervalue our power as human beings. The practice of T'ai Chi and QiGong is designed to unblock the rigid limitations we hold so that the greatest potential within us can flow up and out through our relaxed mind and body.

It's actually very unhealthy for human beings to settle for less than their greatest potential, for *repression of enthusiasm and hope can diminish our health.* Studies reveal that when people give of themselves to make the world a better place, it improves their physical and mental health—kind of an "instant karma," if you will (kudos to John Lennon). And T'ai Chi and QiGong help energize and motivate us for "compassionate action," as T'ai Chi philosophy extols us to aspire to.

Participating in World T'ai Chi and QiGong Day is a way you can expand your T'ai Chi and QiGong journey to include joining with hundreds of thousands of like-minded people worldwide each year to be part of a fun and beneficial global health and healing event known as World T'ai Chi and QiGong Day.

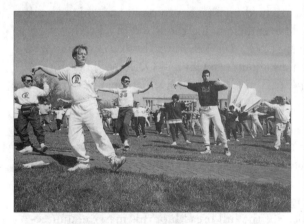

Bill Douglas leading what was reported as "the largest T'ai Chi exhibition outside of China" at the time. This event launched a global annual phenomenon that is now celebrated annually in hundreds of cities in over 70 nations.

Unleash the World-Altering Power Within You!

As we practice T'ai Chi, we realize it changes our lives by showing us that most of what holds us back is not "out there" in the world as much as it is *in our own mental and emotional limitations* in the form of rigidity we've constrained ourselves with unconsciously. As earlier chapters explained, this mental constraint actually affects circulation and health functions over time. But it also holds back our lives. My T'ai Chi and QiGong practice enabled me to open to large, expansive ideas, such as, for example, creating World T'ai Chi and QiGong Day, first by announcing it in the first edition of this book. Then these powerful tools gave me the stress-management techniques needed to endure the stress of actually fulfilling that dream.

> **OUCH!**
>
> When you catch your mind revolving around the negatives of "I can't do this" or "I can't change that," practice the QiGong breathing/energy exercise taught in Part 3. Let your mind and body *let go of everything.* Releasing negatives fills you with hope as you fill with light.

The same T'ai Chi and QiGong energy empowered teachers and organizers in cities worldwide to envision and create massive (and smaller) World T'ai Chi and QiGong Day events locally in over 70 nations that make this global event the historic annual reality it has become. This event has since been officially proclaimed by 22 U.S. governors, and has been recognized as part of past United Nations World Health Organization, and United States

Department of Health & Human Services' events, and by mayors, legislatures, and senates of many states and nations.

The purpose of World T'ai Chi and QiGong Day is twofold: to educate millions worldwide on the profound health and healing benefits of T'ai Chi and QiGong and how they can heal society and save hundreds of billions of dollars annually, and by bringing humanity together across racial, economic, and geopolitical boundaries each year to wrap the earth in a healing wave of energy. In this way we create a vision of what is possible for the world when we focus on health and healing.

The same way T'ai Chi helps us understand that our body is not separate, isolated parts, but a flowing continuum of related networks and energy field, it also helps us understand that we are part of the world, connected to all of humanity. Again, T'ai Chi's Taoist roots speak of this realization, of how we are an integrative part of life, and what is good for the world around us is ultimately good for us.

We are entering an extraordinary time in human history with access to modern *and ancient wonders* to make life better and better. We are learning that by healing ourselves, we heal the world, and vice versa. And today we have access to the best of both modern and ancient sciences. By marrying the dynamic power of our modern Western technological world's information age with the inner peace and clarity that ancient Eastern wisdom has cultivated and refined for us over the last 2,000 years, we may be at the beginning of a wondrous human renaissance where health and clarity merge with limitless potential to *create the world of our dreams.*

Bookmark www.worldtaichiday.org and enjoy its free resources, and get involved in this global movement for health and healing. Encourage friends and family to utilize the many free resources there, where they can sign up for a free email newsletter that offers breaking medical research on T'ai Chi and QiGong, free tutorials, healthy and tasty recipes, and essays on how to get the most out of your T'ai Chi and QiGong journey.

Photos of Past World T'ai Chi and QiGong Day Events

The motto of World T'ai Chi and QiGong Day is "One World … One Breath." Following are a small sampling of the spectacular human art that is World T'ai Chi and QiGong Day. Find past event photos from nearly 70 nations at the Photo Video Gallery of www.WorldTaiChiDay.org.

"One World … One Breath," the official motto of World T'ai Chi and QiGong Day, written in 34 different languages.

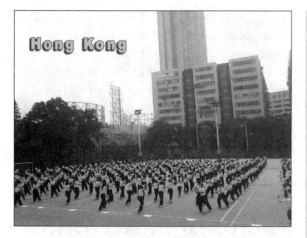

This WTCQD event was sponsored by the Hong Kong Chinese Martial Arts Association.
(Photo courtesy of World T'ai Chi and QiGong Day event organizers in Hong Kong.)

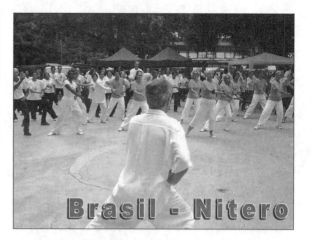

(Photo courtesy of World T'ai Chi and QiGong Day event organizers in Niteroi, Brazil.)

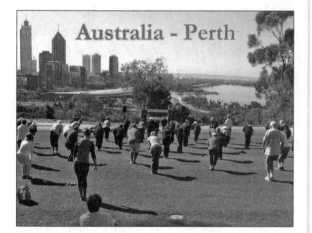

(Photo courtesy of World T'ai Chi and QiGong Day event organizers in Perth Australia.)

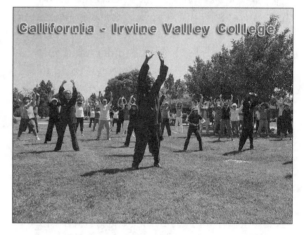

The University of California at Irvine, in conjunction with Professor Shin Lin, holds annual WTCQD events at UCI.
(Photo courtesy of World T'ai Chi and QiGong Day event organizers in Irvine, California.)

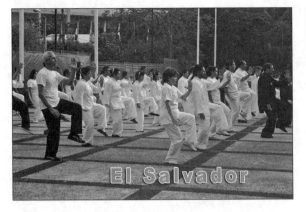

(Photo courtesy of World T'ai Chi and QiGong Day event organizers in San Salvador, El Salvador.)

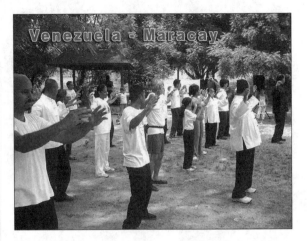

(Photo courtesy of World T'ai Chi and QiGong Day event organizers in Maracay, Venezuela.)

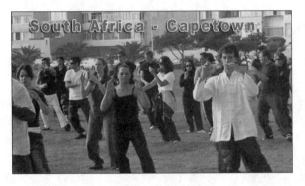

(Photo courtesy of World T'ai Chi and QiGong Day event organizers in Capetown, South Africa.)

The Least You Need to Know

* You have the seeds for wondrous change *within you.*
* Fear limits our ability to expand our mind and world to open up to hopeful visions.
* T'ai Chi and QiGong can help you breathe and relax, and open to limitless possibility.
* Joining in World T'ai Chi and QiGong Day can help change the world by lessening stress and fear, and expanding health and hope.
* Your internal personal world and our collective external world community become limitless as we practice life tools enabling us to relax into the future.

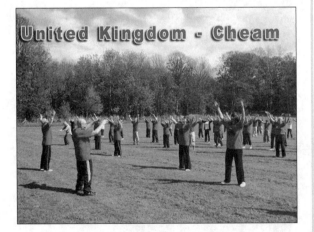

(Photo courtesy of World T'ai Chi and QiGong Day event organizers in Cheam, United Kingdom.)

The T'ai Chi and QiGong Yellow Pages

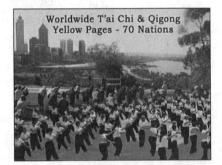

Although two chapters in this book relate to particular T'ai Chi styles (Chapters 13 and 14), the majority of this book is a valuable resource for anyone exploring any style of T'ai Chi or QiGong. In fact, this book is used as a student primer and textbook by many teachers of many different styles worldwide. With that in mind, I created this appendix to expose readers to the many styles and schools in their communities, so you can hit the ground running in beginning your T'ai Chi and QiGong journey now.

For those who can't attend local live classes, the four-hour instructional DVD listed in Appendix C can be a godsend. Its real-time class-like format is similar to attending classes *in the comfort of your own home*. The DVD details the illustrated instructions in Chapter 13, and teaches the Moving QiGong warm-ups in a real-time, relaxing, meditative format. You may also find that after learning at home, it's easier to learn in live classes, even if the styles are different.

In this appendix, you'll find links to the world's most extensive listing of contact information for T'ai Chi and QiGong organizations, schools, and teachers, a list of some of the most popular T'ai Chi and QiGong-related magazines and journals, and links to some of the largest world conferences and congresses on T'ai Chi and QiGong.

National and International T'ai Chi and QiGong Directories, Organizations, and Associations

World T'ai Chi and QiGong Day
www.worldtaichiday.org

The world's most comprehensive, and easily searchable, listing of T'ai Chi and QiGong classes, schools, and organizations in all 50 U.S. states and in over 70 nations worldwide.

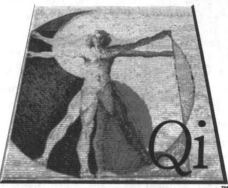

At www.worldtaichiday.org, click on Events/Schools. Due to the volume of listings (for most directories), the authenticity of each listing cannot be verified; rather, the listings are a clearinghouse of information to assist in your search for a school near you, not an endorsement. You are your own best judge of what school or teacher is right for you. Always use discernment when contacting and choosing a school or teacher.

Bookmark or favorite-place www.worldtaichiday.org for continually updated information for all the school listings. You can also join the free email mailing list there to get breaking information on T'ai Chi and QiGong medical research, free video tutorials, and T'ai Chi and QiGong news from the T'ai Chi and QiGong community all around the world.

World Healing Day
World Healing Day offers a directory of the full spectrum of mind-body internal healing arts, including T'ai Chi, QiGong, Yoga, Reiki, Meditation, and more.

Bookmark this website, and you can also join the free email mailing list there for information on the global event, breaking medical research on the mind-body arts, and more.
www.WorldHealingDay.org
www.WorldYogaDay.org
www.WorldReikiDay.org
www.WorldHealingMeditationDay.org

Find Tai Chi
www.FindTaiChi.com

Tai Chi Lifestyle
www.TaiChiLifestyle.com

Canadian Taijiquan Federation
www.canadiantaijiquanfederation.ca

International Tai Chi Association (ITCCA) Italia
www.itcca.it

Hong Kong Chinese Martial Arts Association
www.hkcmaa.com.hk/index_en.html

National QG Assn.—Nationwide and Int'l.
www.nqa.org

World QiGong Federation
www.eastwestqi.com/wqf/wqf.htm

American QiGong Association
www.eastwestqi.com/html/aqa/aqa.html

American Tai Chi and QiGong Association
www.americantaichi.org/

Tai Chi Union for Great Britain
www.taichiunion.com

British Council for Chinese Martial Arts
www.bccma.com

Taijiquan and QiGong Federation for Europe (TCFE)
www.tcfe.org

QiGong Association of America
www.qi.org

Yang Family Tai Chi Association
www.yangfamilytaichi.com/splash.php

Sun Style Association
www.suntaiji.com/sunlutang.html

Tai Chi Chih
www.taichichih.org/

Bookmark www.WorldTaiChiDay.org, and join the free email mailing list there for information and updates on new and emerging associations and directories.

World T'ai Chi and QiGong Conferences and Congresses

World Congress on QiGong—San Francisco
www.eastwestqi.com/wcq/wcq.html

TCM Kongress—Germany
www.tcm-kongress.de/en/index.htm

www.WorldTaiChiDay.org

T'ai Chi and QiGong Magazines and Journals

Qi—The Journal of Traditional Eastern Health and Fitness
www.qi-journal.com/journal.asp

The Empty Vessel: A Journal of Contemporary Taoism
www.abodetao.com/

Tai Chi Chuan Magazine UK
www.taichiunion.com/magazine.php

Taijiquan Journal
www.taijiquanjournal.com/

Kung Fu Magazine
www.kungfumagazine.com/

www.WorldTaiChiDay.org

Suggested Readings

Bach, Richard. *Jonathan Livingston Seagull*. New York: The Macmillan Company, 1970.

Badgley, Laurence, MD. *Healing AIDS Naturally*. Foster City, CA: Human Energy Press, 1987.

Batmanghelidj, F., MD. T*he Body's Many Cries for Water*. Falls Church, VA: Global Health Solutions, Inc., 1997.

Behr, Thomas E., PhD. *The Tao of Sales*. Rockport, MA: Element Books, Inc., 1997.

Benson, Herbert, MD. *The Relaxation Response*. New York: Avon Books, 1975.

Booth, Jennifer. *Wind Blowing Lotus Leaf: The Way of Enlightened Action*. Huntington Beach, CA: Warrior of Light Publications, 1999.

Borysenko, Joan, PhD., and Miroslav Borysenko, PhD. *The Power of the Mind to Heal*. Carlsbad, CA: Hay House, Inc., 1994.

Capra, Fritjof (author of The Tao of Physics). *The Web of Life*. New York: Doubleday, 1996.

Chen Pan Ling. *Chen Pan Ling's Original Tai Chi Chuan Textbook*. New Orleans: Blitz! Design, 1998.

Chopra, Deepak. *Ageless Body, Timeless Mind*. New York: Harmony Books, 1993.

Cohen, Kenneth S. *The Way of Qigong: The Art and Science of Chinese Energy Healing*. New York: Ballantine Books, 1997.

Diller, Lawrence H., MD. *Running on Ritalin: A Physician Reflects on Children, Society, and Performance in a Pill*. New York: Bantam Books, 1998.

Douglas, Bill. *A Conspiracy of Spirits* (T'ai Chi novel). Illumination Corporation publishing, 2011.

Douglas, Bill. *2012 The Awakening* (T'ai Chi novel—Chosen Best Awakening Fiction of the Year). Illumination Corporation, 2010.

Gerber, Richard, MD. *Vibrational Medicine*. Santa Fe, NM: Bear and Company, 1988.

Greene, Brian. *The Elegant Universe: Superstrings, Hidden Dimensions, and the Quest for the Ultimate Theory*. New York, London: W.W. Norton and Company, 1999.

Lasorso, Vincent J. Jr. *Immortal's Gift: A Parable for the Soul*. Cincinnati, OH: White Willow School of Tai Chi, 2000.

Lee, Martin, PhD., with Melinda Emily and Joyce Lee. *The Healing Art of T'ai Chi.* New York: Sterling Publishing Co. Inc., 1996.

Leight, Michelle Dominique. *The New Beauty: East-West Teachings in the Beauty of Body and Soul.* New York: Kodansha America Inc., 1995.

Lipton, Bruce, PhD. *Biology of Belief.* Santa Rosa, CA: Mountain of Love/Elite Books, 2005.

Loupos, John. *Inside Tai Chi: Contemporary Views on an Ancient Art.* Roslindale, MA: YMAA Pub. Center, 2002.

Luk, Charles. *Taoist Yoga, Alchemy and Immortality.* York Beach, ME: Samuel Weisner, Inc., 1973.

Mann, Felix, MB, LMCC. *Acupuncture: The Ancient Chinese Art of Healing.* New York: Random House, 1978.

Mayer, Michael. *Secrets to Living Younger Longer: The Self Healing Path of Qigong, Standing Meditation and Tai Chi.* Orinda, CA: Bodymind Healing Pub., 2004.

McGaa, Ed (Eagle Man). *Mother Earth Spirituality—Native American Paths to Healing Ourselves and Our World.* San Francisco: Harper, 1990.

Moyers, Bill. *Healing and the Mind.* New York: Doubleday, 1993.

Rothstein, Larry, EdD, Lyle H. Miller, PhD., and Alma Dell Smith, PhD. *The Stress Solution.* New York: Pocket Books, 1993.

Sandifer, Jon. *Acupressure for Health, Vitality and First Aid.* Rockport, MA: Element Books Limited, 1997.

Sang, Larry. *The Principles of Feng Shui.* Monterey Park, CA: The American Feng Shui Institute, 1994.

Shanor, Karen Nesbitt, PhD. *The Emerging Mind: New Research into the Meaning of Consciousness,* Based on the Smithsonian Institution Lecture Series. Los Angeles: Renaissance Books, 1999.

Sheldrake, Rupert. *A New Science of Life: Morphic Resonance.* Rochester, VT: Park Street Press, 1995.

Star, Jonathan, trans. *Rumi: In the Arms of the Beloved.* New York: Jeremy P. Tarcher/Putnam, 1997.

Talbot, Michael. *The Holographic Universe.* New York: HarperCollins Publishers, Inc., 1991.

Watts, Alan. *The Way of Zen.* New York: Vintage Books, 1985.

Weil, Andrew, MD. *Healthy Aging: A Lifelong Guide to Your Physical and Spiritual Well-Being.* New York: Rodale, Inc., 2005

———. *Spontaneous Healing.* New York: Ballantine Books, 1995.

Williams, Tom, PhD. *The Complete Illustrated Guide to Chinese Medicine.* Rockport, MA: Element Books, Inc., 1996.

Yang, Dr. Jwing-Ming. *Taijiquan, Classical Yang Style: The Complete Form and Qigong.* Roslindale, MA: YMAA Pub. Center 1999.

Yu-Cheng Huang. *Change the Picture.* Skokie, IL: Yu-Cheng Huang, 1998.

Yutang, Lin. *The Wisdom of Laotse.* New York: The Modern Library, 1948.

Author's Acclaimed Four-Hour, Class-Like DVD

Anthology of T'ai Chi and QiGong: The Prescription for the Future DVD (four hours)

This book's valuable Web Video Support are excerpts from the author's world-acclaimed *fully instructional* four-hour DVD mentioned above, and from Angela's nearly 80-minute *Mulan T'ai Chi* DVD. These programs offer you the experience of studying with us in our live classes.

If you would like a multi-hour, real-time, class-like, in-depth video experience with the author, that will enable you to sink deep into the relaxation aspect of your T'ai Chi practice, you can order his Four-Hour DVD Anthology today at www.SMARTaichi.com.

To order by phone, call 1-913-648-2256 (international) or 1-877-482-4241 (toll-free in the United States). Be sure to state that you are a *CIG to T'ai Chi & QiGong* reader to get the special generous CIG reader discount on the four-hour Anthology DVD.

A few comments from people who've enjoyed Bill's DVD: *Anthology of T'ai Chi & QiGong: The Prescription for the Future.*

An excellent introduction to this ancient art.
—*Book List Magazine* (published by the American Library Association)

The BEST!!!!!!
—E. Young, California

I look forward to my practice and feeling like I'm doing it with a 'friend.' All in all, I get the feeling that Bill really wants people to get T'ai Chi and QiGong, rather than just *make a buck*. I highly recommend him and his instruction to everyone.
—Linda Lyon, California

A must-have for stressed people. Thanks, Bill, for being the guide.
—Johan Pyfferoen, Veurne, Belgium

Your videos are the best T'ai Chi videos I've seen … *easy to follow*.
—Francesca Sato, Rome, Italy

If you want clear instruction, a knowledgeable instructor, and a great product, get this DVD!
—Arthur L. Fleschner, Philadelphia, PA

NOTE: More DVDs by this book's authors and other masters around the world will soon become available through SMARTaichi. com. Join the Free Email Newsletter List at WorldTaiChiDay.org and select "Products" as one of your areas of interest, to be alerted as new resources become available. You can also sign up there to get free World T'ai Chi Day email newsletters on breaking T'ai Chi and QiGong medical research, health tips, healthy diet recipes from author Angela Wong Douglas, and much more. You can also email us with questions at BillDouglas@WorldTaiChiDay.org and at AngelaOrders@aol.com.

Bill Douglas's QiGong Meditation CDs:

Anthology of QiGong: Relaxation Therapy and Mind Expansion: Contains four meditation tracks, including *Introduction to QiGong Breathing, QiGong: Relaxation Therapy, QiGong: Expanding Awareness, and QiGong: An Earth Cleansing.*

QiGong: For Children's Health and Relaxation: Perfect for young children to enjoy at nap time or bedtime, it combines breathing and relaxation techniques with a fanciful flying adventure of the imagination. Teachers and parents will enjoy benefits from it as they too listen along with it.

DVD from co-author Angela Wong Douglas:

Mulan Quan Tai Chi & Moving Qigong— A Feminine Art for Power and Strength DVD (approximately 80 minutes)

Coming soon! Mulan Fan and Mulan Sword DVDs.

Also coming soon! Online advanced T'ai Chi and QiGong instructional videos in all the major styles from some of the world's great masters. To be notified as they come online, join the free email mailing list at www. WorldTaiChiDay.org.

Again, you can order our acclaimed DVD and CD programs today at www.SMARTaichi. com, or via links at Appendix C's Web Video Support where you can get *a very generous CIG reader discount* on the four-hour *Anthology of T'ai Chi & QiGong* DVD (see www.idiotsguides. com/taichi).

abdominal breathing   The QiGong breathing technique whereby the abdominal area, or lower lungs, fills first and then the upper chest fills, fully inflating the lungs. On the exhale, the upper chest relaxes inward as the lungs deflate, followed by the abdominal muscles relaxing inward, allowing the lower lungs to deflate and fully expending the air from the lungs.

acupressure   A massage technique of stimulating the acupuncture points without the use of acupuncture needles.

acupuncture   A medical science that manipulates the flow of Qi, or life energy, through the body to maximize the body's health systems.

acupuncture maps   Diagrams or models to help acupuncturists locate the acupuncture points on the body.

aura   The sometimes-visible aspect of life energy, whether seen with Kirlian photography or with the naked eye.

biofeedback   A computer program often used to train people to relax under stress by showing their blood pressure, heart rate, and so on, while the participant uses relaxation techniques to normalize those indicators.

Bone Marrow Cleansing   A Moving QiGong exercise designed to cleanse the bone marrow of stress that might inhibit the immune system.

Carry the Moon   A Moving QiGong exercise designed to help the spine stay supple, support kidney function, and promote flexibility throughout the frame.

center   The physical, mental, emotional, and spiritual clarity that T'ai Chi and QiGong are designed to cultivate. Modern psychologists call this homeostasis.

Chen style   An ancient T'ai Chi style and the basis of the Yang style.

Chinese Drum, The   A QiGong warm-up for T'ai Chi preparation.

Chinese Medica   The bible of Traditional Chinese Medicine (TCM), encompassing all known knowledge on acupuncture, herbal medicine, and QiGong.

crisis   The Chinese character for *crisis* is made of two characters, the character for *danger* plus the one for *opportunity*.

dan tien   The physical energy center of the body, located approximately 1½ to 3 inches below the navel, near the center of the body.

DHEA (dehydroepiandrosterone)   Adequate dehydroepiandrosterone levels are related to youthfulness and a more functional immune system. QiGong practice is believed to elevate DHEA levels.

Dong Gong   *See* Moving QiGong.

energy meridians   In Chinese, *jing luo*, or channel network. Modern acupuncturists may refer to these meridians as "bioenergetic circuits." These are the paths that Qi moves through to circulate within the body, although they are not physical vessels like veins or arteries. They are energy channels where energy appears to flow more easily through the body's tissue. There are 14 main meridians, and 12 of those are directly associated with bodily organs, such as the heart and liver.

External QiGong   A TCM practice whereby the provider allows his or her Qi, cultivated through internal QiGong practice, to flow, usually from the hands, out into the patient to help the healing process.

fan lao huan tong   In Chinese, this means "reverse old age and return to youthfulness." This is the goal of T'ai Chi and QiGong.

Feng Shui   The Chinese design art for creating flow and balance of energy within homes and other structures.

fight-or-flight response   The body's reflex response to stress that involves elevated blood pressure, increased heart rate, and feelings of subdued panic.

free radicals   Atoms with an extra electron, believed to contribute to the aging process. Regular T'ai Chi practice may reduce the cell damage these free radicals cause.

Grand Terminus   The yin yang symbol, and also the final movement of the Kuang Ping Yang style of T'ai Chi.

holistic   Chinese philosophy that sees the entire universe within each individual part, in much the same way the body's building blocks of DNA coding are contained within each individual cell in the body.

homeostasis   Modern therapists use this term to describe a chemical, emotional, and mental sense of health and well-being. This is what T'ai Chi is designed to promote.

horary clock   TCM's understanding of the ebb and flow of life energy patterns within the body. This understanding is used to treat various conditions using acupuncture, herbal, or QiGong therapy for optimal results.

Horse Stance   The basic stance for T'ai Chi, QiGong, and most martial arts.

hypertension   High blood pressure caused most often by unmanaged stress. High blood pressure is the cause of most heart disease.

I Ching   Also known as *The Book of Changes*, the *I Ching* is an ancient Chinese book of divination. The book is used to tell fortunes or to inspire people to look more deeply into themselves and their lives before making life decisions.

Jing Gong   *See* Sitting QiGong.

Kirlian photography   A photography method that appears to capture images of Qi or life energy.

Kuang Ping Yang style   The 64-movement long form of T'ai Chi brought to the West by master Kuo Lien Ying.

Lao-Tzu The founder of Taoist philosophy.

master One who cultivates a clarity in life, enabling her to be a nurturing force to herself and the world.

Moving QiGong Moving exercises, such as T'ai Chi, that stimulate the flow of Qi through the body.

Mulan Quan style A relatively modern form, rooted in a more ancient style. This may be the most elegant form of T'ai Chi, incorporating both dance and martial arts forms.

postbirth breathing Normal abdominal T'ai Chi breathing.

prebirth breathing A form of breathing that requires the abdominal muscles to draw in on an in-breath and relax out on an exhale.

psychoneuroimmunology The modern science of studying how the mind's attitudes and beliefs affect physical health.

Push Hands A sparring tool and/or a subtle tool for self-awareness, whereby two partners (or opponents) engage in a dancelike exchange, becoming aware of one another's posture and balance. This can be carried to an extreme of pushing the opponent down when he is vulnerable, or merely becoming gently conscious of when he is vulnerable without actually pushing him down.

Qi Life energy. The Chinese character for *Qi* is also the character for air, as in breath.

QiGong "Breath work" or "energy exercise." There are about 7,000 QiGong exercises in the Chinese Medica (the bible of Chinese medicine).

sensei A teacher; a term of respect often used in martial arts circles.

sifu Chinese for "one who has mastered an art." This term applies not only to martial arts; a master chef or artist might be a sifu as well.

sinking Qi Settling the weight of the body into the leg you are shifting onto.

Sitting QiGong Meditative exercises to promote the flow of Qi throughout the body.

Soong Yi-Dien "Loosen up"; also a T'ai Chi instruction to loosen the body, mind, and heart, encouraging the student to be more flexible and adaptable to all changes.

spirit The Latin root of *spirit* is *spir*, "to breathe," similar to the Chinese Qi, or life energy, expressed by the same word as *air*.

stress In TCM, the result of unmanaged stress is blocked energy and is the source of most physical, mental, emotional, and social problems.

T-cells Cells that are believed to support the immune system by consuming viruses, bacteria, and even tumor cells. T'ai Chi practice is believed to boost the body's production of T-cells.

T'ai Chi A moving form of QiGong. Most Moving QiGong forms have only a few simple movements and lack the continuous flow of the many multiple movements that T'ai Chi forms weave together.

T'ai Chi Ch'uan "Supreme ultimate fist" or highest martial art.

Taoism An ancient Chinese philosophy of life that holds that the Tao, the way of life, or the invisible force of nature's laws, can be accessed in states of alert calm. Regular immersion in the effortless power of life energy (through QiGong meditation) is believed to access the Tao for our lives, leading us to the most effortless and meaningful way to live.

Taoist Canon An ancient book that held all the early writing on QiGong, although at that time QiGong was called Tao-yin.

Taoist philosophy   Often thought of as T'ai Chi philosophy because the subtle awareness of self and life energy is so directly applicable to Taoism's goal of getting in touch with the Tao's natural laws and quiet power.

Tao-yin   "Leading or guiding the energy"; another ancient name for QiGong.

To gu na xin   "Expelling the old energy, absorbing the new," which was another name for QiGong used in the past.

Traditional Chinese Medicine (TCM)   The Chinese health sciences that see the body and mind as a holistic entity united by the flow of life energy, or Qi. The three main branches of TCM are acupuncture, herbal medicine, and exercises such as T'ai Chi and QiGong, often used in combination.

Vertical Axis   The postural alignment for T'ai Chi.

Wan Yang-Ming   Philosopher who fused the physical motions of T'ai Chi Ch'uan with the philosophy of Taoism.

Wu style   A formidable martial art form of T'ai Chi popular in many countries.

Yang Lu-Chan   The great grandmaster of Kuang Ping Yang style, who created it after studying the Chen family style.

Yang style   A form of T'ai Chi very popular in the United States and China.

Yellow Emperor's Classic of Chinese Medicine, The   The bible of Chinese Medicine in 200 B.C.E. It stressed that "true medicine" is curing disease before it develops.

yin and yang   The Chinese concepts of universal forces. All things are an eternally flowing interaction of two opposites; the ideal is healthful balance in all things. Yin is internal, dark, feminine, and receptive. Yang is external, light, masculine, and dynamic.

Zang Fu   In Chinese, "solid-hollow." A system that indicates how Qi, or life energy, flows throughout and between organs. It is the model of how the entire body is interlinked by that flow, and shows how treating associated organs or energy meridians can improve others.

zazen   The Zen art of meditation. Directly translated, it means "just sitting."

zen   An oriental art of being here and now, allowing the mind and heart to let go of past and future attachments so one can be fully immersed in the moment.